The
Respiratory
Functions
of Blood

TOPICS IN HEMATOLOGY

Series Editor: Maxwell M. Wintrobe
University of Utah, Salt Lake City

THE RESPIRATORY FUNCTIONS OF BLOOD
Lars Garby and Jerry Meldon

DISORDERS OF RED CELL METABOLISM
Ernest Beutler

In preparation:
TRACE ELEMENTS IN HUMAN METABOLISM
Ananda S. Prasad

The Respiratory Functions of Blood

Lars Garby
and Jerry Meldon

University of Odense
Odense, Denmark

PLENUM MEDICAL BOOK COMPANY
NEW YORK AND LONDON

Library of Congress Cataloging in Publication Data

Garby, Lars.
    The respiratory functions of blood.

    (Topics in hematology)
    Bibliography: p.
    Includes index.
    1. Blood gases. 2. Oxygen transport (Physiology) 3. Carbon dioxide transport
(Physiology) I. Meldon, Jerry, joint author. II. Title. III. Series. [DNLM: 1. Biological
transport. 2. Blood gas analysis. 3. Respiration. 4. Respiration disorders. WH100
G214r]
QP99.3. G3G37   612'.22   77-21980
ISBN 0-306-30998-X

© 1977 Plenum Publishing Corporation
227 West 17th Street, New York, N.Y. 10011

Plenum Medical Book Company is an imprint of Plenum Publishing Corporation

Printed in the United States of America

Foreword

This monograph is the first of a series which is designed to present in depth timely reviews of subjects related to the blood. Insofar as each subject lends itself, the clinical aspects of each topic will be presented as fully as is appropriate, in addition to the basic features. As a consequence, the various monographs should be found useful not solely by hematologists. Depending on the nature of each topic, it is expected that these monographs will be found important by physiologists and specialists in fields other than hematology, as well as by scientists of very diverse interests. The present treatise illustrates this point. Doctors Garby and Meldon have brought together in a most useful way the spectacular advances which have been made in the last decade or two in a field of fundamental biologic importance. They have also brought to the discussion of this subject their own observations and interpretations as well as their profound understanding of the respiratory functions of the blood.

Maxwell M. Wintrobe

Salt Lake City, Utah

Preface

This volume is an attempt to summarize the present state of knowledge of the respiratory functions of blood in health and disease.
Though it deals fairly thoroughly with physicochemical aspects of
the blood's gas transport properties and with the molecular chemistry of hemoglobin, its main emphasis is the gas transport function of
the blood *in vivo* and modes of its disturbance in disease. Thus, the
carriage of oxygen and carbon dioxide by the blood is examined in
the contexts of lung and circulatory function plus the requirements
set by the tissues, as well as disturbances of these systems. Particular
attention is accorded the mechanisms of compensation for such
perturbations which originate in the cardiopulmonary system and
blood itself, and the effects of these responses upon the overall
transport of oxygen.

The book is intended to serve as a relatively comprehensive and
advanced introduction to the physiology of blood gas transport for
clinical and laboratory investigators whose work carries them into
this realm. It should therefore be of relevance to a number of
branches of medicine—hematology, cardiology, anesthesiology,
clinical physiology, and pneumology—and will hopefully be of
interest to molecular biologists, biochemists, and physiologists
whose activities in this field bring in aspects of clinical relevance, and
to chemical and biomedical engineers concerned with problems of
extracorporeal gas exchange.

Acknowledgments

We are indebted to Dr. David Flenley, Edinburgh, and Dr. Simon H. de Bruin, Nijmegen, for valuable discussions; Mrs. Ingeborg Pedersen, Odense, for excellent typing; the Medical Faculty, Odense University, for financial support; and the U.S. National Heart and Lung Institute for a Postdoctoral Fellowship (No. 1 FO2 HL54901) to J. M.

Lars Garby

Jerry Meldon

Odense, Denmark

Contents

Chapter 8
Disturbances of the Respiratory Functions of Blood **207**

Notation

The following is an alphabetical dictionary of symbols employed in the text, along with typical units.

a activity; also a parameter in r–pH^{pl} correlations as defined by equation (5-32).

A_j Adair constants [cf. equation (4-12)]

b parameter in r–pH^{pl} correlations as defined by equation (5-32)

B defined by equation (5-9)

ΔB^{bl} blood base excess concentration, i.e., the difference between the prevailing and standard whole blood B values

c molality in mol/kg water, though c_{Hb} denotes *grams* of hemoglobin per *liter of whole blood*

C defined just prior to equation (4-7)

C_i concentration of species i in mol/liter (M)

$\overline{CO}, \overline{CO_2}$ see $\bar{X}$

D diffusivity in cm^2/sec

$[DPG]_T$ total erythrocyte 2,3-DPG concentration in mmol/liter (cells)

$(DPG)^c$ total erythrocyte 2,3-DPG concentration in mmol/liter (H_2O)

F Faraday's constant; also used to denote free energy

ΔF	defined by equation (4-1); also used to denote free energy of reaction
G	Gibbs free energy
ΔG_I	defined by equation (4-8)
h	hematocrit
$\bar{H}^+$	see $\bar{X}$
Hm	heme monomer
$[i]$	concentration of species i in mol/liter
J_i	flux of species i in mol/cm^2/sec
k, K	equilibrium constants
k_1, k_{-1}	respective association and dissociation rate constants of the reaction $CO_2 + H_2O = H_2CO_3$ (see Chapter 5)
k_{ass}, k_a	association rate constants
k_{diss}, k_d	dissociation rate constants
K_a'	equilibrium constant of overall reaction (2-3)
K_w	equilibrium constant of water ionization reaction
L	capillary length in cm; also a constant defined in the introduction to the Monod–Wyman–Changeux model
m	zero-order O_2 consumption rate constant in mol/cm^3/sec
M	defined by equation (4-29)
$[Mb]$	tissue myoglobin concentration in mol/liter(tissue)
n	number of moles; also used as the Hill parameter in equation (4-34)
N_i^j	local net flow of species i into phase j in mol/cm^3/sec
$\bar{O}_2$	see $\bar{X}$
pCO_2, pO_2	partial pressures (tensions) of CO_2 and O_2 in mm Hg (1 mm Hg = 0.133 kPa)
pK	$-\log_{10} K$
$p(50)$	equilibrium O_2 partial pressure (tension) at 50% hemoglobin saturation
$P_{CO_2}^t$	permeability (Krogh diffusion constant) of CO_2 in tissue in mol/cm^2/sec/(mm Hg/cm)
$P_{HCO_3^-}$	permeability of HCO_3^- in red cell membrane in cm/sec
$P_{O_2}^t$	permeability (Krogh diffusion constant) of O_2 in tissue in mol/cm^2/sec/(mm Hg/cm); in absence of myoglobin, $P_{O_2}^t = D_{O_2}^t \cdot \alpha_{O_2}^t$

q denotes quaternary structure in hemoglobin

q_R respiratory quotient, i.e., ratio of CO_2 production to O_2 consumption rates

Q defined by equation (6-16)

r radial coordinate in cm; also denotes Donnan distribution coefficient defined by equation (5-29)

r_{sv} red cell surface-to-volume ratio in cm^{-1}

R ideal gas constant; also denotes "relaxed" conformation of hemoglobin

S_{Mb}^{bl} defined following equation (6-19)

t number of binding sites in a macromolecule for a given species [see equation (4-1)]; also denotes tertiary structure of hemoglobin

T absolute temperature; also denotes constrained ("taut") conformation of hemoglobin

u velocity of blood through capillary in cm/sec

V fluid volume

x longitudinal (capillary axial) coordinate in cm; also used to denote activity [see equation (4-2)]

$\bar{X}$ number of moles of ligand X bound per mole of macromolecule monomer, except when number of sites are included in equation

z electrical charge

Greek Letters

α solubility coefficient in mol/liter/mm Hg; also denotes normalized ligand concentration [see equation (4-7)] and a hemoglobin chain

β buffer capacity in eq/pH unit; also denotes a hemoglobin chain

η defined in Table X

θ angular coordinate; also used as defined following equation (5-42)

$\mu, \mu^0, \tilde{\mu}$ chemical, standard chemical, and electrochemical potentials

ν charge (valence) of protonated protein [see equation (2-18)]

ρ_{H_2O} defined following equation (5-29)

ρ_i local rate of depletion of species i by chemical reaction in mol/cm^3/sec

τ residence time of blood in systemic capillaries in sec

ϕ defined following equation (5-37)

ϕ_j volume fraction of phase j in blood

Φ electrical potential in volts

ω defined following equation (5-31)

Subscript

cap capillary

diss dissociation

DPG 2,3-diphosphoglycerate

f free (unbound) species

Hm heme monomer

i species i

min minimum

Pr protein

rel relative value

tis tissue

T total amount of particular species in solution

Superscript

a arterial quantity

A alveolar quantity

bl blood

c red cells

c–pl from cells to plasma

ISF interstitial fluid

pl plasma

t tissue

t–pl from tissue to plasma

v venous quantity

Chapter 1

Introduction

The term respiration refers to the gaseous interchange between an organism and its surroundings, the more obvious chemical features of which are the consumption of oxygen and elimination of carbon dioxide. Among the vital steps in the overall process of respiration is the transport of both gases by the blood. Thus it is of fundamental importance that the extent of the blood's uptake and release of each gas, and the rates at which they occur, depend to a large degree upon the physicochemical properties of this medium and that such properties may vary appreciably among individuals. Furthermore, these properties are, themselves, perturbed by the very processes of uptake and release.

Among such variations and perturbations one has, by tradition, received particular attention: the change in the activity of hydrogen ions. Others have also been studied in detail, such as changes in the blood's bicarbonate ion content, shifts of these and chloride ions as well as water between red cells and plasma, and binding of several anions to hemoglobin.

However, it is probably fair to say that what usually is meant by the respiratory functions of the blood is the uptake, binding, and release of oxygen and carbon dioxide only, and moderation of the associated changes in the concentrations of hydrogen ions within the blood. Apart from the latter changes, others may result from perturbations in the production and consumption of protons by the tissues. Although such processes are only indirectly, if at all connected with respiration, they too are traditionally treated under the heading of The Respiratory Functions of the Blood. The present treatise follows that tradition.

The blood's performance of its respiratory functions is strongly linked to the properties of the compartments with which it exchanges matter, i.e., with those of the gas phase in the lung and the liquid phase of the tissues. It depends as well upon its own rate of flow through these regions of exchange. Therefore, the respiratory functions of the blood should be described and analyzed in relation to the characteristics of lung function, tissue function, and circulation. The present treatise attempts to do so and, in this way, departs somewhat from tradition.

Many aspects of the respiratory functions of the blood are now known in considerable detail. However, a comprehensive and critical treatment of all of them would be an undertaking far beyond the capacity of the present authors. Comparative aspects of the biochemistry and physiology of the system are only briefly mentioned and then in rather haphazard fashion. The determination of hemoglobin structure and the increasingly profound understanding of the relationship between structure and function have had very considerable impact upon the sciences of evolution and genetics. These aspects of blood respiratory functions are discussed, but narrowly, in relation to the so-called "abnormal" hemoglobins with abnormal binding of oxygen. Thus, the present account is concerned primarily with the physiological and pathophysiological aspects of the respiratory functions of human blood, and deals with molecular, comparative, and genetic aspects only insofar as they are deemed important for understanding of normal and abnormal function in man.

The respiratory functions of the blood have been the subject of several extensive and thorough monographs and review articles during this century. Sir Joseph Barcroft's *The Respiratory Function of the Blood*, published in 1914, was the first modern account of accumulated knowledge in this field. A notable article on the carbon dioxide carriers in the blood was contributed by D. D. van Slyke to *Physiological Reviews* of 1922. The considerable body of data collected during World War I and the decade following it by J. B. S. Haldane in Oxford, Barcroft and A. V. Hill in Cambridge (England), van Slyke in New York, and L. J. Henderson at Harvard was logically and succinctly synthesized in Henderson's famous monograph, *Blood: A Study in General Physiology*, which appeared in 1928.

Two important works were published in 1935: J. B. S. Haldane and J. G. Priestley's *Respiration*, a text, and F. J. W. Roughton's "Recent work on carbon dioxide transport by the blood," which appeared in *Physiological Reviews*. Roughton again summarized developments in the field of carbon dioxide transport in the 1943 *Harvey Lectures*.

The chemistry of heme proteins was reviewed by Jeffries Wyman in *Advances in Protein Chemistry* of both 1948 and 1964. These two papers witness a clarification of the interactions among different ligands in their binding to hemoglobin in terms of so-called linked functions.

Transport of both carbon dioxide and oxygen was reviewed critically by Roughton in the *Handbook of Physiology, Respiration, Volume I*, published in 1964. The three-dimensional structure of hemoglobin, first at 5.5 Å resolution and, eight years later, at 2.8 Å resolution, and stereochemical explanations for the protein's cooperativity and allosteric interactions were published by Max Perutz and his collaborators at Cambridge (England) in a series of contributions starting in 1960 and summarized in several papers in *Nature* of 1970 and 1972.

Hemoglobin and Myoglobin in Their Reactions with Ligands, a comprehensive text by E. Antonini and M. Brunori, appeared in 1971. The interactions of hemoglobin with hydrogen ions, carbon dioxide, and organic phosphates were dealt with critically by J. V. Kilmartin and L. Rossi-Bernardi in *Physiological Reviews* of 1973.

R. and R. E. Benesch contributed a review of the interactions of red cell organic phosphates with hemoglobin to *Advances in Protein Chemistry* of 1974. In that same year, a review of advances in hemoglobin chemistry and provocative discussion of physiological implications was presented by C. Bauer in *Reviews of Physiology, Biochemistry and Pharmacology*, and O. Siggaard-Andersen's treatise, *The Acid–Base Status of the Blood*, was published in revised form.

A fascinating history of the developments up to 1930 was traced by John Edsall in *The Journal of the History of Biology* of 1972.

Chapter 2

Two Gas Transport Problems

In this chapter, the main respiratory functions of the blood are introduced and outlined from the point of view of the overall demands of the body. While such an approach must undoubtedly carry with it a flavor of teleology, it is a convenient way to summarize the content of current concepts.

Requirements at Rest

Oxygen

A normal resting man consumes about 10 millimoles (mmol) of oxygen each minute. The overwhelming majority of these molecules are used in the reaction

$$2H^+ + 2e^- + \tfrac{1}{2}O_2 = H_2O \qquad (2\text{-}1)$$

which takes place in the mitochondria and provides the free energy necessary for maintenance of ionic gradients, muscular contraction, and chemical synthesis.

The oxygen requirements of the tissues at rest are further characterized by end-capillary oxygen tensions, which in general are substantially above zero. That mixed venous blood has an oxygen tension, pO_2, at rest of no less than 35–40 mm Hg has been construed as indicative of a requirement for the normal functioning of at least some oxygen-consuming reactions within the tissue.

Observations of oxygen consumption and venous blood pO_2 do not, however, provide a clear-cut picture of the relationship between these two variables. A major number of reported observations suggest that most of the oxygen is consumed in reactions whose rates are independent of mixed venous blood pO_2 in the latter's normal range. Thus, in isolated skeletal muscle of dogs, the oxygen consumption has been found (Stainsby and Otis, 1964; Honig *et al.*, 1971; Durán and Renkin, 1974) to be effectively independent of blood flow and, by implication, venous pO_2, as the flow is varied within its normal range. This independence does not, however, appear to be true of small animals, e.g., rats and guinea pigs (Whalen *et al.*, 1973). Moreover, a dependency is at times observed in dogs as well (Durán and Renkin, 1974). The reasons for these discrepancies, which may be illusory, have not been elucidated, but they might be interanimal differences in muscle cell metabolic state prior to experimentation.

Whole-body oxygen consumption in man and larger animals is insensitive to moderate changes in either the blood's hemoglobin concentration or affinity for oxygen, which reduce mixed venous blood pO_2 (Naylor *et al.*, 1972; Riggs *et al.*, 1973; Watkins *et al.*, 1974; von Restorff *et al.*, 1975). It is therefore possible that the high O_2 tension in venous blood at rest reflects a circulating oxygen reserve to be utilized in case of emergency: there is some 30 sec worth of very hard work in the oxygen content of the veins that might well have been crucial to the escape of prehistoric man from a hungry beast. Alternatively, one might explain the high blood flow—and thereby the high venous blood pO_2—by the blood flow-limited transport of some quantity other than oxygen (heat?). In this event though, the high hemoglobin concentration would require explanation.

Still, it is possible that the high resting blood flow and the increase in cardiac output often observed after reductions in hemoglobin concentration or increases in blood affinity for oxygen might be explained by flow-limited transport of oxygen to reactions that consume very little gas but require a high oxygen tension. For example, in the brain both the tryptophane hydroxylase reaction rate and blood flow depend on venous pO_2 far above the range of tensions over which the ATP–ADP-coupled oxygen consumption is blood pO_2 dependent (Davis *et al.*, 1972). Furthermore, microcirculatory flow and capillary density in rat cremaster muscle respond to variations in tissue pO_2 level far above the tensions at which oxygen-consuming mitochondrial reactions are pO_2 sensitive (Prewitt and Johnson, 1976). If it is, in fact, reactions characterized by a low oxygen affinity that "set" blood flow—and thereby the capillary oxygen tension—a whole new field opens up in physiology.

Regardless of the details of the coupling between blood pO_2 and tissue oxygen consumption, the fact remains that the delivery of 10 mmol of oxygen per minute to the tissues takes place with an oxygen tension in mixed venous blood of 35 to 40 mm Hg. Thus, the uptake of that same amount of oxygen in the lungs normally starts with that oxygen partial pressure in the blood.

Normal blood flow through the lungs is about 5 liters/min, while the partial pressure of oxygen in the lung alveoli and arterial blood is between 90 and 100 mg Hg. Both these quantities are maintained by processes that involve expenditure of energy: the first to overcome vascular resistance to blood flow, the second to transport oxygen by convection to the lung alveoli and thus ensure a sufficient gradient of oxygen tension across the alveolar–capillary membrane and saturation of pulmonary capillary blood.

If we maintain that the energetic requirements have priority, i.e., that performance of cardiac and respiratory work be minimal, then *at rest the job of the blood is to take up and deliver oxygen to the extent of 10/5 = 2 mmol/liter for a partial pressure change from 35–40 to 90–100 mm Hg.*

Carbon Dioxide

The demands on the blood to carry carbon dioxide can be expressed in a similar manner. Between 8 and 10 mmol of carbon dioxide are produced every minute through substrate oxidation reactions. Thus, as with oxygen, about 2 mmol of carbon dioxide must be taken up and released per liter of blood during its passage through the tissues and lungs.

The partial pressure of carbon dioxide in the lung alveoli is maintained near 40 mm Hg through the mechanical work of respiration, and that is also the value of $p\mathrm{CO_2}$ in arterial blood. The limits within which the partial pressure of the gas may vary in mixed venous blood are, however, apparently not set by any energy requirement. Instead, they are most probably related to a completely different type of demand of the organism: maintenance of the hydrogen ion concentration in the body fluids within a fairly narrow range. Since blood and whole body fluid pH values are each strongly dependent upon blood $p\mathrm{CO_2}$, the demand upon the blood to transport carbon dioxide is intimately related to the control of hydrogen ion concentration.

A provocative rationalization of the control of $p\mathrm{CO_2}$, and thereby the pH, within the physiologically observed limits has been presented by Rahn *et al.* (1975).

The requirements on the blood to transport carbon dioxide are specified more precisely in what follows. At this stage, we anticipate the results by simply stating that *at rest the capacity of the blood to take up and release carbon dioxide is required to be 2 mmol/liter of blood for a partial pressure change from 40 to ~50 mm Hg.*

Equilibrium Binding Curves

The above-mentioned cardinal properties of the blood regarding $\mathrm{O_2}$ and $\mathrm{CO_2}$ transport are conveniently expressed in terms of the equilibrium binding curves for the two gases. Such curves are simply plots of content per unit volume versus gas partial pressure at chemical equilibrium, and thus explicitly contain the capacities mentioned above. The fact that "Blut ist ein ganz besonderer Saft" (Goethe, *Faust*) is illustrated by a comparison of its $\mathrm{O_2}$ and $\mathrm{CO_2}$ uptake/release properties with those of a simple salt solution of physiological ionic strength.

Binding in a Simple Salt Solution. The uptake of oxygen in a salt solution is for all intents and purposes determined alone by the gas's physical solubility according to Henry's law:

$$[\mathrm{O_2}] = \alpha_{\mathrm{O_2}} p\mathrm{O_2} \qquad (2\text{-}2)$$

where $[O_2]$ is the concentration in solution, α_{O_2} the solubility coefficient, and pO_2 the partial pressure of oxygen. At 37°C, the value of α_{O_2} in a salt solution of physiological composition is approximately 0.0013 mmol/liter/mm Hg. Thus, the amount of oxygen absorbed as its partial pressure increases from 40 to 95 mm Hg is only $0.0013 \times 55 = 0.07$ mmol/liter, about 30 times less than the required 2 mmol/liter.

For carbon dioxide the situation is different because CO_2 reacts chemically with water to form carbonic acid and bicarbonate ion according to

$$CO_2 + H_2O \leftrightharpoons H_2CO_3 \leftrightharpoons HCO_3^- + H^+ \tag{2-3}$$

Bicarbonate ions dissociate further into H^+ and CO_3^{2-}, but the extent of reaction is negligible below a pH of 8. An additional direct reaction of CO_2 with OH^- ions is also negligible under the same conditions.

The total carbon dioxide content of a physiological salt solution at 37°C and pH below 8 may thus be expressed as

$$[CO_2]_T = \alpha_{CO_2} pCO_2 + [HCO_3^-] \tag{2-4}$$

where $\alpha_{CO_2} pCO_2 = [CO_2 \text{ (dissolved)}] + [H_2CO_3]$, and α_{CO_2} has a value of 0.03 mmol/liter/mm Hg. In fact, the concentration of carbonic acid is so small that it may be neglected in such considerations.

On the basis of the electroneutrality constraint, the concentrations of charged species must satisfy

$$[OH^-] + [HCO_3^-] - [H^+] = [M^+] = 0 \tag{2-5}$$

where $[M^+]$, the *net* charge concentration (e.g., in milliequivalents per liter) due to nontitratable cations and anions, is zero in a solution initially derived from salts of strong acids and bases.

(Practically speaking, the hydrogen ion concentration is not a measurable quantity. What is usually referred to as the experimentally determined pH is a measure of proton *activity*. Therefore, the quantity $[H^+]$ should henceforth be taken to imply 10^{-pH}. Since in essentially all situations of physiological interest $[H^+]$ is negligible in electroneutrality considerations, the discrepancy between proton concentration and activity poses no difficulty here.)

Equilibrium of the above reactions and ionization of water dictate the following two relationships:

$$\frac{[H^+][HCO_3^-]}{\alpha_{CO_2}pCO_2} = K_a' \tag{2-6}$$

$$[H^+][OH^-] = K_w \tag{2-7}$$

where K_a', the apparent* acid dissociation constant of carbonic acid, is $10^{-6.1}$ mol/liter, and K_w is $10^{-13.6}$ (mol/liter)^2.

The above relationships may be combined to give

$$[HCO_3^-] = \frac{K_a'\alpha_{CO_2}pCO_2}{[H^+]} = \frac{K_a'\alpha_{CO_2}pCO_2}{(K_w + K_a'\alpha_{CO_2}pCO_2)^{1/2}} \tag{2-8}$$

The result for $pCO_2 = 40$ mm Hg is $[CO_2]_T = (1.2 \times 10^{-3} + 0.03 \times 10^{-3})M = 1.23$ mM, and pH = 4.5. When such a solution is titrated at $pCO_2 = 40$ mm Hg with, for example, NaOH to the normal arterial plasma pH, 7.40, its total carbon dioxide concentration increases by virtue of the additional bicarbonate to 25.1 mM. If pCO_2 is then raised to 50 mm Hg, $[HCO_3^-]$ remains practically unchanged at 23.9 mM, while $\alpha_{CO_2}pCO_2$ increases by 0.3 mM, so that $[CO_2]_T$ increases to 25.4 mM. At the same time, the pH decreases to 7.30.

The increase in total carbon dioxide concentration in going from 40 to 50 mm Hg pCO_2, 0.3 mM, is roughly one-sixth that required. In order to raise $[CO_2]_T$ to 27.1 mM, it is necessary to increase pCO_2 to 107 mm Hg. This will change the pH from 7.40 to 6.97, a value much too low to be accepted. The carbon dioxide binding curve of such a solution is illustrated in Figure 1.

Uptake and Release in the Presence of an Oxygen and Proton Binding Protein. The problem of providing the blood with an exchange capacity of the required magnitude for both oxygen and carbon dioxide was solved through the evolution of a molecule to which both oxygen and protons could be bound. For reasons made clearer as we proceed, a protein molecule was the logical choice.

---

*The constant is an apparent one in that the expression in the denominator is the sum of dissolved CO_2 and carbonic acid concentrations. The true dissociation constant of carbonic acid is several hundred times greater.

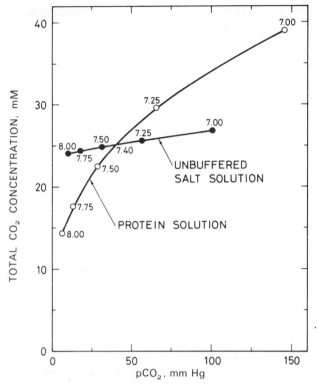

Figure 1. Carbon dioxide binding curves in a physiological sodium chloride/ bicarbonate solution (●) and in the same solution with 2 mM of a protein with 25 proton binding sites per molecule, each with an acid dissociation constant of 10^{-7} M (○). Numerical values correspond to the prevailing pH.

For a protein molecule binding one molecule of oxygen, the reaction may be written

$$Pr + O_2 \rightleftharpoons PrO_2 \qquad (2\text{-}9)$$

and the equilibrium oxygen binding curve obtained from the following relationships:

$$[PrO_2]/[Pr][O_2] = k \qquad (2\text{-}10)$$

$$[Pr]_T = [Pr] + [PrO_2] \qquad (2\text{-}11)$$

$$[O_2]_T = [O_2] + [PrO_2] \qquad (2\text{-}12)$$

where [Pr] and [PrO$_2$] are the molar concentrations of deoxygenated protein and protein–oxygen complex, respectively; k the association constant; and [Pr]$_T$ and [O$_2$]$_T$ the respective total concentrations of protein and oxygen.

The equilibrium oxygen binding curve is thus expressed by

$$[O_2]_T = [O_2] + \frac{k[O_2]}{1 + k[O_2]}[Pr]_T \qquad (2\text{-}13)$$

Let $k' = k\alpha_{O_2}$ and assume that [PrO$_2$] $\gg$ [O$_2$] for oxygen tensions below 100 mm Hg. The binding curve then reduces, in the pO_2 range of interest, to

$$[O_2]_T = \frac{k'pO_2}{1 + k'pO_2}[Pr]_T \qquad (2\text{-}14)$$

An oxygen release capacity of 2 mmol/liter for a change in oxygen tension from 95 to 40 mm Hg is then obtained whenever

$$2 \times 10^{-3} = [Pr]_T \left\{ \frac{95k'}{1 + 95k'} - \frac{40k'}{1 + 40k'} \right\} \qquad (2\text{-}15)$$

The value of k' that minimizes the required total protein concentration may be determined by differentiation of the term in brackets of (2-15) with respect to k' and equating the resulting expression with zero. Substitution of this value of k' into (2-15) yields a value for [Pr]$_T$ of 9.4 mM.

A protein required to remain within the vascular bed must have a molecular weight of some 50,000 to 100,000, which at a concentration of 10 mM corresponds to some 500–1000 g/liter. Such a solution would likely have a viscosity at least 10 times that of human whole blood and require considerable energy expenditure to circulate. It is therefore not difficult to imagine Nature's search for a protein molecule able to bind more than a single molecule of oxygen.

A macromolecule binding more than one molecule of ligand can be constructed according to either of two fundamentally different principles: (1) the binding sites are independent of each other, (2) the binding sites are not independent, but rather interact in such a manner that the affinity of each site for ligand depends upon whether or not the other site(s) are occupied. In the case of independent binding, the shape of the binding curve will always be characterized by a decreasing slope as the free ligand concentration rises. If, in addition, the sites are identical, then the binding curve is denoted by an expression analogous to (2-14), where k' is the intrinsic binding constant common to all sites and $[Pr]_T$ the molar concentration of binding sites.

Obviously then, an oxygen release capacity of 2 mmol/liter for a pO_2 change from 95 to 40 mm Hg may be obtained with a total protein concentration of $9.4/n$ mM, where n is the number of such identical binding sites per molecule. With four binding sites, the protein concentration becomes 2.35 mM, which by coincidence is the concentration of hemoglobin in normal human whole blood. The associated binding curve is the lower of the two hyperbolas illustrated in Figure 2. With eight binding sites and the same protein concentration, the higher of the two hyperbolas in Figure 2 is derived. Such a solution allows the exchange of 4 mmol of oxygen per liter when its partial pressure falls from 95 to 40 mm Hg.

For reasons that are not obvious, Nature did not select oxygen-carrying molecules with independent binding sites in higher animals. Instead, a protein accommodating four molecules of oxygen was developed, with binding sites exhibiting a very special type of interdependence, namely *positive cooperation*. Thus, during the successive binding of oxygen molecules, the affinity of unoccupied binding sites to oxygen generally increases, the result being an S-shaped binding curve, as shown in Figure 2. Such a form of the binding curve, first described in the classical paper by Bohr *et al.* (1904), is particularly well suited to the requirements of the body during muscular work and is impossible to obtain with independent binding sites. The required exchange capacity for oxygen is achieved with a protein concentration of 2.0 to 2.5 mM. It remained for evolution to solve the viscosity problem—and others as well (see below)—by confining these molecules within an envelope in the shape of a biconcave disk, some 90 μm^3 in volume.

The carbon dioxide exchange problem might have been solved in similar fashion, i.e., through binding of CO_2 to the same or some

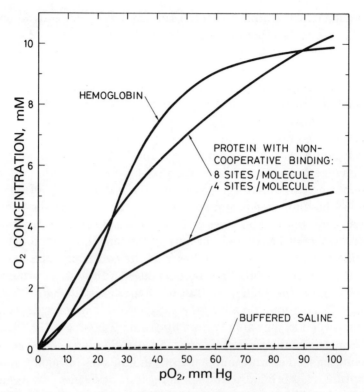

Figure 2. Oxygen binding curves in: buffered saline (broken line); 2.35 mM solutions of proteins with independent O_2 binding sites and optimal binding constant for O_2 transport at rest: four sites per molecule (lower hyperbola), eight sites per molecule (upper hyperbola); 2.35 mM hemoglobin solution (sigmoid).

other protein molecule. However, the properties of the oxygen-binding protein obviated this. It sufficed to provide this protein with proton binding sites, such that reactions (2-3) are coupled with the set of reactions

$$Pr - (H^+)_m \rightleftharpoons Pr - (H^+)_{m-1} + H^+ \qquad (2\text{-}16)$$

The solution's carbon dioxide binding curve now differs strikingly from that obtained in the absence of protein. Equations (2-4) and (2-6) are unchanged (insofar as we have not yet considered binding of CO_2 to the protein), but the electroneutrality condition is now

$$[M^+] + z[Pr]_T - [HCO_3^-] = 0 \qquad (2\text{-}17)$$

where $[Pr]_T$ is the concentration of proton binding sites, z the average charge per site, and $[H^+]$ and $[OH^-]$ may be neglected.

If we consider a protein containing independent proton binding sites each with the same acid dissociation constant, K mol/liter, then

$$[H^+][Pr^{\nu-1}]/[HPr^\nu] = K \qquad (2\text{-}18)$$

where $[Pr^{\nu-1}]$ is the total concentration of sites from which protons have dissociated, $[HPr^\nu]$ the concentration of undissociated sites, and ν is either zero (e.g., a carboxyl group) or unity (e.g., an amino group).

The final required relationship expresses the conservation of protein mass:

$$[Pr]_T = [Pr^{\nu-1}] + [HPr^\nu] \qquad (2\text{-}19)$$

Let us now consider a system that, as before, exhibits a pH value of 7.40 at $p\,CO_2 = 40$ mm Hg, and thus a simultaneous bicarbonate concentration of 23.9 mM. Moreover, let us assign to K the value 10^{-7} mol/liter, which by virtue of its proximity to $[H^+]$ implies near-maximal buffering in the pertinent range of pH. If we now require a 2 mmol/liter change in $[CO_2]_T$ when $p\,CO_2$ is raised to 50 mm Hg, then $[HCO_3^-]$ must increase to 25.6 mM, which implies a pH = 7.33. Assuming the protein is anionic, i.e., $\nu = 0$, then the values of z, or $-1/(1 + 10^{7-\text{pH}})$, at the pH values of 7.40 and 7.33, are, respectively, -0.715 and -0.681. Substitution of these and the corresponding $[HCO_3^-]$ values into equation (2-17) yields a value for $[Pr]_T$, the concentration of proton binding sites, of 50 mM. Thus with a total protein concentration of 2.0 to 2.5 mM, 20–25 proton binding sites per molecule afford the solution the capacity to bind carbon dioxide as demanded with a very small shift in pH. The binding curve is shown in Figure 1.

A Question of Rate. Of the two reactions (2-3), the hydration of dissolved carbon dioxide is intrinsically so slow that the flux of CO_2

from tissue would be expected to effect a large increase in pCO_2 along the capillary. This is apparently inimical to the maintenance of normal tissue function. In order to accelerate the reaction in the blood, evolution introduced into the red cells a catalyst, carbonic anhydrase. This enzyme is present in the erythrocytes at a concentration of only 1 g/liter, but increases the rate of hydration by a factor on the order of 10,000.

Requirements during Exercise

The situation described above refers to resting conditions. During muscular exercise, the relative increase in oxygen consumption is much greater than the increase in cardiac output. For example, muscular exercise requiring 100 mmol of oxygen per minute, i.e., ten times the amount at rest, is typically accompanied by only a fourfold increase in cardiac output. If we maintain the view that this phenomenon is an expression of a "primary requirement," it follows that the oxygen exchange capacity must now be $100/20 = 5$ mmol/liter for a decrease in oxygen tension from 95 to some 27 mm Hg. The importance of the S-shaped oxygen binding curve obtained through positive cooperativity is obvious. As seen in Figure 2, 5 mmol of oxygen is released per liter of blood when the oxygen tension goes from 95 to 27 mm Hg (compared with less than 3 mmol for the solution of the protein with four independent sites), and this value is quite insensitive to moderate changes in arterial oxygen tension. The carbon dioxide uptake under these conditions effects an increase in the pCO_2 of mixed venous blood to about 55 mm Hg, and a change in pH of only 0.1 unit.

The reaction between oxygen and hemoglobin is strongly exothermic; thus the release of oxygen molecules from hemoglobin is accompanied by an uptake of heat from the surroundings. It follows from le Chatelier's principle that an increase in temperature decreases the affinity of hemoglobin for oxygen. The additional heat produced by the muscle cells during work, and transmitted to the blood, thereby facilitates the transfer of oxygen from blood to tissues. This effect, and a similar one due to lower pH values, may be quite large and is discussed in more detail in Chapters 4 and 6.

Some Further Requirements

Regulation

The integrated gas transport system, i.e., the respiratory, circulatory, and blood systems, must meet demands that vary considerably under changing physiological and pathophysiological conditions. Short- and long-term adaptations are therefore to be anticipated. Furthermore, disturbances in one or several parts of the total system may be expected to provoke compensating changes in other parts. The processes of adaptation and compensation are usually subsumed under the general heading Regulation, a subject we treat rather extensively in what follows in the remainder of this volume.

As we have seen, the gas transport properties of the blood system depend primarily on the concentration of binding sites for oxygen and protons as well as the affinities of these sites. Both characteristics are subject to regulation. The hemoglobin concentration is regulated through the so-called erythropoietin system, which by negative feedback processes controls the rate of production of red cells. The affinities of both the oxygen and proton binding sites of the hemoglobin molecule are susceptible to change as a result of special properties of the protein molecule: when modifying "effector" molecules or ions bind to hemoglobin, a change in its affinity for both species results.

The second sort of transport regulation is intimately connected with those features of the hemoglobin molecule responsible for cooperativity. It is characteristic of the blood that all transported species, i.e., oxygen, carbon dioxide, and protons, are also effector molecules. Thus, oxygen is an effector with respect to proton and carbon dioxide binding, protons modify oxygen and carbon dioxide binding, and carbon dioxide is an effector with respect to oxygen and proton binding. A fourth important effector molecule is 2,3-diphosphoglycerate (2,3-DPG), an intermediate of the glycolytic reaction sequence in the red cells.

Darwinian Evolution in the Genealogy of Hemoglobin

The preceding outline of the respiratory functions of the blood was written in the context of an analysis of overall body requirements for gas transport. For purposes of simplicity in exposition, it was assumed that through evolution a protein molecule has been developed whose oxygen and proton binding properties were geared to the requirement of minimizing the energy expenditure for gas transport. It is of some interest to note that recent work on evolution in the genealogy of hemoglobin provides evidence that such may very well have been the case. Goodman *et al.* (1975) have shown that mutations that improved hemoglobin function in the very same terms as used in the previous sections were accepted at faster rates in the first vertebrates, while the rates decreased after functional opportunities had been exploited. Furthermore, residue positions in the molecule that acquired cooperative functions changed more rapidly than other positions. Such a pattern can be explained by positive selection for more optimal function according to Darwin, and is therefore difficult to reconcile with the theory of random fixation of selectivity neutral mutations.

Why Red Cells?

A characteristic feature of the blood—and one that has profound effects on its ability to transport oxygen and carbon dioxide—is its heterogeneity: blood is a suspension of red cells in plasma. Both "respiratory" proteins, i.e., hemoglobin and carbonic anhydrase, are confined to the red cells, which are further characterized by a boundary of highly specific permeability. The construction of this separate phase in mammals, whose blood exhibits a high oxygen-carrying capacity, solved a number of technical problems.

In the first place, relatively simple mechanisms could be evolved so as to protect the iron atoms in hemoglobin from oxidation. Although the immediate environment of these atoms within the hemoglobin molecule is favorable to the maintenance of iron in its ferrous form,* there remains a definite tendency to release elec-

---

*The problem of assigning oxidation states or numbers to the iron atoms in hemoglobin is not straightforward. It is discussed in more detail in Chapters 4 and 7.

trons. When that occurs, the electronic configuration of the iron atoms is fundamentally altered. The sixth coordination site, normally free to be occupied by an oxygen molecule, is instead filled by a water molecule or hydroxyl ion to yield ferric hemoglobin (methemoglobin). This compound does not bind oxygen molecules under physiological conditions.

The red cell glycolytic system continuously generates hydride ions, H^-, through the formation of reduced nicotinamide adenine dinucleotide, NADH (see further, Chapter 7). The production of these ions furnishes sufficient electrons to reduce the iron atoms, which are simultaneously and spontaneously oxidized at a rate of about 1–3% per day, and thus to maintain some 99% of them in their oxygen binding form at all times. This would be all the more difficult were the hemoglobin molecules circulating freely in plasma. The mechanisms of iron oxidation and its protection therefrom are of considerable clinical importance, since there are circumstances in which the production of electrons can only keep pace with oxidation when the steady-state concentrations of methemoglobin are considerably in excess of 1%. These are discussed in somewhat more detail in Chapters 7 and 8.

A second problem solved by inclusion of the two "respiratory" proteins within red cells is related to the general phenomenon of proteolytic and oxidative denaturation of protein molecules. Circulating proteins are apparently constantly exposed to processes of this nature and, as a result, exhibit fractional turnover rates between 5% (γ_G-globulin) and 40% (haptoglobin) per day. In contrast, the fractional turnover of hemoglobin is only 1% per day under normal circumstances. Thus, only some 0.1 mmol of hemoglobin need be synthesized each day so as to maintain the total circulating amount at 10 mmol. This relatively low turnover is clearly a result of (1) prevention by the red cell membrane of contact between hemoglobin (as it does carbonic anhydrase) molecules and proteolytic enzymes, and (2) the membrane's ability to survive "wear and tear" in the circulation for about 120 days. Both properties are intimately connected with energy-dependent renewal of membrane lipid components and thus with the production of adenosine triphosphate, ATP, by red cell glycolysis (see further, Chapter 7).

The red cell interior is, however, shielded neither from changes in the oxidation–reduction potential in the plasma nor from substances that can bridge otherwise precluded electron transfers within the cell. Prevention of oxidative denaturation of hemoglobin (and carbonic anhydrase) molecules, whether the oxidation occurs via methemoglobin as an intermediate or some other mechanism, involves reaction products of the glycolytic system in the red cells. The mechanisms are discussed in more detail in Chapter 7.

Separation of the two respiratory proteins from the plasma by a phase boundary also impermeable to the phosphorylated intermediates of glycolysis—a necessary requirement of that process—promoted the evolution of a specific mechanism for the control of hemoglobin oxygen affinity. One of the shunt pathways of glycolysis, the diphosphoglycerate pathway (see Chapter 7), involves a metabolite whose concentration far exceeds what might be envisaged as necessary for the function, in the glycolytic system, of production of ATP and reduced nicotinamide adenine dinucleotides. However, at such a concentration the metabolite, 2,3-DPG, is a powerful allosteric effector toward hemoglobin, serving to regulate the latter's affinity for oxygen. This system is described in more detail in the following chapters.

Red cells have a very high concentration of hemoglobin, ~ 330 g/liter; the viscosity of the fluid inside the cells is therefore ~ 7 cP, or six times that of plasma. The red cell membrane is, however, quite deformable and may also move about the contents of the cell. Furthermore, its outer surface offers a minimum of friction. The result is that the effective viscosity of blood flowing through large vessels, i.e., more than, say, 1 mm in diameter, is not much— perhaps 40%—greater than that of a homogeneous solution containing the same amount of hemoglobin as whole blood. In smaller vessels, the effective viscosity is much *smaller*. This is because the distribution of red cells and plasma in these vessels is such that the cells flow in an axial stream, "lubricated" by a layer of plasma, i.e., the Fåhraeus–Lindquist effect (1931). The blood vessels constituting the greater proportion of vascular hydraulic resistance have diameters much below 1 mm, and the effective viscosity in these vessels is less than one-half that in the larger. The net effect upon overall viscosity of enclosing hemoglobin solution in red cells has been calculated to be a decrease in the pressure necessary to circulate the blood of a dog, from a value of 140 to one of 100 mm Hg (Snyder, 1973). This estimate is in very good agreement with the results of the classical experiments of Whittaker and Winton (1933).

There are thus considerable advantages in confining the blood's respiratory proteins to a separate phase. The costs of this arrangement may be calculated to be quite small. Red cells consume glucose at a rate of about 1 mmol/liter/hr, corresponding to a total cost of some 30 kcal/day. The cost of forming the peptide bonds of the nonhemoglobin proteins of the red cells, renewed at a rate of only 1% per day, is negligible by comparison with the maintenance costs of 30 kcal/day. Thus, only some 1–2% of the whole-body energy expenditure is used to maintain this arrangement. The cost of circulating the blood is much higher, roughly 10% of the whole-body energy requirement at rest.

Chapter 3

Physical Relationships in Blood–Tissue Gas Transport

In the previous chapter we discussed, in a qualitative way, certain general properties of the blood that are of importance in its gas transport function. In this chapter, we take the further steps of (1) placing this function of the blood in relation to the entire gas transport system and (2) deriving, from the laws of physics, quantitative relations among the relevant properties of this system that govern the transfer of oxygen to metabolizing tissue as well as carbon dioxide removal from it. Our goal is an evaluation of the particular importance of the prevailing values of those properties of *the blood* associated with the execution of this function, and of how these properties are coordinated with the functioning of the entire transport system. This chapter serves furthermore as an introduction to the more detailed analysis that appears in Chapters 5 and 6.

The transport system is essentially a device for bringing the tissue cells into communication with the atmospheric source of oxygen and sink for carbon dioxide. Mechanical work of breathing ensures that oxygen and carbon dioxide tensions are about 100 and 40 mm Hg, respectively, in the lung alveoli; mechanical work of the heart circulates the blood between the lungs and the remainder of the organism. As discussed in the previous chapter, the physicochemical properties of the blood can be interpreted as having been selected so as to minimize this work.

The blood's uptake and delivery of oxygen and carbon dioxide occur at the level of the capillaries in direct contact with the lung alveoli and the metabolizing tissues. It is within these microvessels that the gas transport properties of the blood are activated. The physical structures surrounding the respective capillary networks of the lungs and systemic tissue differ fundamentally, and this is reflected in the associated physics of gas transport. The alveolar capillaries are surrounded by a gas phase, while the immediate environment of the systemic capillaries is the heterogeneous fluid phase consisting of the oxygen-consuming and carbon-dioxide-producing cells plus extracellular fluid.

Transport across the *alveolar*-capillary membrane promotes equilibration of the blood at the partial pressures of oxygen and carbon dioxide in the alveoli. Establishment of near-alveolar gas *tensions* in the blood during the course of passage through the lungs is ensured by the fact that the relaxation times associated with gas diffusion across the membrane are small by comparison with the duration of blood passage. In addition, the transfer of requisite *amounts* of oxygen and carbon dioxide per unit of blood is contingent upon there being an adequate hemoglobin concentration and oxygen affinity, together with rapid chemical reaction and translocation of several species *within* the blood.

The oxygen tension at the capillary–*tissue* interface must be so high as to guarantee the maintenance of the O_2 tension within the tissue despite metabolism and diffusional resistance, above some minimum value necessary for oxidative metabolism to proceed. Ensuring that tension *throughout* the capillary demands, besides a high arterial oxygen tension, a suitable combination of blood flow rate, hemoglobin concentration, hemoglobin oxygen affinity, and rates of chemical reaction and translocation within the blood. The uptake of carbon dioxide—in amounts determined by the stoichiometry of metabolic reactions—is ensured simply by the solubility of carbon dioxide in blood. Confinement of the CO_2 tensions and pH of the blood and tissues to within relatively narrow limits is ensured by certain unique chemical properties of the blood.

The analysis of capillary–tissue exchange involves an examination of the distinct but coupled processes occurring within the tissues and the blood. The conventional approach treats the tissue as a single unstirred phase—a mathematical justification for which is given by Forster (1967)—wherein diffusion and chemical reaction are the prevailing phenomena. In the steady state, the rates of these two processes must balance, i.e., *the rate at which the diffusional flux of dissolved gas decreases with respect to position in tissue is equal to the rate at which the gas is depleted by reaction.* This is expressed mathematically by the following equation:

$$D_i^t \nabla^2 C_i^t = \rho_i^t \qquad (3\text{-}1)$$

where D_i^t is the diffusion coefficient (assumed independent of direction), C_i^t the concentration, and ρ_i^t the rate of consumption of species i in the tissue t.

If one adopts the cylindrical coordinate system illustrated in Figure 3, then $\nabla^2 C$ may be taken to imply

$$\frac{1}{r}\frac{\partial}{\partial r}\left(r\frac{\partial C}{\partial r}\right) + \frac{1}{r^2}\frac{\partial^2 C}{\partial \theta^2} + \frac{\partial^2 C}{\partial x^2}$$

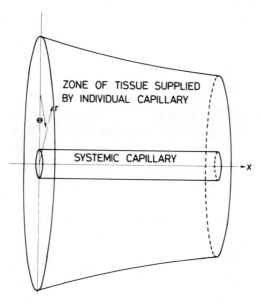

Figure 3. Diagram of assumed capillary and tissue geometries, with cylindrical coordinate system indicated.

Of the two gaseous species O_2 and CO_2, only the former need be treated for the purpose of determining the net fluxes of both. This is because (1) we make the usual assumption that the oxygen diffusivity and the parameters of oxygen consumption can be treated as independent of intratissue variations in pCO_2 and related quantities such as pH; and (2) the flux of CO_2 from tissue is calculated directly from the oxygen flux into tissue on the basis of stoichiometry, i.e., the so-called *respiratory quotient.*

The term $\rho_{O_2}^t$ includes metabolic oxygen consumption and, in the presence of diffusible myoglobin, rates of combination and dissociation of oxygen from that protein. At this stage, it suffices to consider metabolism only, postponing the more complex case of simultaneous myoglobin-facilitated oxygen transport until the more rigorous analysis in Chapter 6.

Assuming that the diffusion coefficient is effectively position-independent in tissue, that the only significant oxygen fluxes are those along the coordinate directed radially outward from the capillary, and that tissue oxygen tension and concentration obey Henry's law, equation (3-1) may assume the following form:

$$\frac{\alpha_{O_2}^t D_{O_2}^t}{r} \frac{d}{dr}\left(r\frac{dp O_2^t}{dr}\right) = \rho_{O_2}^t \qquad (3\text{-}2)$$

where $\alpha_{O_2}^t$ is the solubility coefficient for oxygen in tissue.

The behaviors of both the real-life system and the solution to the analogous mathematical description given above depend on the conditions at the boundaries that enclose the relevant tissue volume. Here we conveniently take the volume to be that which is supplied with oxygen from a single capillary. The boundary conditions necessary for the integration of equation (3-2) then are those stipulating two physical constraints at the radial extremities of that volume [as is consistent with the dimensionality and order of equation (3-2)].

It is generally agreed that there is no appreciable resistance to the transfer of gas at the capillary–tissue interface. Thus the gas partial pressures in the blood and tissue phases are essentially equal along this boundary, i.e.,

$$p O_2^t = p O_2^{bl}, \qquad r = r_{cap} \qquad (3\text{-}3)$$

The other radial extremity is, by definition, characterized by the vanishing of gas fluxes. Since the fluxes are purely diffusional, the partial pressure gradients must also vanish along this surface, i.e.,

$$dp O_2^t/dr = 0, \qquad r = r_{tis} \tag{3-4}$$

The solution to equation (3-2) is now completely determined if one specifies an expression for the oxygen consumption rate $\rho_{O_2}^t$. For most physiological systems of interest, $\rho_{O_2}^t$ is believed to obey Michaelis–Menten functionality with respect to $p O_2^t$. Nonetheless, the limiting case of zero-order (saturation) kinetics is both a reasonable and attractive choice by virtue of the facts that (1) such kinetics are reported to prevail down to extremely low (less than 1 mm Hg) oxygen tensions, and (2) a simple analytical solution to equation (3-2) is derivable for such a case.

We therefore replace $\rho_{O_2}^t$ in equation (3-2) with the constant m, which denotes the rate of metabolic oxygen consumption per unit of tissue volume. The solution, first given by Krogh (1918–1919b), is then

$$p O_2^t = p O_2^{bl} - \frac{m}{\alpha_{O_2}^t D_{O_2}^t}\left(\frac{r_{tis}^2}{2}\ln\frac{r}{r_{cap}} - \frac{r^2 - r_{cap}^2}{4}\right) \tag{3-5}$$

As expected, $p O_2^t$ expressed by (3-5) is a decreasing function of r in the latter's allowable domain, $r_{cap} \leqslant r \leqslant r_{tis}$. The minimum value, $(p O_2^t)_{min}$, is related to r_{tis} by

$$(p O_2^t)_{min} = p O_2^{bl} - \frac{m}{\alpha_{O_2}^t D_{O_2}^t}\left(\frac{r_{tis}^2}{2}\ln\frac{r_{tis}}{r_{cap}} - \frac{r_{tis}^2 - r_{cap}^2}{4}\right) \tag{3-6}$$

Thus, given tissue physicochemical parameters m, α, and D, plus capillary radius r_{cap}, one has in equation (3-6) a relationship among $p O_2^{bl}$, r_{tis}, and $(p O_2^t)_{min}$. The first four parameters can be—and traditionally have been—assumed constant along the capillary–tissue axial coordinate x. However, $p O_2^{bl}$ and either one of or both r_{tis} and $(p O_2)_{min}$ are subject to continuous variation with x.

The variations in $p O_2^{bl}$ are intimately related to the *in vivo* oxygen affinity of hemoglobin, as discussed in depth below. Tissue radius r_{tis} is a function of the volume density and orientations of the capillaries, plus blood flow directions and distribution within them.

For example, if the capillaries are identical and parallel, and subject to uniform perfusion, then symmetry considerations define r_{tis} as a constant equal to one-half the distance between the axes of adjacent capillaries. This limiting geometric case, often referred to as the "Krogh cylinder," has frequently been adopted for the analysis of tissue oxygenation, and owes its appeal to the associated mathematical simplicity. In this framework, wherein r_{tis} is fixed, the value of $(pO_2)_{min}$, as calculated from (3-6), decreases along the length of the capillary by the same amounts as does pO_2^{bl}.

On the other hand, morphological studies indicate that capillary networks are generally not so neatly arranged. Evidence of countercurrent flows and skew orientation has prompted the development of more complex theoretical models. The particular goal of most such analyses has been the estimation of tissue pO_2 profiles with such precision as to allow either the anticipation of tissue hypoxia or a test of the validity of proposed capillary network models by comparison of the theoretical profiles with experimentally obtained *in vivo* pO_2^t histograms. The significance of changes in blood properties has in most studies been accorded secondary consideration.

For the particular goal of evaluating the relative importance of various factors in the blood's performance of its respiratory functions, the tissue model selected is rather less critical. The one adopted here, and detailed in Chapter 6, is a modification of the Krogh cylinder approach by the assignment of a constant value (zero) to $(pO_2^t)_{min}$ from which are calculated r_{tis} values that decrease along the length of the capillary as a function of pO_2^{bl}. As such, we return to Krogh's relationship between blood and tissue oxygen tensions.

Equation (3-5) indicates that tissue oxygen tensions in a cylindrical disk of tissue perpendicular to the capillary axis are determined by the blood pO_2 at the center. A more rigorous analysis admitting the possibility of significant diffusion in tissue along the axial coordinate would lead to a more complex relationship, i.e., dependence of the pO_2^t value at any point upon the complete pO_2^{bl} profile. Whatever the level of complexity, however, pO_2^t must always be an *increasing* function of pO_2^{bl}, and it is therefore of primary interest to be able to calculate the oxygen tension profile within the capillary.

The partial pressure of oxygen in the blood entering the capillaries of most organs, the arterial pO_2, is determined by the partial pressure in the alveolar gas phase, equilibration of pulmonary blood with that pressure, venous–arterial shunting as it might occur, and transport of oxygen across precapillary vessels. Within the systemic capillary, the saturation of hemoglobin must decrease from the value determined by the arterial pO_2 and, inasmuch as oxyhemoglobin represents nearly all the oxygen content of the blood, the decrease is directly proportional with the amount of oxygen released to tissue. Given the rapidity of oxygen–hemoglobin equilibration, the corresponding pO_2^{bl} value at any axial location is then effectively determined by the prevailing saturation and the whole blood oxygen-binding curve.

It is worthwhile at this point to emphasize that the respective transport processes occurring in the blood and tissue phases are coupled, i.e., neither may be regarded as proceeding independently of the other since, as already stated, (1) the tissue pO_2 depends upon that in the blood, and (2) the blood pO_2 depends, via the hemoglobin saturation with oxygen, upon tissue oxygen consumption. This physical reality is reflected in the theoretical analysis, where the equations describing tissue and blood phenomena must be solved *simultaneously*. This same interdependence is manifested at the level of oxygen–hemoglobin interaction in that the flux of oxygen to tissue is governed by blood pO_2, the *amount* released is reflected by the saturation, and the two blood properties are linked via the whole blood oxygen-binding curve; thus the coupling of phenomenological, mass conservation, and chemical equilibrium relationships.

The equilibrium relationship between pO_2^{bl} and hemoglobin oxygen saturation $\bar{O}_2$ varies significantly with the prevailing red cell pH and concentration of 2,3-DPG, $[DPG]_T$, temperature, and to a lesser extent, pCO_2. Certainly $[DPG]_T$ and, as a reasonable approximation at least at rest, the temperature may be assumed effectively constant during steady-state gas transport. On the other hand, that very process is responsible for positional variations in both the pCO_2 and pH of circulating blood. Accurate estimation of the pO_2^{bl} profile therefore requires simultaneous determination of the local pCO_2 and pH.

Calculation of blood pH and $p\text{CO}_2$ profiles is based upon a knowledge of the kinetics of the important chemical reactions involving protons and CO_2, and insertion of these data into a set of species conservation relations. Separate equations for plasma and red cell concentrations are required for those ionic species that distribute themselves between the two phases according to thermodynamic and electroneutrality constraints.

The conservation relations in the blood differ from equation (3-2) insofar as radial diffusion is not believed to be a rate-limiting process, and convection (bulk flow) predominates. The assumption of negligibly small radial concentration variations means that diffusive fluxes between red cells and plasma and between plasma and tissue enter explicitly rather than through boundary conditions. Expressed verbally, the material balance states:

The rate of change of concentration of a particular species with respect to the time of passage along a capillary is proportional to the algebraic sum of boundary fluxes and internal reaction rates and inversely proportional to blood flowrate.

Taking the capillary to be a right-circular cylinder (as shown in Figure 3) and the hematocrit and flowrate to be constant, then the same relationship is expressed mathematically by

$$\pi r_{\text{cap}}^2 \phi_j u \frac{dC_i^j}{dx} = \pi r_{\text{cap}}^2 N_i^j - \pi r_{\text{cap}}^2 \phi_j \rho_i^j \tag{3-7}$$

where C_i^j is the concentration, N_i^j the net inward diffusive flow at the phase boundary and ρ_i^j the rate of depletion by chemical reaction, all in reference to species i in phase j; ϕ_j is the volume fraction of phase j; and u is the linear velocity of the blood (assumed to be constant and identical in both phases).

For the erythrocyte phase, this reduces to

$$u \frac{dC_i}{dx} = -(r_{\text{sv}} J_i^{\text{c-pl}} + \rho_i^c) \tag{3-8}$$

while the corresponding plasma relation is given by

$$u \frac{dC_i^{\text{pl}}}{dx} = \frac{h}{1-h} r_{\text{sv}} J_i^{\text{c-pl}} + \frac{2 J_i^{\text{t-pl}}}{(1-h) r_{\text{cap}}} - \rho_i^{\text{pl}} \tag{3-9}$$

where r_{sv} is the ratio of erythrocyte surface to volume and h the hematocrit (expressed as a fraction). Superscript c refers to erythrocytes and pl to plasma, while J is a flux; thus J_i^{c-pl} refers to the transmembrane flowrate per unit of membrane area of species i from erythrocytes to plasma, and J_i^{t-pl} to the flowrate per unit of interfacial area from tissue to plasma.

Insofar as u, r_{sv}, h, and r_{cap} are constants, the integration of equations (3-8) and (3-9) necessitates supplementary expressions for J_i^{c-pl}, J_i^{t-pl}, and ρ_i^j only, plus boundary conditions amounting to the complete set of concentrations at $x = 0$ (the arterial end of the capillary). Transmembrane fluxes can be expressed as functions of permeabilities and species concentrations. Chemical reaction data are described in detail in the ensuing chapters. The fact that most reactions of interest are extremely rapid justifies the assumption that they attain effective local equilibrium. Similarly, the great permeability of red cell membrane to gases allows the identification of plasma and red cell gas tensions. These considerations allow appreciable reduction in mathematical complexity.

In the steady state, the only significant net species fluxes between tissue and plasma are those of O_2 and CO_2. All other relevant components that distribute themselves between the blood and tissue either exist in a state of quasi-equilibrium across the blood–tissue interphase, or flow in negligible amounts—as, for example, the flows of acid and base associated with digestion and excretion.

As stated earlier, the fluxes of O_2 and CO_2 are related by the stoichiometry of tissue metabolic reactions, i.e., the flux of CO_2 is equal to the negative of that of O_2 multiplied by the respiratory quotient. Furthermore, the flux of O_2 must be equal in magnitude to the rate of oxygen diffusion in the tissue, at the capillary–tissue interface, i.e.,

$$J_{O_2}^{t-pl} = D_{O_2}^t \alpha_{O_2}^t (dp\,O_2^t/dr)_{r=r_{cap}} \qquad (3\text{-}10)$$

Thus, whereas the dynamics of tissue transport processes depend upon the blood oxygen *tension* profile, the simultaneous processes within the blood are responsive to the diffusive *flows* into and out of the tissue.

The solution to the above set of equations constitutes then the main step toward attainment of the goals set out at the introduction to this chapter. As indicated, this requires a knowledge of the kinetics and equilibria of blood-gas chemistry, the kinetics of O_2 diffusion and reaction in tissue, and a model of the capillary network. The physicochemical parameters of blood gas transport are detailed in the following two chapters; pertinent geometry is discussed in connection with the further development of the model of capillary–tissue exchange in Chapter 6.

By way of recapitulation, the conservation relationships for oxygen, the species of primary interest, can be written in integral form so as to account for the following overall balance:

The rate of loss of O_2 from the blood = the rate of diffusion of O_2 into the tissue at the capillary–tissue interface = the rate of consumption of O_2 in the tissue.

For a capillary of length L, the balance is expressed mathematically by

$$\pi r_{cap}^2 h u [Hm]^c (\bar{O}_2^a - \bar{O}_2^v)$$

$$= -2\pi r_{cap} D_{O_2}^t \alpha_{O_2}^t \int_0^L (dp\,O_2^t/dr)_{r=r_{cap}}\, dx$$

$$= 2\pi \int_0^L \int_{r_{cap}}^{r_{tis}} \rho_{O_2}^t r\, dr\, dx \tag{3-11}$$

where $[Hm]^c$ is the erythrocyte hemoglobin concentration (expressed as moles of heme per liter of cells), $\bar{O}_2$ the fractional saturation of heme sites with oxygen, and superscripts a and v denote arterial and venous conditions, respectively. The hemoglobin oxygen affinity is the unwritten factor which relates $\bar{O}_2$ to blood pO_2, the latter being a primary determinant of the tissue pO_2 profile.

An analogous relation describes the overall transport of CO_2. A factor expressing the CO_2 content per unit of blood volume—accounting for physically dissolved gas, bicarbonate, and carbamino hemoglobin—replaces the $h[Hm]^c \bar{O}_2$ term; the term accounting for O_2 diffusional flux is multiplied by the negative of the respiratory quotient, and the same is true for the metabolic term.

Finally, an analysis of the processes occurring in the lung would contain the same equations for blood transport. The alveolar side would be represented simply by quasi-steady-state gas tensions, while the fluxes between the blood and alveoli would be proportional to the differences between the partial pressures in the respective phases. In this monograph we have, perhaps arbitrarily, considered the systemic capillaries to be the location at which the primary demand upon the blood, i.e., supply of oxygen to metabolizing tissue, is made. Therefore, the model detailed in Chapter 6 treats lung function in a less rigorous manner than it does capillary–tissue exchange.

Chapter 4

Blood as a Physicochemical System—I

Hemoglobin and Its Interaction with Ligands

The analysis in the previous chapter placed the respiratory functions of the blood in relation to the total system of transport of oxygen and carbon dioxide and suggested those physicochemical properties of the blood that are the main determinants of its gas transport function. These properties include the equilibrium and kinetic characteristics of:

1. Oxygen and carbon dioxide binding to hemoglobin, and CO_2 hydrolysis.
2. The distribution of carbon dioxide, oxygen, and protons between red cells and plasma.

Accordingly, in this chapter an account is given of the interactions of hemoglobin with oxygen and carbon dioxide and how these interactions are influenced by binding of other ligands. The equilibria and rates of CO_2 hydrolysis and translocation of relevant species between red cells and plasma are dealt with in the following chapter. Throughout, the treatise is limited to those aspects of the system that are believed to be of physiological and clinical interest.

The interaction between hemoglobin and its ligands is a classical field of endeavor and the one in the field of the respiratory functions of the blood that has developed most rapidly during the last decade. In the first place, the binding curves of oxygen and carbon dioxide of whole blood and the effects thereupon of physiological and pathophysiological perturbations have been determined to a very considerable degree of accuracy. Second, spectacular advances in the knowledge of the function of hemoglobin on a molecular level have to a very large extent clarified the molecular mechanisms underlying these binding curves. A number of different contributions from various fields and groups of investigators have led to this latter achievement, the most important being the full exploitation of the techniques of X-ray crystallography by Max Perutz and his collaborators at Cambridge, England.

Hemoglobin Structure

There are at least six genes that control globin synthesis in normal man, resulting in the formation of six structurally different polypeptide chains. They are designated α, β, γ, δ, ε, and ζ. All normal and most abnormal hemoglobin molecules are tetramers consisting of two different pairs of polypeptide chains, each chain forming a monomeric subunit. The amino acid sequences of the α, β, γ, and δ chains are shown in Table I.

Table I
Amino Acid Sequences of Human Hemoglobin α, β, γ, and δ Chains[a]

	NA			A1														
	1	2	3	A1	2	3	4	5	6	7	8	9	10	11	12	13	14	15
α	Val	—		Leu	Ser	Pro	Ala	Asp	Lys	Thr	Asn	Val	Lys	Ala	Ala	Try	Gly	Lys	Val
β	Val	His	Leu	Thr	Pro	Glu	Glu	Lys	Ser		Ala	Val	Thr	Ala	Leu	Trp	Gly	Lys	Val
γ	Gly	His	Phe	Thr	Glu	Glu	Asp	Lys	Ala		Thr	Ile	Thr	Ser	Leu	Trp	Gly	Lys	Val
δ	Val	His	Leu	Thr	Pro	Glu	Glu	Lys	Thr		Ala	Val	Asn	Ala	Leu	Trp	Gly	Lys	Val

A	AB																
16	1	B1	2	3	4	5	6	7	8	9	10	11	12	13	14	15	16
Gly	Ala	His	Ala	Gly	Glu	Try	Gly	Ala	Glu	Ala	Leu	Glu	Arg	Met	Phe	Leu	Ser
Asn	—	—	Val	Asp	Glu	Val	Gly	Gly	Glu	Ala	Leu	Gly	Arg	Leu	Leu	Val	Val
Asn	—	—	Val	Glu	Asp	Ala	Gly	Gly	Glu	Thr	Leu	Gly	Arg	Leu	Leu	Val	Val
Asn	—	—	Val	Asp	Ala	Val	Gly	Gly	Glu	Ala	Leu	Gly	Arg	Leu	Leu	Val	Val

Table I—continued

C1	2	3	4	5	6	7	CD 1	2	3	4	5	6	7	8	D1	2	3
Phe	Pro	Thr	Thr	Lys	Thr	Tyr	Phe	Pro	His	Phe	—	Asp	Leu	Ser	His	—	—
Tyr	Pro	Trp	Thr	Gln	Arg	Phe	Phe	Glu	Ser	Phe	Gly	Asp	Leu	Ser	Thr	Pro	Asp
Tyr	Pro	Trp	Thr	Gln	Arg	Phe	Phe	Asp	Ser	Phe	Gly	Asn	Leu	Ser	Ser	Ala	Ser
Tyr	Pro	Trp	Thr	Gln	Arg	Phe	Phe	Glu	Ser	Phe	Gly	Asp	Leu	Ser	Ser	Pro	Asp

4	5	6	7	E1	2	3	4	5	6	7	8	9	10	11	12	13	14
—	—	—	Gly	Ser	Ala	Gln	Val	Lys	Gly	His	Gly	Lys	Lys	Val	Ala	Asp	Ala
Ala	Val	Met	Gly	Asn	Pro	Lys	Val	Lys	Ala	His	Gly	Lys	Lys	Val	Leu	Gly	Ala
Ala	Ile	Met	Gly	Asn	Pro	Lys	Val	Lys	Ala	His	Gly	Lys	Lys	Val	Leu	Thr	Ser
Ala	Val	Met	Gly	Asn	Pro	Lys	Val	Lys	Ala	His	Gly	Lys	Lys	Val	Leu	Gly	Ala

E15	16	17	18	19	20	EF1	2	3	4	5	6	7	8	F1	2	3	4
Leu	Thr	Asn	Ala	Val	Ala	His	Val	Asp	Asp	Met	Pro	Asn	Ala	Leu	Ser	Ala	Leu
Phe	Ser	Asp	Gly	Leu	Ala	His	Leu	Asp	Asn	Leu	Lys	Gly	Thr	Phe	Ala	Thr	Leu
Leu	Gly	Asp	Ala	Ile	Lys	His	Leu	Asp	Asp	Leu	Lys	Gly	Thr	Phe	Ala	Gln	Leu
Phe	Ser	Asp	Gly	Leu	Ala	His	Leu	Asp	Asn	Leu	Lys	Gly	Thr	Phe	Ser	Gln	Leu

F5	6	7	8	9	FG1	2	3	4	5	G1	2	3	4	5	6	7	8
Ser	Asp	Leu	His	Ala	His	Lys	Leu	Arg	Val	Asp	Pro	Val	Asn	Phe	Lys	Leu	Leu
Ser	Glu	Leu	His	Cys	Asp	Lys	Leu	His	Val	Asp	Pro	Glu	Asn	Phe	Arg	Leu	Leu
Ser	Glu	Leu	His	Cys	Asp	Lys	Leu	His	Val	Asp	Pro	Glu	Asn	Phe	Lys	Leu	Leu
Ser	Glu	Leu	His	Cys	Asp	Lys	Leu	His	Val	Asp	Pro	Glu	Asn	Phe	Arg	Leu	Leu

G9	10	11	12	13	14	15	16	17	18	19	GH1	2	3	4	5	6	H1
Ser	Cys	Cys	Leu	Leu	Val	Thr	Leu	Ala	Ala	His	Leu	Pro	Ala	Glu	Phe	Thr	Pro
Gly	Asn	Val	Leu	Val	Cys	Val	Leu	Ala	His	His	Phe	Gly	Lys	Glu	Phe	Thr	Pro
Gly	Asn	Val	Leu	Val	Thr	Val	Leu	Ala	Ile	His	Phe	Gly	Lys	Glu	Phe	Thr	Pro
Gly	Asn	Val	Leu	Val	Cys	Val	Leu	Ala	Arg	Asn	Phe	Gly	Lys	Glu	Phe	Thr	Pro

2	H3	4	5	6	7	8	9	10	11	12	13	14	15	16	17	18	19
Ala	Val	His	Ala	Ser	Leu	Asp	Lys	Phe	Leu	Ala	Ser	Val	Ser	Thr	Val	Leu	Thr
Pro	Val	Gln	Ala	Ala	Tyr	Gln	Lys	Val	Val	Ala	Gly	Val	Ala	Asn	Ala	Leu	Ala
Glu	Val	Gln	Ala	Ser	Trp	Gln	Lys	Met	Val	Thr	Gly	Val	Ala	Ser	Ala	Leu	Ser
Gln	Met	Gln	Ala	Ala	Tyr	Gln	Lys	Val	Val	Ala	Gly	Val	Ala	Asn	Ala	Leu	Ala

20	H21	22	23
Ser	Lys	Tyr	Arg
His	Lys	Tyr	His
Ser	Arg	Tyr	His
His	Lys	Tyr	His

[a] Listed from N-terminal to C-terminal end. Notation is that for sperm whale myoglobin. Deletions in a chain are indicated by dashes. (From Dickerson and Geis, 1969.)

The blood of a normal adult man contains at least six different species of hemoglobin molecules as listed in Table II. They all have the same principal structure and function, and differ only in detail. As indicated in Table II, hemoglobin A (A for adult) makes up more than 90% of the total hemoglobin concentration in a normal adult man. Throughout most of this chapter, we deal with the structure and function of hemoglobin A only. Embryonic and fetal hemoglobins are discussed separately in a later section of this chapter and the so-called abnormal hemoglobins are treated in Chapter 8.

Hemoglobin A has the composition $\alpha_2\beta_2$ and a molecular weight of 64,400. There are 141 amino acids in each of the α chains and 146 in each of the β chains. The primary structures, i.e., the amino acid sequences, of the chains are shown in Table I and Figure 4. The secondary structure, i.e., the extended or helically coiled conformation of the polypeptide chains, is shown schematically in Figures 4 and 5. As indicated in the figures, most of the amino acid residues are in the α-helix conformation. The tertiary structure, i.e., the folding of the secondary structure, and the quaternary structure, i.e., the sterical arrangement of the four monomers or subunits in the tetramer, have been revealed to a considerable extent by X-ray crystallography and are illustrated in Figures 5–9. There is little doubt that these structures are the same, or very nearly so, within intact red cells.

Within each subunit or chain, the general arrangement of the amino acid residues is such that hydrophobic or nonpolar residues are directed toward the inside of the subunit so as to leave hydrophilic or polar groups sticking out into the solvent. This arrange-

Table II
Hemoglobin Species Found in the Blood of Normal Adult Man

Hemoglobin	Structure	Percent of normal adult hemolysate
A	$\alpha_2\beta_2$	92
A_2	$\alpha_2\delta_2$	~ 2–3
A_{IA}	Not known	~ 1
A_{IB}	Not known	~ 2
A_{IC}	$\alpha_2(\beta\text{-N-hexose})_2$	~ 4
F	$\alpha_2\gamma_2$	~ 1

ment explains the high solubility of the tetramer in water—a necessary property in view of the extremely high concentration of these molecules in red cells: 330 g/liter. The stability of folding appears to depend much more on hydrophobic than on van der Waals or electrostatic interactions (Chotia and Janin, 1975).

The contacts between different subunits (see Figures 5 and 7) have been elucidated in appreciable detail (see Fermi, 1975): In general, contacts between dissimilar chains are essentially hydrophobic in nature, while those between similar chains are essentially polar. The interactions that maintain the tertiary and quaternary structures, though individually not much stronger than thermal energy levels, are many: the stability of the structure is largely entropic in origin.

The two α and two β chains delimit a central cavity (Figures 6 and 9). This is filled with water and several polar residues.

X-ray crystallographic studies have established that two different arrangements of the subunits within the tetramer are much more stable than all others. One of these two quaternary conformations predominates when the sixth coordination site of the iron atom in the heme groups is saturated with ligand, e.g., oxygen, and the other predominates when these binding sites are vacant. These structures have been denoted as *oxy* and *deoxy*, respectively (Figures 8 and 9). The differences between them are due to changes in the interchain contacts $\alpha_1\beta_2$ and $\alpha_2\beta_1$, and these in turn are due to changes in subunit tertiary structure. The transition from the deoxy to the oxy structure that follows saturation with oxygen has been ascribed to structural changes linking the position of the iron atom relative to the plane of the porphyrin ring to the tension of the bond linking iron and histidine F8 (Figures 4 and 11), and to subsequent changes in tertiary structure. The salient feature of these structural changes is that they work both ways: Changes in quaternary and/or tertiary structure induced by factors other than saturation of heme iron may affect the position of iron in the porphyrin ring and so change the affinity of this binding site. These mechanisms are discussed in more detail in a later section of this chapter.

The presence of two structurally different conformations and their relation to ligation at the hemes was demonstrated already in 1938 by Haurowitz. He showed that when oxygen was introduced

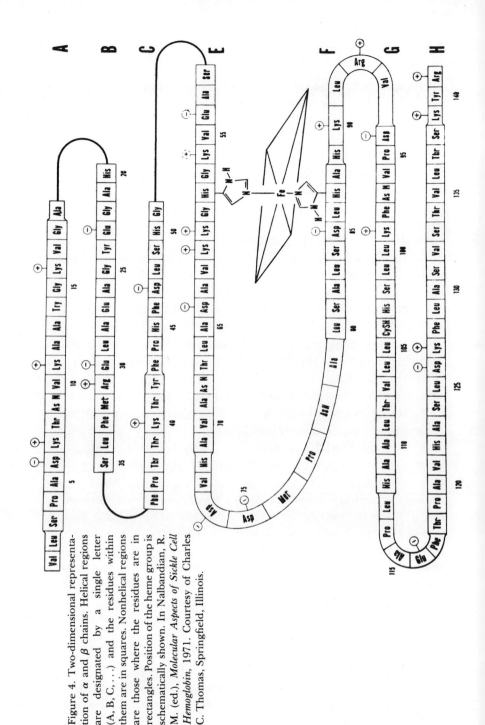

Figure 4. Two-dimensional representation of α and β chains. Helical regions are designated by a single letter (A, B, C, ...) and the residues within them are in squares. Nonhelical regions are those where the residues are in rectangles. Position of the heme group is schematically shown. In Nalbandian, R. M. (ed.), *Molecular Aspects of Sickle Cell Hemoglobin*, 1971. Courtesy of Charles C. Thomas, Springfield, Illinois.

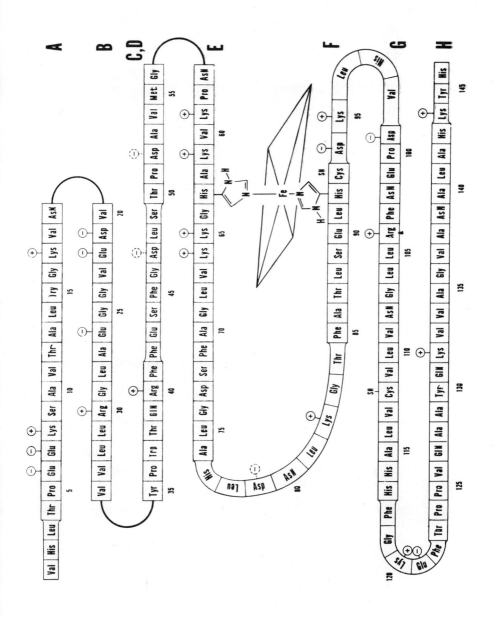

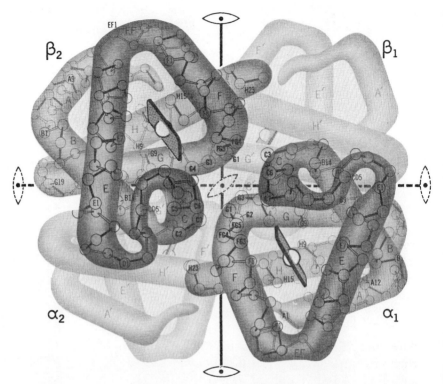

Figure 5. The folding and packing of chains in hemoglobin. The true symmetry axis (solid line) is vertical. One pseudoaxis (dashed line) is horizontal; the other rises directly out of the page. The residues that participate in the $\alpha_1\beta_2$ interchain contacts are labeled in bold type in large circles. [From R. E. Dickerson and I. Geis, *The Structure and Action of Proteins*, W. A. Benjamin, Inc., Menlo Park. Copyright 1969 by Dickerson and Geis.]

into solution, crystals of deoxygenated hemoglobin need to disintegrate before new—and different—crystals of oxyhemoglobin can be formed. Haurowitz' conclusion with respect to the mechanism of this phenomenon is worthy of note. In speaking of the recrystallization, he concludes, obviously stimulated by the papers of Pauling (Pauling, 1935; Coryell *et al.*, 1937), that it is "vermutlich auf eine Änderung der zwischen den Hämgruppen wirksamen Kräfte zurückzuführen."

The stereochemical relations between the two conformations have been identified in great detail by the Cambridge school, though only a few of the highlights are mentioned here. The greatest

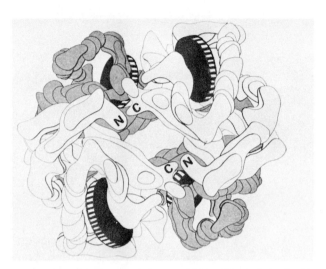

Figure 6. A model of hemoglobin at low resolution. The α chains in this model are light, the β chains dark, and the heme groups black. [After M. F. Perutz. The hemoglobin molecule. Copyright ©1964 by Scientific American, Inc. All rights reserved.]

difference between the two states is the wider separation of the β chains in the unliganded form. This is illustrated in Figures 8 and 9 and also indicated in Table III. The separation is engendered by a symmetrical rotation of the two subunit pairs $\alpha_1\beta_1$ and $\alpha_2\beta_2$. These pairs rotate so closely together that there is not much change in the contacts between the subunits of each pair. On the other hand, there is much more displacement in the contacts between chains α_1 and β_2

Table III

Distances (in Å) between Iron Atoms in Liganded (Oxy-) and Unliganded (Deoxy-) Hemoglobin[a]

Iron atoms		Deoxyhemoglobin	Oxyhemoglobin
Fe_1–Fe_2	β_1–β_2	39.9	34.4
Fe_3–Fe_4	α_2–α_1	34.9	36.0
Fe_1–Fe_3	α_2–β_1	24.7	25.0
Fe_2–Fe_4	α_1–β_2	24.6	25.0
Fe_1–Fe_4	α_1–β_1	36.9	35.0
Fe_2–Fe_3	α_2–β_2	36.9	35.0

[a]See Figures 5 and 9. (From Perutz, 1969.)

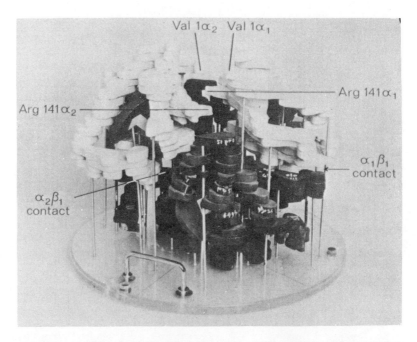

Figure 7. Model of oxyhemoglobin representing the electron density at 5.5 Å resolution. α subunits are white, β subunits black. The disks represent heme. The model shows the positions of the N- and C-terminal residues of the chains facing the internal cavity and the contacts between unlike subunits. [From M. J. Perutz and L. J. Ten Eyck, *Cold Spring Harbor Symp. Quant. Biol.* **36**, 296, 1971. Reproduced by permission.]

and between α_2 and β_1. The contact between α_1 and β_2 is dovetailed so that the CD region of one chain fits into the FG region of the other: In the liganded form, the side branch of threonine C3α fits into a notch formed by the main branch of valine FG5β. In the unliganded form, this same notch is occupied by the side branch of threonine C6α, i.e., the one protruding from the next turn of the C6 helix. Stereochemically, these two relative positions appear to be much more stable than others. On these grounds, intermediate forms are considered unlikely.

The two quaternary conformational states discussed above are defined by X-ray crystallographic data describing the distances between the iron atoms and above-mentioned contacts. The question of whether there might be other quaternary conformations in

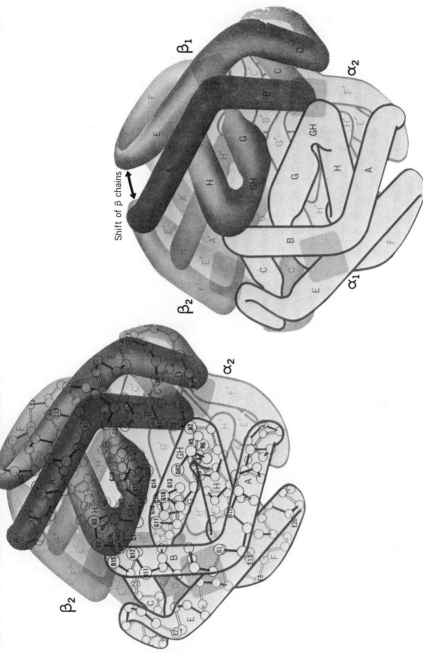

Figure 8. The hemoglobin molecule seen from the right in Figure 5. Left: oxyhemoglobin; right: deoxyhemoglobin. [From R. E. Dickerson and I. Geis, *The Structure and Action of Proteins*, W. A. Benjamin, Inc., Menlo Park. Copyright 1969 by Dickerson and Geis.]

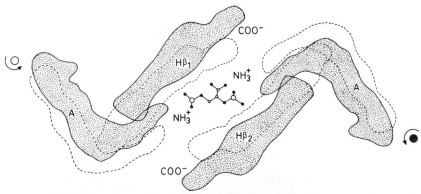

Figure 9. Projection of part of the electron density maps of oxy (---) and de-oxyhemoglobin (—) at 5.5 Å resolution, showing the N- and C-terminal portions of the β chains grouped around the twofold axis of symmetry, which is normal to the plane of the paper. In relation to Figure 5, the molecule is viewed from the bottom and the parts seen here are near the top. On oxygenation, the N-terminals move apart and the H helices close up, making less space for the DPG molecule. The circular arrows indicate the positions of the axes about which the β subunits rotate during deoxygenation. [From M. J. Perutz, *Nature (London)* **237**, 495, 1970. Reproduced by permission.]

solutions of hemoglobin has not yet been settled (see Perutz *et al.*, 1976; see also p. 87).

Under physiological conditions with respect to ionic strength, pH, and temperature, both quaternary conformations are quite stable with respect to their dissociation into dimers: $\alpha_2\beta_2 = 2\alpha\beta$. In the unliganded state, the dissociation constant for this reaction is extremely low, on the order of 10^{-10}–10^{-12} mol/liter. By contrast, liganded tetramer dissociates much more appreciably ($K_{diss} \approx 10^{-6}$ M). However, even at full ligand saturation, the dissociation into dimers is so small in the intact red cell that there are practically no dimers at all. Furthermore, no monomers exist under these conditions. When hemoglobin appears in the plasma *in vivo*, however, the situation is very different. Here, the concentration is usually quite low, on the order of 10^{-4} mM tetramer, in contrast to 5 mM tetramer in the red cells. At the former condition, there must be significant amounts of dimer. The dimers bind to one of the plasma proteins—haptoglobin—for recycling of hemoglobin constituents, a process that is of considerable physiological and clinical importance. Dimer formation also appears necessary for the passage of hemoglobin across the glomerular membrane in the kidney.

The heme groups (Figure 10) are embedded in pockets between helices E and F (Figures 4, 5, and 11). The edge containing the polar propionic acid groups is near the surface, while the remainder of the heme is buried deep inside the protein, where its surroundings are highly hydrophobic. Apparently the hydrophobic nature of the pocket is essential for maintaining the iron in its ferrous state: The low dielectric constant in this surrounding supposedly inhibits the charge separation that must occur upon oxidation (Wang *et al.*, 1958; Wang, 1958). There is only one covalent bond between the heme and the globin subunit: that connecting iron with N_ε in histidine F8. There are in addition, however, a large number of van der Waals contacts. In the α and the β chains, respectively, 18 and 20 amino acids make contact with the respective

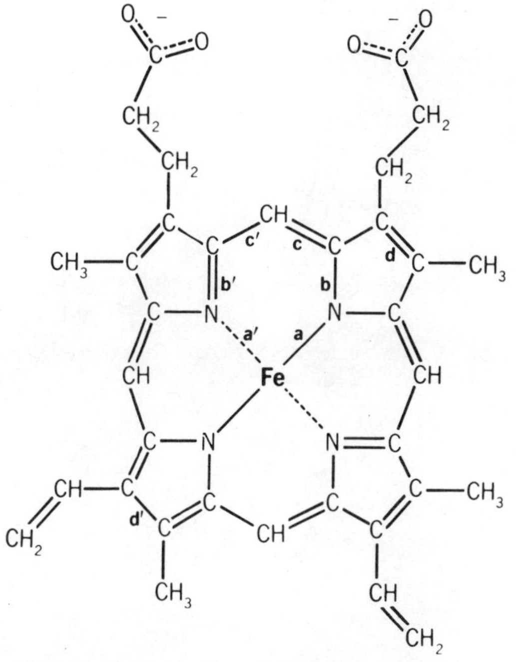

Figure 10. A schematic representation of the heme group. The porphyrin ring is unsaturated and has many delocalized π electrons. The backbone has fourfold symmetry with bonds a and a', b and b', c and c', and d and d' being equivalent. [From R. E. Dickerson and I. Geis, *The Structure and Action of Proteins*, W. A. Benjamin, Inc., Menlo Park, Copyright 1969 by Dickerson and Geis.]

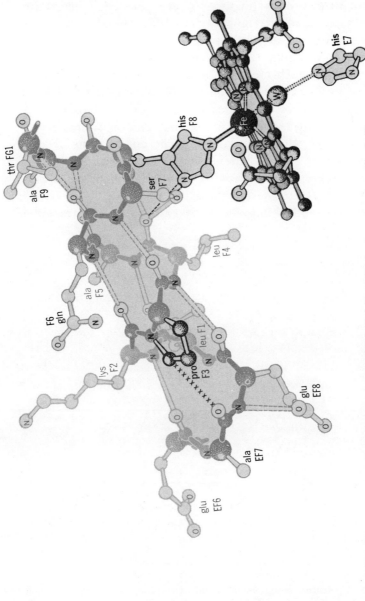

Figure 11. The heme environment. With a water or oxygen molecule at W, the iron atom is octahedrally coordinated. There are hydrogen bonds from the carbonyl of Leu F4 to the hydroxyl of Ser F7 and to the other ring nitrogen of His F8. His F8 is number 87 in the α chains and 92 in the β chains. His E7 is 58 in the α chains and 63 in the β chains. His E7 is 58 in the α chains and 63 in the β chains. [From R. E. Dickerson and I. Geis, *The Structure and Action of Proteins,* W. A. Benjamin, Inc., Menlo Park. Copyright 1969 by Dickerson and Geis.]

hemes (for details, see Fermi, 1975). The affinity of the α chains for heme is higher than that of the β chains (Bunn and Jandl, 1966, 1968; Winterhalter and Deranleau, 1967).

The ligand binding site on the distal side of the heme, i.e., that directed toward histidine E7, is wide enough in the α chain to accommodate ligand without much interaction with neighboring amino acid residues. A water molecule hydrogen-bonded to histidine E7 must, however, be displaced (Fermi, 1975). Similarly, in binding to the iron of the β chains, the ligand must displace the methyl group of valine E11β (Perutz, 1970).

The tetramer molecule measures approximately $55 \times 50 \times 60$ Å and therefore occupies a volume of approximately 180×10^{-9} μm^3. The concentration of hemoglobin in normal red cells is about 330 g/liter of packed cells. Thus, the $\sim 300 \times 10^6$ molecules in one red cell encompass about 60% of the 90 μm^3 total volume. At least half of *that* volume is solvent water since the latter is known to constitute about 70% of the total red cell volume (cf. p. 114). Since there is on the average between 10 and 20 Å, or very little space between adjacent hemoglobin molecules in red cells (Damaschun *et al.*, 1975), one might anticipate that, quite apart from the complication of dimer formation, the properties of hemoglobin in dilute solutions might not be the same as those prevailing in intact cells. This problem is discussed further on pp. 96–99.

Ligand Binding and Conformational States

The outstanding characteristic of the hemoglobin molecule is that it reversibly binds oxygen, carbon dioxide, protons, and 2,3-diphosphoglycerate (2,3-DPG) when the concentrations of these species vary within their physiological and pathophysiological ranges. In fact, all the important functions of the molecule known at the present time may be reduced to the phenomena of reversible binding of these four components.

Binding of small molecules and ions to hemoglobin is determined by the affinities of the respective binding sites. The sites for the four main ligands have largely been identified and are discussed in some detail in a following section. Oxygen binds to the iron atoms in the heme groups. Protons bind mainly to imidazolyl groups of histidine residues. Carbon dioxide binds to the four N-terminal valines. 2,3-DPG binds with each of its phosphate groups to positively charged residues located about the entrance to the central cavity between the β chains, as well as to one or two as yet unidentified sites.

The affinity of a binding site to a ligand is determined not only by the atomic composition at the site but also by the exact positioning of the atoms close to the site. For example, the proton affinity of a nitrogen atom in an imidazole group depends very much upon how the carbon 4 atom in the ring is bound; in imidazole, the acid dissociation constant at 25°C is approximately 10^{-7} M, in 4-methylimidazole it is three times less and in histidine ten times larger. Both the atomic composition and configuration of the different ligand binding sites in hemoglobin depend upon the composition and temperature of the medium. Therefore, the affinities are subject to alteration under physiological conditions.

However, even in the same medium at constant temperature, the hemoglobin molecules, though of identical chemical composition and primary structure, assume different tertiary and quaternary structures. This phenomenon is a consequence of the randomness of molecular behavior. The distribution of molecules among the different possible states (e.g., with respect to tertiary and quaternary structure) may be described according to statistical thermodynamics in terms of the energies associated with the different states: Molecules in states associated with a higher energy are less abundant than molecules with a lower energy.

As mentioned already, the hemoglobin molecule can exist in at least two different quaternary conformations. The predominant conformation when the heme iron atoms are unliganded is characterized by, among other things, the presence of inter- and intrasubunit salt bridges, which afford it a constrained or taut (T) configuration. The contribution of these bonds, shown in Figure 12, to the total stabilization energy of the T structure is still not quite clear, partly because estimates of the bond energy of individual salt bridges indicate only that the value is between 1 and 2 kcal and partly because there is uncertainty about their total number (cf. Fermi, 1975). The total energy difference between the two structures under physiological conditions in the absence of 2,3-DPG is about 6 kcal (see p. 70), i.e., rather lower than can be expected solely on the basis of the bonds shown in Figure 12.

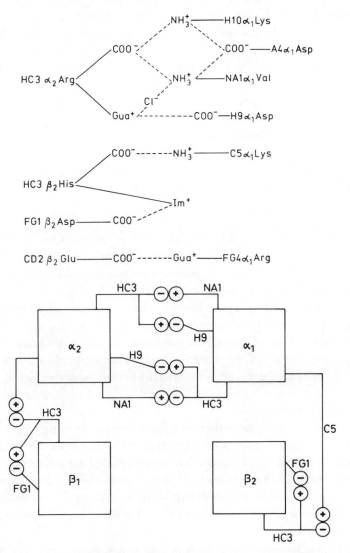

Figure 12. Inter- and intrasubunit salt bridges. [From M. J. Perutz (1976), "Structure and Mechanism of Haemoglobin." In: *Br. Med. Bull.* Vol. 32, No. 3, pp. 195–208. Reproduced by permission.]

The other conformation is obtained when the heme iron atoms are liganded: The salt bonds are broken so as to give the tetramer a relaxed (R) quaternary structure.

As does the tetramer, the subunits also exist in at least two conformations. The stereochemical relation between these two conformational states is not so well known but must be intimately related to ligand binding and the formation and breaking of the salt bridges mentioned above. The probability that a given subunit is in a given tertiary conformation is determined, as with the tetramer, by the intrinsic properties of the subunit and by medium composition and temperature, but also, to an unknown extent, by the tertiary conformation of neighboring subunits and, to a large extent, by the quaternary conformation of the tetramer.

Considering quaternary and tertiary conformations only, the hemoglobin molecule may be denoted by

$$[\alpha^{s_1}\alpha^{s_2}\beta^{s_3}\beta^{s_4}]^S, \qquad \text{where } s_i = \text{r or t} \quad \text{and} \quad S = \text{R or T}$$

There are thus 2×16 possible conformational states in which any hemoglobin molecule may exist. In principle, each of the possible states has, with its own stereochemical configuration, its own particular set of affinities toward ligands. This underlies the phenomenon of *preferential binding*. The *macroscopic* affinity toward any of the ligands must therefore depend upon the *intrinsic* affinity of each state as well as the distribution of molecules among the respective states. An extreme case in which the molecule or a subunit in the molecule is exclusively in one state in the absence of ligand and in another state when ligand is bound is called *induced-fit binding* (Koshland *et al.*, 1966).

Through the phenomenon of preferential binding to certain conformations, ligand association equilibria are *coupled* to conformational equilibria. Thus the two processes of ligand binding and conformational change may be represented by the scheme shown in Figure 13. It should be noted that this scheme is simplified considerably by the neglect of variations in relative subunit positions within the tetramer.

In the two-state models, it is assumed that the tetramer may exist in but two quaternary structures and the subunits in two

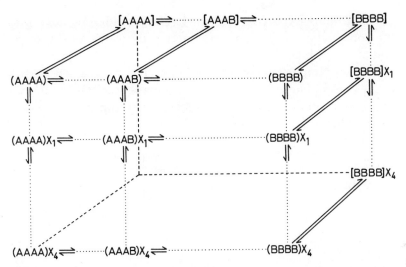

Figure 13. A generalized two-state model for the interaction between hemoglobin and oxygen. R ↔ T transitions are denoted by bracket changes and r ↔ t transitions by A–B interchange.

tertiary structures. The quaternary transitions are represented by the notation R ↔ T and tertiary transitions by t ↔ r.

The scheme in Figure 13 also illustrates the interactions between conformations, i.e., the *allosteric interactions*. The term allosteric (from Greek ἄλλος, another, different; στερεός, solid, cubic: of a different shape) was introduced by Monod and Jacob (1961) to describe the effect of an inhibiting or activating agent upon the action of an enzyme in terms of the structural alterations, i.e., allosteric transition, induced in the latter by the binding of the former. In the hemoglobin molecule, one can distinguish between two types of allosteric interactions:

(1) that between the quaternary structure of the molecule and tertiary structure of each individual subunit—for example, the transition (AAAA) → (AAAB) may be followed by the transition (AAAB) → [AAAB] because the state [AAAB] is preferred to the state (AAAB); and

(2) that between the tertiary equilibria of neighboring subunits—for example, the state (ABBB) might be preferred to (AABB) following transition from (AAAB) to (AABB).

The indirect coupling of ligand binding at different sites due to the combination of preferential binding, conformational change, and allosteric interaction may also be illustrated as in Figure 14.

A most important consequence of allosteric transitions relates to the *energy* of ligand binding to a macromolecule. The total work required to saturate a macromolecule with t binding sites is (Wyman, 1964, 1967)

$$\Delta F = t \cdot RT \ln x_m \qquad (4\text{-}1)$$

where x_m is the ligand activity which divides the area of the binding curve, plotted in semilogarithmic coordinates, into two equal parts, i.e.,

$$\int_{x=0}^{x=x_m} \bar{X} d \ln x = \int_{x=x_m}^{x=\infty} (t - \bar{X}) \, d \ln x \qquad (4\text{-}2)$$

where $\bar{X}$ is the number of moles of ligand X bound per mole of macromolecule.

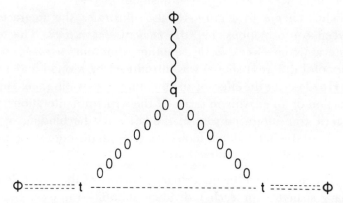

Figure 14. Schematic representation of the indirect coupling of ligand binding at different sites. The symbols q and t represent the quaternary conformations of the molecule and the tertiary conformation of a subunit, respectively, while φ represents the occupancy (i.e., vacant or occupied) of a ligand binding site. The notations 00000 and – – – – – represent molecular constraints (q–t interactions) and nearest neighbor constraints (t–t interactions), respectively, while ⌇⌇⌇ and = = = = = represent preferential ligand binding to different quaternary and tertiary conformations, respectively. (From Herzfeld and Stanley, 1974.)

For an allosteric system in which the macromolecule assumes several discrete conformational forms, Wyman (1967) has shown that $(1/x_m)^t$ is the weighted average of the several $(1/x_{mi})^t$ values. For example, in the case where there are but two allosteric forms, in relative amounts ν_1 and ν_2, and each form contains four binding sites, the total work of saturating the macromolecule with ligand is

$$\Delta F = RT \ln x_m^4 = -RT \ln \left[\frac{\nu_1}{x_{m1}^4} + \frac{\nu_2}{x_{m2}^4} \right] \qquad (4\text{-}3)$$

In the absence of allosteric transitions between the two forms, the work is

$$\Delta F^* = RT\nu_1 \ln x_{m1}^4 + RT\nu_2 \ln x_{m2}^4 \qquad (4\text{-}4)$$

The difference $\Delta F^* - \Delta F$ expresses the decrease in the work required to saturate the macromolecule with ligand that results from the allosteric transition between the two conformations. It is given by

$$\Delta F^* - \Delta F = RT \ln \left\{ \left(\frac{x_{m2}^4}{x_{m1}^4} \right)^{\nu_2} \left[1 + \nu_2 \left(\frac{x_{m1}^4}{x_{m2}^4} - 1 \right) \right] \right\} \qquad (4\text{-}5)$$

In the limiting cases where $\nu_2 = 0$ or 1, the difference $\Delta F^* - \Delta F = 0$; this is also true when $x_{m1} = x_{m2}$. In all other cases, the difference is positive, which leads to the term "positive cooperativity."

Molecules and ions that affect the affinity of the macromolecular system toward another species are called *effector ligands*. It is clear from the foregoing discussion that when such species exhibit preferential binding to one of the quaternary or tertiary conformations, the affinity of the macromolecule is modified by a shift in the conformational equilibria and thus the value of $\Delta F^* - \Delta F$. Such species are called *allosteric effectors*.

The Monod–Wyman–Changeux Model

The scheme in Figure 13 may be greatly reduced by introducing certain simplifying assumptions concerning the pathways. For example, the probability of a certain state's existence may be taken to be vanishingly small. We have already mentioned the fact that the oxygen-liganded form of hemoglobin exists almost exclusively in the R conformational state. Constraints of this type are discussed in the following sections of this chapter. At this stage, we only wish to point out that such seemingly complicated phenomena as cooperativity of oxygen binding and effects of, e.g., protons on the oxygen affinity, can easily be explained by the combination of the three—physically quite simple—phenomena of preferential binding, conformational change, and allosteric interaction. To demonstrate this, we derive here the ligand binding function for one of the most simply constructed representations: the now classical model of Monod *et al.* (1965).

The Monod–Wyman–Changeux (MWC) model assumes two quaternary conformations of the molecule, T and R. In the absence of ligand, their thermodynamic equilibrium is defined by the ratio $L = [T]/[R]$, where [T] and [R] are the concentrations of the two conformations. In each conformation there is one ligand binding site on each subunit. Furthermore, the subunits have the same conformation within each quaternary state; this is the so-called symmetry assumption. The binding sites are all identical, i.e., binding is described by a single intrinsic equilibrium association constant for each state.

For four subunits, the scheme in Figure 13 reduces accordingly to

$$
\begin{array}{ccc}
(AAAA) & \rightleftharpoons & [BBBB] \\
X\downarrow\uparrow & & \downarrow\uparrow X \\
(AAAA)X & & [BBBB]X \\
\downarrow\uparrow & & \downarrow\uparrow \\
\vdots & & \vdots \\
X\downarrow\uparrow & & \downarrow\uparrow X \\
(AAAA)X_4 & & [BBBB]X_4
\end{array}
$$

where (AAAA) denotes the T state and [BBBB] the R state. Note that, consistent with the assumptions, conformations [AAAA] and (BBBB) are forbidden.

For each state, we thus have four binding equations. They are represented as follows, where P stands for (AAAA) or [BBBB] and K_p for K_T or K_R, the *intrinsic* binding constants for each state:

$$P + X \rightleftharpoons PX, \qquad [PX_1] = K_P[X] \cdot 4[P]$$

$$PX + X \rightleftharpoons PX_2, \qquad [PX_2] = K_P[X] \cdot \tfrac{3}{2}[PX]$$

$$PX_2 + X \rightleftharpoons PX_3, \qquad [PX_3] = K_P[X] \cdot \tfrac{2}{3}[PX_2] \qquad (4\text{-}6)$$

$$PX_3 + X \rightleftharpoons PX_4, \qquad [PX_4] = K_P[X] \cdot \tfrac{1}{4}[PX_3]$$

The apparent—or macroscopic—binding constants in equations (4-6), i.e., the values defined by $[PX_1]/[X] \cdot [P]$, $[PX_2]/[X] \cdot [PX]$, etc., are seen to differ from the intrinsic—microscopic—binding constants K_P. This difference is a matter of definition. The intrinsic binding constant for a ligand that binds to several sites on a macromolecule is that which would be obtained if one could measure the extent of the reaction at a single site in the absence of the others. This is generally impossible. However, since the model under discussion assumes the equivalence of binding sites and absence of interactions among them, the relation between intrinsic and apparent binding constants is readily obtained from statistical considerations. For example, in the reaction $[P] + [X] \rightarrow [PX_1]$, governed by the apparent binding constant $[PX_1]/[X][P]$, there are four sites available for binding X but only one from which bound X may dissociate. Therefore, $[PX_1]/[X] \cdot [P]$ must be four times larger than K_P. Similarly, $[PX_2]/[X] \cdot [PX_1]$ must be 3/2 times K_P, since there are three sites available for binding X but only two from which X dissociates.

The total concentration of molecules in the T state is

$$[T] + [TX_1] + [TX_2] + [TX_3] + [TX_4]$$

while that of molecules in the R state is

$$[R] + [RX_1] + [RX_2] + [RX_3] + [RX_4]$$

Thus, the fractional saturation of the protein with ligand, $\bar{X}$, is equal to

$$\frac{[TX_1] + 2[TX_2] + 3[TX_3] + 4[TX_4] + [RX_1] + 2[RX_2] + 3[RX_3] + 4[RX_4]}{4\{[T] + [TX_1] + [TX_2] + [TX_3] + [TX_4] + [R] + [RX_1] + [RX_2] + [RX_3] + [RX_4]\}}$$

Substituting for [T], [TX₁], etc., and [R], [RX₁], etc., by means of (4-6), and defining $\alpha = K_R[X]$ and $C = K_T/K_R$, the above expression for $\bar{X}$ may be transformed into

$$\bar{X} = \frac{LC\alpha(1+C\alpha)^3 + \alpha(1+\alpha)^3}{L(1+C\alpha)^4 + (1+\alpha)^4} \tag{4-7}$$

where L, as defined previously, is equal to the ratio of the concentrations of unliganded protein in the two conformations.

The oxygen binding curve expressed by (4-7) contains only three parameters, L, C, and K_R, but unfortunately belongs to a class of mathematical relations in which the parameters are highly "redundant" (Reich and Zinke, 1974). This means that a large number of sets of these three parameters can be found that lead to practically identical binding curves, and therefore unique solutions for the parameter values cannot be obtained without additional independent information.

The MWC model may be shown to imply that the slope of a plot of equilibrium data in $\ln(\bar{X}/1-\bar{X})$ vs. $\ln[X]$ coordinates (a "Hill" plot) approaches unity as [X] approaches both zero and infinity (see Figure 15). The two limiting tangents intersect the x axis at values of

$$\ln[X] = \ln\{(L+1)/(LC+1)\} - \ln K_R$$

and

$$\ln\{(LC^3+1)/(LC^4+1)\} - \ln K_R$$

respectively. If, as appears reasonably well approximated in the oxygen–hemoglobin system: (1) L and $LC \gg 1$, then the first intercept is essentially equal to $-\ln K_T$, and (2) LC^3 and $LC^4 \ll 1$, then the second is essentially equal to $-\ln K_R$.

A measure of cooperativity in ligand binding, i.e., of the extent to which the *macroscopic* affinity changes during successive saturation of binding sites, is ΔG_I, the "energy of interaction," defined as the difference between the standard free energies of reaction of the first and fourth ligands. Thus, if the observed *macroscopic* binding constants for these reactions are, respectively, k_1 and k_4, the interaction energy is

$$\Delta G_I = RT \ln(16k_4/k_1) \tag{4-8}$$

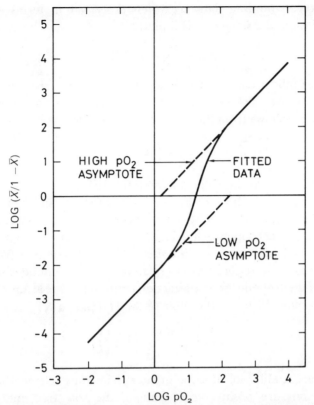

Figure 15. A plot of hemoglobin saturation with oxygen, expressed as $\log(\bar{X}/1-\bar{X})$, versus the logarithm of oxygen tension, as required by the Monod–Wyman–Changeux model. The limiting tangents intersect the x axis at values corresponding to $-\log(K_T)$ and $-\log(K_R)$.

where 16 is the statistical factor relating the observed and intrinsic binding constants. In the case of independent binding sites, $k_1 = 16k_4$ and $\Delta G_I = 0$, i.e., there is no cooperation.

In the MWC model, it can be shown (Bunn and Guidotti, 1972) that

$$\Delta G_I = RT \ln \frac{(1+LC^4)(1+L)}{(1+LC^3)(1+LC)} \qquad (4\text{-}9)$$

Thus, the value of ΔG_I may, in principle, be obtained from the limiting tangents to the oxygen binding curve, as described above.

Oxygen binding data are often described in terms of the parameter n, the slope of a Hill plot, i.e.,

$$d \ln \frac{\bar{X}}{1 - \bar{X}} = nd \ln[\text{X}] \qquad (4\text{-}10)$$

because of the usual near-constancy of n observed in the range of $\bar{X}$ from 0.2 to 0.8. If we denote by $[\text{X}]_{1/2}$ the oxygen partial pressure at $\bar{X} = 0.5$, it follows from the above definition that

$$\frac{\bar{X}}{1 - \bar{X}} = \left(\frac{[\text{X}]}{[\text{X}]_{1/2}} \right)^n \qquad (4\text{-}11)$$

which is known as the Hill equation (Hill, 1910).

The value of Hill's constant n is often used as an index of the degree of cooperativity of ligand binding: the higher the value of n, the greater the cooperativity. The general relation between n and the interaction between binding sites is, however, complex. Wyman (1967) has derived the following relationship between the *minimum* value of the free energy of interaction realized per site at any degree of saturation, $\bar{X}$, and n, the slope of the Hill plot at $\bar{X}$:

$$\Delta F_I = \frac{RT}{\bar{X}(1 - \bar{X})} \left(1 - \frac{1}{n} \right)$$

Thus, a Hill plot of slope greater than unity tells us that the interactions are positive (cooperative); the *true* free energy of interaction is not necessarily related to n in such a simple manner.

From equations (4-7) and (4-10) there can be derived an explicit relationship among n, C, and $\alpha_{1/2}$ [L may be eliminated by setting $\bar{X} = 0.5$ and $\alpha = \alpha_{1/2}$ in equation (4-7)]. However, as shown by Bunn and Guidotti (1972), experimental data are *not* entirely consistent with the predicted relationship.

The theory underlying the MWC model takes cognizance of the fact that an allosteric effector regulates ligand binding through preferential binding to one of the quaternary conformations. Consider an effector at a concentration I that binds to the T conformation with an intrinsic dissociation constant K_{IT} and to the R conformation with a constant K_{IR}. The allosteric constant L_I in the presence of effector is then

$$L(1 + I/K_{IT})^4 / (1 + I/K_{IR})^4$$

where L is the constant in the absence of effector. If $K_{IT} < K_{IR}$, i.e., if binding to the T state is preferred, then $L_I > L$ and sigmoidicity is increased.

In its basic form as developed here, the MWC model is an oversimplification of the true hemoglobin–oxygen system. In particular, the symmetry assumption, i.e., that the tertiary conformations are uniquely coupled to quaternary conformations, is almost certainly incorrect (see Perutz *et al.*, 1976). Modifications of the MWC model are discussed later.

Adair's Intermediate Compound Hypothesis

Establishment of the correct stoichiometry for the reaction of hemoglobin with oxygen led Adair (1925) to propose a scheme comprising the intermediate compounds HbO_2, $Hb(O_2)_2$, etc.:

$$O_2 + Hb(O_2)_{j-1} \rightleftharpoons Hb(O_2)_j, \qquad j = 1, 2, 3, 4$$

This implies the following equilibrium relationship:

$$\bar{O}_2 = \frac{\sum_j j A_j (pO_2)^j}{4[1 + \sum_j A_j (pO_2)^j]} \tag{4-12}$$

where the A_j consist of empirically derivable binding constants.

Although the physical model underlying this scheme is no longer accepted, the binding expression is a practical way of describing oxygen binding data insofar as they can be fitted—with very small deviations—to data obtained in a large variety of experimental situations. However, like those in the MWC model, the parameters in the Adair model are highly redundant and therefore not generally determined with high precision.

Linked Functions

The interaction between hemoglobin and its ligands may be shown to obey certain fundamental and theoretically grounded rules. These relate the binding of one ligand to that of another, and thus form the concept of "linked functions." In recent years, they have been of profound importance to the understanding of several phenomena observed in the hemoglobin–ligand system. However, inasmuch as they are purely thermodynamic in nature, they provide no information on mechanism.

In order to elucidate the concept, we choose a salt solution containing hemoglobin and oxygen and assume that, of the ions present, only protons affect the interaction between hemoglobin and oxygen. We consider variations in the chemical potentials of oxygen and of protons, denoted by μ_{O_2} and μ_{H^+}, respectively. They are obviously related to two other quantities: the molar bindings of oxygen and protons to hemoglobin, i.e., $\bar{O}_2$ and $\bar{H}^+$. Since there are no other components present that affect the interactions between hemoglobin, oxygen, and protons, we may write

$$d\bar{O}_2 = \left(\frac{\partial \bar{O}_2}{\partial \mu_{O_2}}\right)_{\mu_{H^+}} \cdot d\mu_{O_2} + \left(\frac{\partial \bar{O}_2}{\partial \mu_{H^+}}\right)_{\mu_{O_2}} \cdot d\mu_{H^+} \qquad (4\text{-}13)$$

$$d\bar{H}^+ = \left(\frac{\partial \bar{H}^+}{\partial \mu_{H^+}}\right)_{\mu_{O_2}} \cdot d\mu_{H^+} + \left(\frac{\partial \bar{H}^+}{\partial \mu_{O_2}}\right)_{\mu_{H^+}} \cdot d\mu_{O_2} \qquad (4\text{-}14)$$

The terms $(\partial \bar{O}_2/\partial \mu_{O_2})_{\mu_{H^+}}$ and $(\partial \bar{H}^+/\partial \mu_{H^+})_{\mu_{O_2}}$ are *direct binding coefficients* that relate the change in molar binding of one component to the change in chemical potential of the same species in unbound form. On the other hand, the coefficients $(\partial \bar{O}_2/\partial \mu_{H^+})_{\mu_{O_2}}$ and $(\partial \bar{H}^+/\partial \mu_{O_2})_{\mu_{H^+}}$ express the mutual interaction of oxygen and protons in their binding to hemoglobin. The question at hand is the relationship between the latter two partial derivatives. A derivation of that relationship has kindly been made available to the authors by Professor G. A. J. van Os (personal communication). We have chosen to reproduce it here with minor modification:

The total Gibbs free energy of the equilibrated solution containing hemoglobin (Hb), oxygen (A), and protons (B) plus additional species (i) that do not bind to Hb may be expressed as

$$G = n_{Hb} \cdot \mu_{HbA_\alpha B_\beta} + n_A \cdot \mu_A + n_B \cdot \mu_B + \sum n_i \mu_i \qquad (4\text{-}15)$$

where:

n_{Hb} = number of moles of heme monomer in solution

n_A, n_B = the numbers of moles of *unbound* O_2 and protons

$HbA_\alpha B_\beta$ = effective formula of protein monomer to which are bound an average of α moles of O_2 (i.e., $\alpha = \bar{O}_2$) and β moles of H^+ (i.e., $\beta = \bar{H}^+$)

$\mu_{HbA_\alpha B_\beta}$ = chemical potential of $HbA_\alpha B_\beta$

μ_A, μ_B = chemical potentials of unbound O_2 and H^+

n_i, μ_i = corresponding quantities for nonbinding species

In the equilibrium condition, the ligands have distributed themselves between Hb and solvent water in such a way that G is at a minimum. This means that

$$(\partial G/\partial\alpha)_\beta = 0 = (\partial G/\partial\beta)_\alpha$$

The expression for G may be differentiated as indicated above to yield

$$n_{\text{Hb}} \cdot \left(\frac{\partial\mu}{\partial\alpha}\right)_\beta + \mu_{\text{A}} \cdot \left(\frac{\partial n_{\text{A}}}{\partial\alpha}\right)_\beta = 0 = n_{\text{Hb}} \cdot \left(\frac{\partial\mu}{\partial\beta}\right)_\alpha + \mu_{\text{B}} \cdot \left(\frac{\partial n_{\text{B}}}{\partial\beta}\right)_\alpha$$

where $\mu_{\text{HbA}_\alpha\text{B}_\beta}$ has been abbreviated as μ.

Since a virtual displacement of a differential amount of ligand from free solution to Hb (or vice versa) does not change the total amount of that ligand in solution, it follows that

$$(dn_{\text{A}} = -n_{\text{Hb}} \cdot d\alpha)_\beta, \qquad (dn_{\text{B}} = -n_{\text{Hb}} \cdot d\beta)_\alpha$$

and therefore that

$$(\partial\mu/\partial\alpha)_\beta = \mu_{\text{A}}, \qquad (\partial\mu/\partial\beta)_\alpha = \mu_{\text{B}}$$

Since at constant Hb concentration μ is a function of α and β, we may write

$$d\mu = (\partial\mu/\partial\alpha)_\beta \, d\alpha + (\partial\mu/\partial\beta)_\alpha \, d\beta \qquad (4\text{-}16)$$

and therefore

$$d\mu = \mu_{\text{A}} \, d\alpha + \mu_{\text{B}} \, d\beta$$

which is an exact differential equation. It is therefore true that

$$(\partial\mu_{\text{A}}/\partial\beta)_\alpha = (\partial\mu_{\text{B}}/\partial\alpha)_\beta$$

which translates into

$$(\partial \log p\text{O}_2/\partial\bar{\text{H}}^+)_{\bar{\text{O}}_2} = -(\partial p\text{H}/\partial\bar{\text{O}}_2)_{\bar{\text{H}}^+} \qquad (4\text{-}17)$$

In order to arrive at the desired practical relationship we consider instead the Legendre transform $(\mu - \mu_{\text{A}}\alpha - \mu_{\text{B}}\beta)$. If we differentiate this function and combine the result with the expression for $d\mu$, the result is

$$d(\mu - \mu_{\text{A}}\alpha - \mu_{\text{B}}\beta) = -\alpha \, d\mu_{\text{A}} - \beta \, d\mu_{\text{B}} \qquad (4\text{-}18)$$

which is again an exact differential equation. Cross differentiation now yields*:

$$(\partial \bar{O}_2/\partial p\,H)_{p\,O_2} = -(\partial \bar{H}/\partial \log p\,O_2)_{pH} \qquad (4\text{-}19)$$

It may similarly be shown that

$$(\partial \bar{H}^+/\partial \bar{O}_2)_{pH} = (\partial \log p\,O_2/\partial p\,H)_{\bar{O}_2} \qquad (4\text{-}20)$$

and the analysis may easily be extended to include any number of ligands.

When such linkage arises exclusively from equilibria among various macromolecular conformations, it is termed *allosteric linkage*. This is naturally of special relevance to hemoglobin and has been dealt with comprehensively by Wyman (1967, 1968).

The Molecular Basis of Ligand Binding, Conformational Change, and Allosteric Interaction of the Hemoglobin Molecule

The chemical and stereochemical basis of ligand binding, conformational change, and allosteric interaction of the hemoglobin molecule has been elucidated to a considerable extent during recent years (see Perutz *et al.*, 1969, 1976; Perutz, 1970, 1972; Kilmartin and Rossi-Bernardi, 1973; Edelstein, 1971, 1975; Shulman *et al.*, 1975) and is still a field of intensive research. We shall deal here with the main features only.

Oxygen

As mentioned previously, the hemoglobin tetramer assumes predominantly one quaternary conformation, the *deoxy* conformation, in the absence of oxygen, and another, the *oxy* conformation, when the four hemes are liganded with oxygen. Under physiological conditions with respect to hemoglobin concentration, pH, $p\,CO_2$,

---

*The acceptance of this relation in the years between the two World Wars has not yet been adequately traced (see, however, Edsall, 1972). The original derivation of a similar relation by Adair (1923) is in rather abbreviated form and therefore difficult to judge.

2,3-DPG concentration, temperature, and ionic strength, the ratio of the prevalences of the two conformations is about $2 \cdot 10^4$ in the absence of oxygen, and the reciprocal of that value, $5 \cdot 10^{-5}$, when all the sites are occupied (Garby *et al.*, unpublished results; see Figure 18).

Isolated subunits have the same oxygen affinity as the tetrameri-cally bound subunit that binds the last oxygen molecule. That tetramer appears to be predominantly in the R state and to have no constraints upon the last subunit with respect to binding of oxygen. The oxygen affinity of subunits in the tetrameric T state is, however, much lower. In the progressive binding of oxygen brought about by increasing pO_2, one must visualize a molecular transition from the T to the R structure and thus a gradual increase in the overall affinity to oxygen.

In order to clarify cooperativity of oxygen binding in terms of this simple two-state model, we must identify stereochemical grounds for the low oxygen affinity of the T state compared to the R state, and the mechanisms of conformational change, including breaking of the salt bridges shown in Figure 12. In so doing, we must also take into account the experimental observation that dimers bind oxygen with the same high affinity as isolated subunits and without cooperativity (Ackers *et al.*, 1976).

Perutz (1970, 1972; see also Perutz *et al.*, 1974a,b,c, 1976) has suggested a mechanism based upon the following reversible chain of events: Subunit structure determines the tension of the bond between histidine F8 and iron; this tension determines the exact position of the iron atom in the plane of the porphyrin ring and this position determines the affinity of the iron atom for oxygen. Binding of an oxygen molecule to iron changes the effective size of the iron atom and reverses the chain of effects. We outline the salient features of this mechanism below.

Iron in heme is either five or six coordinated, i.e., it can accommodate electron orbitals from five or six neighboring atoms (ligands). Four of these are the nitrogen atoms of the four pyrrol rings in protoporphyrin, shown in Figure 10. Formally, these nit-rogen atoms are not identical, insofar as two have hydrogen ions bound. However, because of resonance in the porphyrin structure, the four interactions are in fact identical. Binding of ferrous iron makes the heme moiety neutral. The fifth ligand is the N_ε in the imidazolyl group of histidine F8 (Figure 11).

The sixth coordination site is vacant in deoxyhemoglobin and the iron atom is, somewhat misleadingly, said to be unliganded. In this condition, the ligand field of the iron atom is so weak that it cannot overcome the electron-pairing repulsion energy of the electrons in the d orbitals. Consequently, four of the six electrons in the d orbitals are unpaired and thus contribute to the magnetic moment. This contribution is conceived of as being due to the individual but parallel spins of the unpaired electrons; the structure is said to be in a *high spin state*. In this state, the relatively high occupancy of the d_x2-d_y2 and the d_z2 orbitals, which lie in the same plane as the bond, produces a bonding distance between the center of the iron atom and the nitrogen atoms in porphyrin of 2.18 Å. This distance is considerably larger than the 2.0 Å between the center of the ring and the nitrogen atoms. The iron atom is therefore ~ 0.6 Å from the plane of the porphyrin ring (see Fermi, 1975).

In oxyhemoglobin, an oxygen molecule is attached to the iron atom at the sixth coordination site. This increases the strength of the ligand field to the extent that its stabilization energy is large enough to overcome the electron-pairing repulsion energy. Consequently, all the electrons in the d orbitals are paired and the structure is said to be in *a low spin state*. In this state, with relatively low occupancy of the high-energy orbitals, the iron atom is "smaller," and the bond length to the nitrogen atoms in the porphyrin ring so close to the physical separation that the iron atom is all but accommodated in the plane of the ring.

The structure of the Fe–oxygen bond is still unresolved. It is generally accepted as having considerable double-bond character, with electrons in two low-energy d orbitals contributing to the bonding. Controversy revolves about the orientation of the oxygen relative to the heme plane and the extent of electron transfer from iron to oxygen. By convention, the electrons in the heme are "divided" among the atoms, with the iron atom in the ring usually assigned the oxidation number $+2$. Upon binding of oxygen there is significant transfer of electron density from iron to dioxygen, but just how this occurs is not yet clear. Moreover, there is debate as to the extent of transfer, and the nature of the bonding has been characterized both as mostly covalent, with a bonding order of 1.5 between Fe–O and O–O, and as mostly ionic, i.e., as between ferric iron and O_2^-.

Hoard (1966) was the first to suggest that binding of oxygen is accompanied by significant movement of the iron atom relative to the porphyrin ring's plane and also that this might promote changes in globin structure. It remained for Perutz to develop a detailed scheme of how displacements induced by oxygenation might make the quaternary R structure more probable.

When an oxygen molecule reacts with the iron atom, it is accommodated between the porphyrin ring and the two residues, histidine E7 and valine E11 (see Figures 5, 8, and 11). The change in electron distribution discussed above forces the iron to move toward the plane of the porphyrin ring and away from histidine F8. This bond, however, cannot be stretched, and so the F helix must move. The latter movement is directed inward, toward the center of the molecule, and narrows the pocket between helices F and H. As a result, penultimate tyrosine HC2, which in the T state is most frequently in this pocket, is forced to move out. In doing so, the tyrosine must pull along the HC3 residue—arginine in the α chains and histidine in the β chains. This breaks the salt bridges between arginine HC3 in one α chain and both valine NA1 and aspartate H9 in the other α chain, and those between histidine HC3β and aspartate FG1β and between histidine HC3β and lysine C5α (see Figures 12 and 16). The constraints affording the T structure its stabilization energy are thus broken in stepwise fashion, thus increasing the probability of the R structure.

A model for the sequence of events is shown schematically in Figure 17. Here, two important modifications of the Monod–Wyman–Changeux model—suggested by Perutz (1970, 1972)—must first be mentioned. In the first place, Perutz does not assume that the tertiary and quaternary conformations are completely coupled. The binding of oxygen to a subunit in the T structure is influenced by finite constraints imposed by the salt bridges, which in turn stabilize the quaternary T structure. The quaternary R

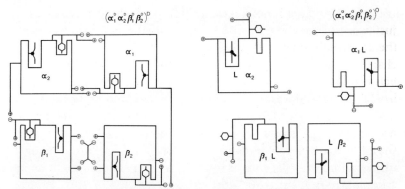

Figure 16. Diagrammatic representation of the tertiary and quaternary configurations of unliganded (A) and liganded (B) hemoglobin (see also Figure 12). The position of 2,3-DPG between the β chains in deoxyhemoglobin is indicated. [From M. J. Perutz, *Nature (London)* **237**, 495, 1970. Reproduced by permission.]

structure has no constraints of this type. Perutz further assumes that the binding of oxygen to a subunit is of the induced-fit type, so that once the subunit has bound oxygen, it assumes the *oxy* tertiary structure. The constraints upon the quaternary T structure

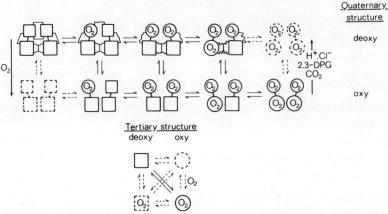

Figure 17. Diagrammatic sketch of the allosteric mechanisms of hemoglobin. The smaller subunits represent the α, the larger ones the β subunits. The clamps between them represent salt bridges; those between the β subunits represent 2,3-DPG. Unstable forms have been drawn in dashed lines. Loosening of salt bridges on ligand binding is indicated by wavy lines. The order of oxygenation and salt bridge rupture is arbitrary. [From M. J. Perutz (1976), "Structure and mechanism of haemoglobin." In: *Br. Med. Bull.* Vol. 32, No. 3, pp. 195–208. Reproduced by permission.]

imposed by that subunit are increased because the subunit is now in the "wrong" conformation.

The assumptions of Perutz for oxygen binding may be given a mathematical expression *formally* identical to that generated by the Monod–Wyman–Changeux model, i.e., equation (4-7) (Herzfeld and Stanley, 1974). However, the *physical content* of the parameters L, K_R, and K_T are different. In the MWC model, L expresses the difference in energy between the two conformations, which arises from an intrinsic energy difference, E_q, plus the sum of the differences in energy between the tertiary conformations of the subunits. In the Perutz picture, L expresses the same intrinsic energy difference plus a difference in energy attributable to quaternary–tertiary constraints, mainly salt bridges, so that

$$L = \exp[(E_q + E'_{qt})/RT]$$

Furthermore, in the Perutz scheme, K_R and K_T are induced-fit binding constants to subunits in the deoxy conformation that differ in oxygen affinity because of quaternary–tertiary constraints, i.e.,

$$K_R = K, \qquad K_T = K \exp[-(E'_{qt} + E''_{qt})/4RT]$$

where E''_{qt} is the contribution due to the wrong conformation.

In the Perutz scheme, there is no cooperativity in the binding of oxygen to the R structure. It has not yet been resolved whether there is cooperation, through t↔t interactions, in oxygenation of the T structure.

According to this somewhat oversimplified scheme, cooperativity arises as a result of a highly specific interplay between positive and negative free energy changes involving many interactions. The transition of the tetramer from the low- to the high-affinity form is associated with a positive free energy change. Part of the free energy of oxygen binding to the low-affinity structure is converted into and stored in tertiary conformational alterations. The net gain in free energy is delocalized throughout the molecule in such a way that the following oxygen molecules find their binding site in a more favorable state.

An energy diagram is shown in Figure 18. The energy values have been calculated from oxygen binding data of whole blood and

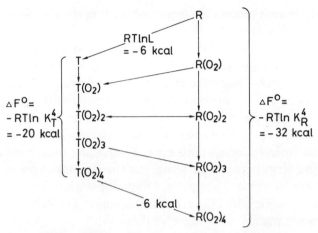

Figure 18. An energy diagram illustrating cooperativity of oxygenation of the hemoglobin tetramer (see text).

concentrated solutions at 37°C, pH^c = 7.20, and pCO$_2$ = 40 mm Hg, and refer to the situation in the absence of 2,3-DPG (Garby, Groth, and de Verdier, unpublished observations). The value of 6 kcal for the difference in energy between the two conformations in the absence of ligand may be accounted for by the salt bridges in Figures 12 and 16. Note that the difference in energy between the two oxygenated structures, E''_{qt}—due mainly to the contribution of wrong tertiary conformations—is very similar in magnitude to E'_{qt}.

The precise sequence of events in the scheme of Figure 17 is not yet known. However, it is probable that the α chains are the first to become oxygenated (Perutz, 1970; Gibson, 1973; Mansouri and Winterhalter, 1973; Ho, 1974), although this appears to be subject to variation with the 2,3-DPG activity of the medium (Ho, 1974). The relation between subunit tertiary structure and tetramer conformation, and the stage at which most molecules change from a quaternary T structure to a quaternary R structure are other unknowns.

Thus, there are two mechanisms to account for the low affinity of the subunits in the quaternary T state:

(1) Tension of the heme iron–histidine F8 bond, which opposes the movement of the iron toward the plane of the porphyrin ring;

according to recent results (Perutz *et al.*, 1976) this mechanism may be the dominant one in the α subunits.

(2) Steric hindrance at the ligand binding sites, which is present in all subunits.

The first mechanism would manifest itself in the allosteric constant L as well as in K_T. As to the second, steric hindrance vanishes upon ligand binding, and the changes in tertiary structure associated with it are opposed by the constraints of the quaternary T structure.

Though the main events described here most likely provide a rather accurate picture of what happens when hemoglobin binds oxygen, some doubts have been expressed concerning the cause-and-effect relationships. According to Perutz (1972), there is a one-to-one relationship between the spin state of the iron atoms and the quaternary structure, so that the two characteristics of the molecule are causally related as in a see-saw: "Changes in quaternary structure alter the tension between the heme-linked histidine and porphyrin rings, which changes the bond lengths and affects the spin state of the heme, and vice versa" (Perutz, 1972). This concept has been questioned by Edelstein, Gibson, and co-workers (Hensley *et al.*, 1975; Edelstein and Gibson, 1975), who point out that there are several instances in which spin state and conformation are not related. In their view, the spin state of the iron, while influencing spectra and the precise orientation of the heme, is of no relevance *per se* to ligand binding and conformational change.

In any event, the affinity of the hemoglobin molecule toward oxygen depends markedly upon the distribution of hemoglobin molecules among the possible conformational states and therefore upon the medium composition and temperature. As will be seen, protons, carbon dioxide, and 2,3-DPG all act as allosteric effector ligands, which, whether indirectly or directly, tend to stabilize the T structure by preferential binding.

Protons

Protons bind reversibly to a large number of sites in the hemoglobin molecule. The ionizable groups and the approximate pK

values are shown in Table IV. In the physiological pH range 6.8–7.8, the great majority of the most active sites belong to the imidazolyl groups of some 20 histidine residues (Janssen *et al.*, 1972), since their pK values lie near the physiological pH. There are in all 38 histidine residues in the tetramer, but nearly half are "masked" and therefore not titratable.

The overall affinity to protons, like that to oxygen, depends upon the distribution of hemoglobin molecules among the possible conformational states and therefore on the composition and temperature of the medium. The buffer capacity of purified oxyhemoglobin in 0.1 M KCl and at 25°C is between 8 and 10 equivalents/mol of tetramer in the physiological pH range (Rollema *et al.*, 1975; see Figure 19), which is considerably lower than that of partially purified oxyhemoglobin at the same temperature and ionic strength (Antonini *et al.*, 1965). The difference is almost certainly due to the presence of 2,3-DPG, ATP, and their Mg complexes in the latter preparation, since the value at 37°C reported by Antonini *et al.* is practically identical to that for erythrocyte fluid (Figure 19) obtained by Siggaard-Andersen (1974).

Table IV

Ionizable Groups in Human Hemoglobin and Their Approximative pK Values (Modified after Roughton, 1964)[a]

Group	Number	pK
α-Carboxyl (terminal)	4	3–4
Carboxyl (aspartic and glutamic)	56	4.3–4.7
Imidazolyl (histidine)	38	5.7–8.1[b]
α-Amino (terminal)	4	7.0–7.9[c]
Sulfhydryl (-SH cysteine)	6	>11[d]
ε-Amino (lysine)	44	10–11[e]
Phenolic (tyrosine)	12	>11[e]
Guanidinic (arginine)	12	~12

[a] Note that several pK values depend on the degree of ligand binding (see text) and that the numbers refer to all groups, whether titratable or not.
[b] Upper limit is for deoxyhemoglobin (Kilmartin *et al.*, 1973).
[c] Lower limit is for oxyhemoglobin (Garner *et al.*, 1975).
[d] β93-SH groups only (Janssen *et al.*, 1974).
[e] Janssen *et al.* (1974).

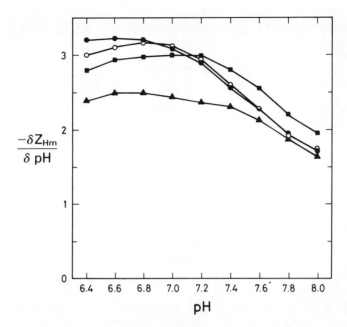

Figure 19. The buffer capacity of human oxyhemoglobin. ▲, purified hemoglobin in 0.1 M KCl at 25°C (Rollema *et al.*, 1975); ■, ●, partially purified hemoglobin in 0.25 M NaCl at 25 and 37°C, respectively (calculated from Antonini *et al.*, 1965); O, erythrocyte fluid at 37°C (after Siggaard-Andersen, 1974).

The isoelectric point of purified hemoglobin is 7.25 in 0.1 M KCl at 25°C (Rollema *et al.*, 1975). It is rather lower at 37°C but is not accurately known; nor is ΔH_I, the apparent heat of ionization, of purified hemoglobin. The value of ΔH_I for partially purified hemoglobin, and probably erythrocyte fluid (see above), in the pH range 6–8 is between 6 and 7 kcal/mol (Antonini *et al.*, 1965).

At 37°C and physiological ionic strength, the overall affinity to protons depends primarily upon the activities of oxygen, 2,3-DPG, ATP, carbon dioxide, and protons, and possibly the hemoglobin concentration as well. Titration curves of oxy- and deoxygenated human erythrocyte fluid, each at $p\mathrm{CO}_2 = 0$, are shown in Figure 20. From the slopes, the corresponding buffer capacity per mole of hemoglobin tetramer is about 12 equivalents/pH unit at physiological red cell pH. Its variation with pH and the concentration of 2,3-DPG is shown in Figure 21. At high carbon dioxide tensions, the

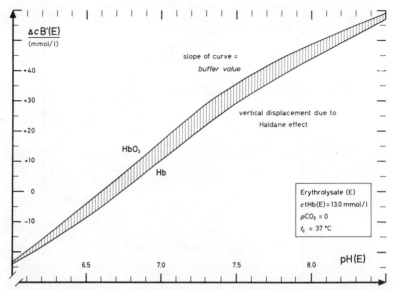

Figure 20. Titration curves at $p CO_2 = 0$ and 37°C for human erythrolysate ([Hm] = 13.0 mM), oxygenated (HbO$_2$) as well as deoxygenated (Hb). The ordinate shows the change in concentration of strong base, the abscissa the pH. The zero point on the ordinate was arbitrarily chosen as the point where the HbO$_2$ curve intersects the pH = 6.6 line. [From O. Siggaard-Andersen: *The Acid–Base Status of the Blood.* Munksgaard, Copenhagen, 1974. Reproduced by permission.]

four N-terminal α-amino groups exist partly as carbamate and the buffer capacity is thereby altered, as discussed in more detail in the next chapter.

The buffer capacity of the contents of intact red cells at 0°C has been determined by Dalmark (1975) to be 10 equivalents/mole of tetramer. This value is in agreement with the data of Siggaard–Andersen (1974) and of Antonini *et al.* (1965), if one applies the temperature correction suggested by the data of the latter investigators.

As suggested in Figure 20, there is a release of protons to the medium when hemoglobin is oxygenated. This is the phenomenon discovered by Christiansen, Douglas, and Haldane in 1914, and often called the "Haldane effect." Christiansen and her co-workers showed that carbon dioxide was released when Haldane's own blood was oxygenated at constant $p CO_2$, and they suggested that this effect was a result of a release of protons from oxygenated hemoglobin: "It

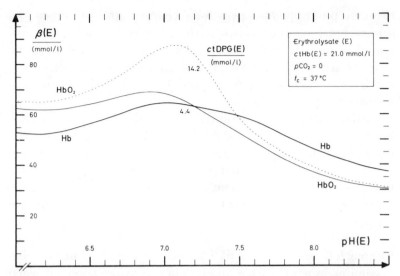

Figure 21. The buffer value of erythrocyte fluid ([Hm] = 21.0 mM) at $pCO_2 = 0$ as a function of pH at 37°C. The solid curves are derived from the slopes of the titration curves in Figure 20. The dotted curve represents the buffer value of oxygenated erythrocyte fluid with a threefold increase in 2,3-DPG concentration. [From O. Siggaard-Andersen: *The Acid–Base Status of the Blood.* Munksgaard, Copenhagen, 1974. Reproduced by permission.]

may be that the oxy-hemoglobin is more acid." As was realized later, probably first by Adair (see p. 64; see also Edsall, 1972), this dependence of proton binding upon the degree of oxygenation is actually required by application of the laws of linked function (see p. 61) to the very early data of Bohr *et al.* (1904). The latter group demonstrated that carbon dioxide decreases the affinity of hemoglobin for oxygen. More recent data (see pp. 96–98) have revealed that the simultaneous change in pH must have been the dominant factor. The protons liberated upon oxygenation are often called Bohr or Haldane protons.

The origin and mechanism of release of the Bohr protons are explained to a considerable extent by the already mentioned events surrounding the breakage of salt bridges when, upon oxygenation, hemoglobin molecules undergo a transition from the T to the R structure (Perutz, 1970). According to Figure 12, the protons of both valine NA1α and histidine HC3β are involved in a salt bridge between positively and negatively charged groups. When the bridges break upon oxygenation, the protons become less strongly bound. The associated change in pK is from 7.8 to 7.0 for the α-amino groups (Garner *et al.*, 1975) and from approximately 8.1 to 7.2 for the imidazolyl groups (Kilmartin *et al.*, 1973*a*; see also Kilmartin, 1974).

Most Bohr protons arise from the residues just mentioned. Perutz (1970) suggested that histidine H5α might also be involved through the formation, in the T state, of a salt bridge with the neighboring carboxyl of aspartic acid H9α. In the R state the same histidine is near the guanidinium group of arginine B12β, and the transition would be expected to change the pK value of histidine in the appropriate direction.

de Bruin *et al.* (1973, 1974*a*) have shown that the uptake of protons following addition of 2,3-DPG to oxygenated hemoglobin maximizes in a pH range lower than the range observed when 2,3-DPG is added to deoxygenated hemoglobin (see further p. 88). If it is assumed that 2,3-DPG binds at the same site in each conformation, it can be deduced that the ionization constants of the involved groups differ in the two states. These groups (discussed in the section on 2,3-DPG) therefore contribute Bohr protons.

Chloride ions also affect the affinity of hemoglobin toward protons. de Bruin *et al.* (1974*b*) and Rollema *et al.* (1975) have provided data indicating that chloride ions bind to positively charged groups in both oxy- and deoxy-hemoglobin. The affinity toward chloride ions is greater in the deoxy state; as such, chloride ions are allosteric effectors by virtue of preferential binding, just as are protons, carbon dioxide, and 2,3-DPG. Binding of chloride increases the pK values of the positively charged groups and therefore causes more protons to be bound. These join the list of Bohr protons. One oxygen-linked site of chloride ion binding is that shown in Figure 12; the others have not yet been identified with certainty, but are most probably identical to the oxygen-linked 2,3-DPG binding site(s) (Chiancone *et al.*, 1975; see also the section on 2,3-DPG).

In the absence of carbon dioxide and 2,3-DPG, but under physiological conditions with respect to temperature, pH (= 7.20), and chloride concentration, 2.0 protons are released when one tetramer molecule binds four oxygen molecules (Figure 22). The number decreases on either side of this pH value. Oxygenation of hemoglobin in the presence of carbon dioxide and 2,3-DPG leads to the values shown in Figure 22. The mechanisms underlying these phenomena are fairly well known and discussed in greater depth in the next two sections.

Since, according to Perutz (1970), the $T \rightarrow R$ transition is intimately related to the previously mentioned rupture of salt bridges, and the latter is (at least in the absence of carbon dioxide and 2,3-DPG) a principal source of Bohr protons, one would expect a rather strong correlation between the $T \rightarrow R$ stabilizing energy (or cooperativity of oxygen binding) and the Bohr effect. For the simple mechanism of the Monod–Wyman–Changeux model the relation may be derived on the basis of equations (4-9) and (4-11). However, the result is not consistent with data gathered by Bunn and Guidotti (1972), who therefore proposed that proton and oxygen binding sites might also be linked to one another within each subunit.

The precise relationship between bindings of protons and oxygen molecules has not yet been determined. Application of the reciprocal (linked functions) relationship to oxygen binding data at 37°C and different physiological pH and $p\mathrm{CO}_2$ values (Garby *et al.*, 1972; Arturson *et al.*, 1974*d*) has shown excellent agreement with the direct measurements of oxygen-linked proton binding shown in Figure 22, i.e.,

$$\int_0^1 \frac{\partial \log p\mathrm{O}_2}{\partial \mathrm{pH}} \, d\bar{\mathrm{O}}_2 = \Delta \bar{\mathrm{H}}^+ (\Delta \bar{\mathrm{O}}_2 = 1)$$

The reciprocal relationship may, of course, also be integrated over narrower saturation ranges. The above-mentioned data indicate that at cellular $\mathrm{pH} \cong 7.15$, in the absence of CO_2 and 2,3-DPG, about 1.4 protons are released upon binding of the first two oxygen molecules and 0.6 upon binding of the last two. Thus, under these conditions, where oxygen molecules show only slight preference for α chains (Ho, 1974), the relation between oxygen and proton binding is saturation-dependent. A similar relationship was also

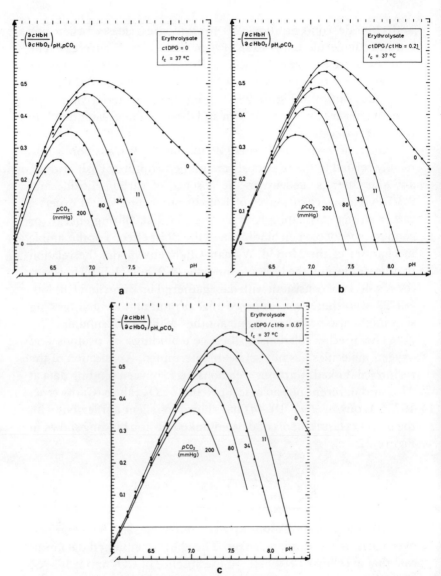

Figure 22. The Haldane coefficient of human erythrocyte fluid at 37°C as a function of pH for various values of pCO_2 and 2,3-DPG concentration ([DPG]/[Hm] = 0 (a), 0.21 (b), 0.67 (c)). The hemoglobin concentration of the titrated fluid was 11.2–14.1 mmol of heme per liter. The values are for a change in oxygen saturation from zero to one hundred percent. [From O. Siggaard-Andersen: *The Acid–Base Status of the Blood.* Munksgaard, Copenhagen, 1974. Reproduced by permission.]

found by Meier *et al.* (1974), Hlastala and Woodson (1975) and by Tyuma and Ueda (1975).

One interpretation of the latter phenomenon is that there must be more conformational change when the first two oxygen molecules bind. However, it is unlikely that the $T \rightarrow R$ transitions behave in this fashion. In fact, the best estimates for the relative number of $T \leftrightarrow R$ transitions for $\bar{O}_2$ changing from 0.0 to 0.5 are below 0.5 (Herzfeld and Stanley, 1974; Garby *et al.*, in preparation). Thus, if the phenomenon is linked to conformational change, it must include $t \leftrightarrow r$ transitions independent of $T \leftrightarrow R$ transitions. This would be consistent with the suggestions of Bunn and Guidotti (1972) referred to above.

Observation of the Bohr effect in valency hybrids (tetramers in which either the two α or two β chains are frozen in the liganded state) and the effect thereupon of organic phosphates (Rollema *et al.*, 1976) also indicate that proton release upon oxygenation is related more to the molecule's ligation state than to its quaternary structure.

Carbon Dioxide

Carbon dioxide combines with amino groups of hemoglobin to form carbamate according to the following reactions:

$$HbNH_3^+ \quad \rightleftharpoons HbNH_2 + H^+ \qquad (4\text{-}21)$$

$$HbNH_2 + CO_2 \rightleftharpoons HbNHCOOH \qquad (4\text{-}22)$$

$$HbNHCOOH \rightleftharpoons HbNHCOO^- + H^+ \qquad (4\text{-}23)$$

Of these reactions, the last is shifted almost completely to the right in the physiological pH range.

The amino-acid residues responsible for carbamate formation have been identified as the four N-terminal α-valines (Kilmartin and Rossi-Bernardi, 1969, 1971). Human hemoglobin has also 44 ε-amino groups of lysine (see Table IV) but their proton affinity, i.e., the pK of reaction (4-21), appears to be so large as to preclude a significant contribution to the total carbamate at physiological pH.

The macroscopic affinity of the α-amino groups toward carbon dioxide depends not only on the proton activity of the medium, i.e., through reactions (4-21) and (4-23), but also on the activities of oxygen and 2,3-DPG. There is, furthermore, a decrease in oxygen-linked carbamate formation with increasing hemoglobin concentration (Baumann *et al.*, 1975).

Oxygen affects the affinity toward carbon dioxide allosterically, as is reflected by the dependence of the equilibrium constants of the above reactions on $\bar{O}_2$ (see below). This clarifies:

(1) the effect of carbon dioxide on the oxygen affinity of hemoglobin at constant pH, first shown by Adair (1925) and later confirmed by Næraa *et al.* (1963, 1966); and

(2) the difference in the degrees of CO_2 absorption, at constant pH and pCO_2, into oxygenated and deoxygenated bloods (Rossi-Bernardi and Roughton, 1967).

The detailed stereochemical explanation is not quite clear but seems to be that in the T state only, the carbamino groups form a salt bridge with an α-NH_3^+ in the vicinity of the N-terminal valines.

Binding of 2,3-DPG also involves the α-amino groups of valines $Na1\beta$ (see the section on 2,3-DPG), so there is direct competition between 2,3-DPG and carbon dioxide for the β chain α-amino groups. This explains the effect of 2,3-DPG upon oxygen-linked carbamino binding, first shown by Bauer (1969, 1970).

Perella *et al.* (1975*a*) measured carbon dioxide binding at 37°C to the oxy and deoxy forms of hemoglobin in concentrated solutions free of 2,3-DPG. At pH = 7.20 and pCO_2 = 40 mm Hg, 0.25 moles of CO_2 were found to associate with 1 mol of hemoglobin tetramer in the oxy conformation, and 0.80 mol/mol in the deoxy conformation. At pH = 7.40, the values were 0.40 and 1.27, respectively.

Perella *et al.* (1975*b*) (see also Kilmartin *et al.*, 1973*b*) measured, furthermore, carbon dioxide binding at 37°C to the oxy and deoxy forms of specifically carbamylated hemoglobins at a total tetramer concentration of 3.5 mм. At pH = 7.4, pCO_2 = 40 mm Hg, and in the absence of 2,3-DPG, the degree of association to the oxy forms of both $\alpha_2\beta_2^c$ and $\alpha_2^c\beta_2$ (c = carbamylated) was calculated to be ~0.25 mole CO_2 per mole of tetramer. The values for the deoxy forms of $\alpha_2\beta_2^c$ and $\alpha_2^c\beta_2$ were 0.42 and 0.85, respectively. These data show that, at least under the conditions chosen, each chain exhibits oxygen-linked carbon dioxide binding, with that of the β chains dominant. The presence of twice as much 2,3-DPG as tetramer had no effect upon the reaction of CO_2 with the oxy forms of either hybrid, nor with the deoxy form of $\alpha_2\beta_2^c$. However, binding to the deoxy form of $\alpha_2^c\beta_2$ decreased to 0.45 mol/mol tetramer.

The data of Perella *et al.* (1975*b*) for the separate extents of carbamino formation with α and β chains may be summed to give values of: (1) 0.50 and 1.27 for the respective oxy and deoxy, DPG-free tetramers and (2) 0.50 and 0.87 in the presence of twice as much 2,3-DPG as tetramer. These values are reasonably consistent with those of Bauer and Schröder (1972) determined in whole blood of normal 2,3-DPG content at the same (erythrocyte) pH: respectively, 0.35 and 0.88 mol/mol oxy and deoxy tetramer. For pH = 7.20, Bauer and Schröder indicate oxy and deoxy values of 0.14 and 0.48. This last pair of values, together with the corresponding data of Perella *et al.* (1975*a*), agree with the notion that at lower pH, where 2,3-DPG binds more avidly to each conformation, there is a correspondingly greater inhibition of carbamino formation as well.

The interpretation of these data in terms of reaction pK values is a growing possibility. Garner *et al.* (1975) estimated the pK values (pK_z) of reaction (4-21) at 26°C for the oxy and deoxy forms of the respective chains as follows: p$K_z(\alpha, \text{oxy}) = 6.95$, p$K_z(\alpha, \text{deoxy}) = 7.79$, p$K_z(\beta, \text{oxy}) = 7.05$, p$K_z(\beta, \text{deoxy}) = 6.84$. Thus, the proton affinity of the α-chain valines shows an increase, while that of the β-chain valines shows a small decrease upon deoxygenation. Morrow *et al.* (1976) have estimated the overall pK values (pK_c) at 30°C for the combined reactions (4-22) and (4-23) to be p$K_c(\alpha, \text{oxy}) = 5.4$, p$K_c(\alpha, \text{deoxy}) = 4.8$, p$K_c(\beta, \text{oxy}) = 5.8$, p$K_c(\beta, \text{deoxy}) = 4.7$. Thus, the CO_2 affinity of each nonprotonated amino group increases substantially upon deoxygenation.

The integrated *oxygen-linked* binding of CO_2, i.e., ΔCO_2 for $\Delta \bar{O}_2 = 1$, at $pCO_2 = 40$ mm Hg and pH = 7.20, is thus 0.55 mol/mol tetramer in the absence of 2,3-DPG (Perella *et al.*, 1975*a*) and 0.34 mol/mol tetramer at a 2,3-DPG concentration of 5 mM in red cells (Bauer and Schröder, 1972). These values are in very good agreement with those calculated from the carbon-dioxide-linked oxygen affinity of whole blood reported by Arturson *et al.* (1974*d*), through the linked functions $(\partial \log pO_2 / \partial \log pCO_2)_{\bar{O}_2}$ and $(\partial \overline{CO}_2 / \partial \overline{O}_2)_{pCO_2}$; that is,

$$-\int_0^1 \frac{\partial \log pO_2}{\partial \log pCO_2} \, d\bar{O}_2 \cong \Delta \overline{CO}_2 \ (\Delta \bar{O}_2 = 1)$$

The available data are shown in Figure 23.

The relationship between release of CO_2 and binding of oxygen is saturation-dependent (Garby *et al.*, 1972; Arturson *et al.*, 1974*d*; Hlastala and Woodson, 1975; see Figure 24). At physiological red cell pH (7.20) and 2,3-DPG concentration (5 mM), differential oxygen-linked CO_2 binding decreases from a value of 0.15 at 15%

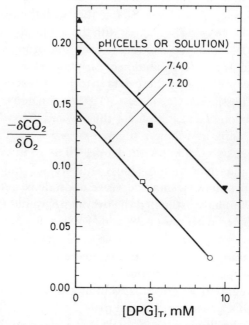

Figure 23. Oxygen-linked carbamino binding at $pCO_2 = 40$ mm Hg and constant pH and $[DPG]_T$ in concentrated hemoglobin solutions ($\triangle$, $\blacktriangle$, $\blacktriangledown$) and in intact cells ($\bigcirc$, $\square$, $\blacksquare$). Filled symbols denote pH = 7.40 and open symbols denote pH = 7.20. $\triangle$ and $\blacktriangle$ (Perella *et al.*, 1975*a*); $\blacktriangledown$ (Perella *et al.*, 1975*b*); $\square$ and $\blacksquare$ (Bauer and Schröder, 1972); and $\bigcirc$ (Arturson *et al.*, 1974*d*). Values refer to a change from fully deoxygenated to fully oxygenated hemoglobin.

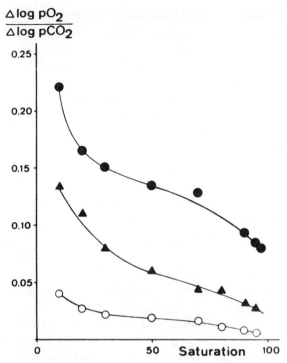

Figure 24. The relation between $\Delta \log pO_2 / \Delta \log pCO_2$ and oxygen saturation at $pH^c = 7.20$ for the pCO_2 difference 22–77 mm Hg at different red cell 2,3-DPG concentrations. ●, $[DPG]_T = 1.2$; ▲, $[DPG]_T = 5.0$; ○, $[DPG]_T = 9.0$ mmol/liter. [From Arturson, Garby, Wranne, and Zaar. *Acta Physiol. Scand.* 1974, **92**, 332. Reproduced by permission.]

oxygen saturation to 0.06 and then 0.025, at 50 and 90% oxygen saturations, respectively.

Saturation dependence of oxygen-linked carbon dioxide binding is also indicated by the results of Baumann, Bauer and Haller (1975) for sheep hemoglobin solutions free of 2,3-DPG. This conclusion can be drawn from a comparison of their data for the effects of CO_2 upon: (1) the relationship between $p(50)$ and pH, and (2) the number of protons released upon *iso*-pH oxygenation of deoxygenated hemoglobin. With 1.3 mM tetramer solutions in the pH range 6.8 to 7.5 and $pCO_2 = 0$, they found a constant $(\partial \log pO_2 / \partial pH)_{\bar{O}_2 = 0.5}$ value of -0.45, and the same value for the integrated oxygen-linked proton binding, i.e., $(\Delta\bar{H}^+/\Delta\bar{O}_2)_{pH}$ over the $\bar{O}_2$ interval from 0 to 1. At $pCO_2 = 60$ mm Hg, $(\partial \log pO_2/\partial pH)_{\bar{O}_2=0.5}$ was again constant over the same pH range, but at the value of -0.21, whereas $(\Delta\bar{H}^+/\Delta\bar{O}_2)_{pH}$ varied from -0.29 at pH 7.0 to -0.12 at pH 7.4.

According to linked functions theory, the derivative or "point" values, $(\partial \log pO_2/\partial pH)_{\bar{O}_2}$ and $(\partial\bar{H}^+/\partial\bar{O}_2)_{pH}$ must be equal at the same set on conditions, at least in the absence of 2,3-DPG (see p. 64). These point values can only equal $(\Delta\bar{H}^+/\Delta\bar{O}_2)_{pH}$ by coincidence, or if the point value is independent of $\bar{O}_2$. Conversely, inequality of $(\partial \log pO_2/\partial pH)_{\bar{O}_2=0.5}$ and the integral value, $(\Delta\bar{H}^+/\Delta\bar{O}_2)_{pH}$, is proof that the latter's point value is saturation dependent, i.e., $\bar{H}^+$ is a nonlinear function of $\bar{O}_2$. If we discount the possibility of a coincidence in the absence of CO_2, then we are led to conclude that the presence of CO_2 upsets the linearity of the $\bar{H}^+ - \bar{O}_2$ relationship.

Now, this effect of CO_2 must be tied in with carbamino reactions, which are intrinsically associated with proton binding–release (reactions 4-21–4-23). It is also theoretically possible that carbamino formation at one site causes, allosterically, a change in pK at one or more other amino acids. In any event, it is most likely that the saturation dependence of oxygen-linked proton binding observed by Baumann *et al.* in the presence of CO_2 is an expression of saturation-dependent oxygen-linked CO_2 binding.

It is also of considerable interest to note that at very low hemoglobin concentrations, 0.03 mM, Baumann *et al.* found that the *shape* of the oxygen binding curve was essentially independent of pCO_2. This suggests that oxygen-linked CO_2 binding is independent of $\bar{O}_2$ under these conditions (cf. p. 99).

Direct confirmation of CO_2 binding to β chain α-amino groups has been achieved by Arnone (1974) through X-ray crystallography. There was, however, no evidence in Arnone's preparation of binding to the α-chain α-amino groups. This finding is puzzling in view of the clearcut evidence of CO_2 reaction with $\alpha_2\beta_2^c$ in the experiments of Perella *et al.* (1975*b*).

As may be inferred from reactions (4-21)–(4-23), formation of carbamate from $-NH_2$ is accompanied by release of a single proton, while formation from $-NH_3^+$ involves release of two. Rossi-Bernardi and Roughton (1967) determined an effective value of ~ 1.5 for binding at constant pH under physiological conditions. For *oxygen-linked* carbamation at constant pCO_2 and pH, the situation differs because of oxygen-linked changes in pK_c and pK_z.

Oxygen-linked formation of carbamate induces a release of protons, which may be estimated from the expression

$$\frac{[\partial \bar{H}^+/\partial \bar{O}_2]_{pH,[DPG]_T,pCO_2=0} - [\partial \bar{H}^+/\partial \bar{O}_2]_{pH,[DPG]_T,pCO_2}}{[\partial \bar{CO}_2/\partial \bar{O}_2]_{pH,[DPG]_T,pCO_2}}$$

(This assumes that the Bohr protons associated with oxygen-linked binding of *DPG* are insensitive to variations in pCO_2 and that use of the reciprocal relations at constant $[DPG]_T$ introduces negligible error.)

Values of the numerator may be obtained from Figure 22, and those of the denominator at $pCO_2 = 40$ mm Hg from Figure 23. Under physiological conditions, the release of, again, 1.5 protons per CO_2 molecule is thereby calculated to be a result of oxygen-linked carbamino formation, roughly independent of oxygen saturation level (Garby *et al.*, 1972; Klocke, 1973). Figure 25 illustrates the dependence of the Bohr coefficient on pCO_2.

2,3-Diphosphoglycerate

2,3-DPG associates with each quaternary conformation, less extensively to the oxy state, under physiological and most pathophysiological conditions. This explains the effect of 2,3-DPG on the oxygen affinity of hemoglobin, discovered by Benesch and Benesch (1967) and Chanutin and Curnish (1967). It is probable that the sole explanation for the binding difference is the varying DPG affinity of the binding site between the two β chains, as shown in Figure 26. The entrance to this site is much narrower in the R state (Perutz, 1970). Other binding sites for 2,3-DPG exist, but whether or not they exhibit preferential binding has not yet been firmly established.

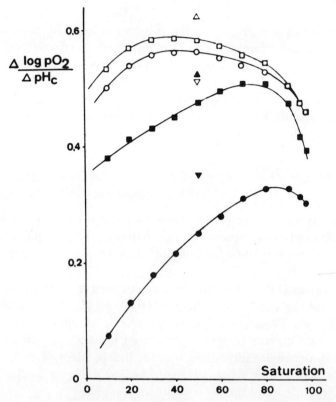

Figure 25. The relation between $\Delta \log pO_2/\Delta pH^c$ and the oxygen saturation for various values of pCO_2 and red cell 2,3-DPG at $pH^c \cong 7.20$. $\square$, $[DPG]_T = 9.3$ mmol/liter and $pCO_2 = 22$ mm Hg; $\bigcirc$, $[DPG]_T = 9.4$ mmol/liter and $pCO_2 = 77$ mm Hg; $\blacksquare$, $[DPG]_T = 1.75$ mmol/liter and $pCO_2 = 22$ mm Hg; $\bullet$, $[DPG]_T = 1.27$ mmol/liter and $pCO_2 = 77$ mm Hg; $\triangle$, $\triangledown$, $[DPG]_T = 2.9$ and 0 mmol/liter, respectively, and $pCO_2 = 0$ mm Hg; $\blacktriangle$, $\blacktriangledown$, $[DPG]_T = 3.4$ and 0 mmol/liter, respectively, and $pCO_2 = 32$ mm Hg. [From Arturson, Garby, Wranne, and Zaar. *Acta Physiol. Scand.* 1974, **92**, 332. Reproduced by permission.]

The precise manner in which 2,3-DPG exerts its effect upon the oxygen affinity of hemoglobin has not yet been clarified. Stabilization of the T state might be achieved by movement of the proximal histidine and heme iron away from the side to which oxygen must bind; the lower affinity would then be a result of either pure steric hindrance or a diminished tendency of the iron in that state to donate π electrons to dioxygen (Maxwell and Caughey, 1976). Effects of 2,3-DPG independent of quaternary conformational

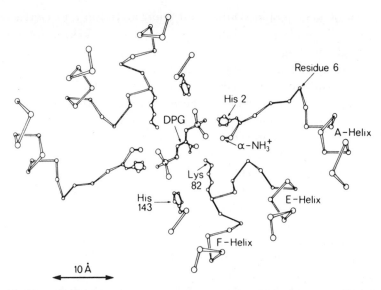

Figure 26. Sketch of DPG binding to human deoxyhemoglobin. DPG binds with the basic residues of the central cavity to form salt bridges with valine 1 and histidines 2 and 143 of both β chains, and with lysine 82 of one β chain. [From A. Arnone. *Nature (London)* **237**, 146, 1972. Reproduced by permission.]

change can also be visualized, though the relation between binding of 2,3-DPG and changes in quaternary structure is another unknown. Recent evidence (Perutz *et al.*, 1976) indicates that binding to oxyhemoglobin of inositolhexaphosphate—which presumably acts very similarly to 2,3-DPG—results in a change from the R to another state *not* identical to the T state.

The 2,3-DPG affinities of both quaternary conformations vary with pH, pCO_2, and temperature, as well as hemoglobin concentration (see p. 99). Under physiological conditions, the association constant for binding to the oxy form of the tetramer is ~100 liters/mol and that to the deoxy tetramer ~3000 liters/mol (Garby and de Verdier, 1971; Berger *et al.*, 1973; Gerber *et al.*, 1973; Udkow *et al.*, 1973; Hamasaki and Rose, 1974). If only one binding site is involved, then under physiological conditions there is no induced-fit binding of 2,3-DPG to hemoglobin.

Changes of 2,3-DPG concentration in the range 25–30 mM, and at otherwise physiological conditions, have no effect on the oxygen affinity of hemoglobin (Duhm and Kim, in Duhm and Gerlach, 1974). This result may be interpreted as being due to saturation of the single binding site in each conformation, or to the balancing effects at more than one oxygen-linked site.

As mentioned previously, the effect of 2,3-DPG on the oxygen affinity of β chains appears to be larger than the effect on α chains, since the nearly random oxygenation of hemes in the absence of 2,3-DPG changes to preferential binding to α chains in its presence (Ho, 1974).

Binding of 2,3-DPG to both oxy and deoxy conformations is pH dependent (Garby *et al.*, 1969; Udkow *et al.*, 1973). The linked functionality is seen most clearly in experiments where proton uptake upon addition of 2,3-DPG to oxy- and deoxyhemoglobin is measured by back titration (Kilmartin, 1973; de Bruin *et al.*, 1973, 1974a; de Bruin and Janssen, 1973; see Figure 27). In the oxy conformation, the extent of protonation coupled to the reaction of 2,3-DPG maximizes at a pH of ~6.5, whereas in the deoxy conformation it maximizes within the range 7.1–7.6.

On the basis of experiments in which the reactions in Figure 27 were studied at varying concentrations of 2,3-DPG, de Bruin *et al.* (1974a) showed that the proton uptake by both Hb and HbO_2 could be described with one single association constant for DPG binding to each form. At pH 6.8 and 25°C, the proton uptake per molecule of 2,3-DPG bound was found to be larger for HbO_2 than for Hb.

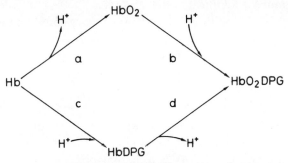

Figure 27. A schematic illustration of the binding–release of protons accompanying the binding of oxygen and 2,3-diphosphoglycerate to hemoglobin. $\Delta \bar{H}^+(a) + \Delta \bar{H}^+(b) = \Delta \bar{H}^+(c) + \Delta \bar{H}^+(d)$. (Adapted from deBruin *et al.*, 1973.)

Under physiological and most pathophysiological conditions, the net result of reactions of 2,3-DPG and protons with oxygenated and deoxygenated hemoglobin is that an increased 2,3-DPG level is associated with an increased Bohr effect (Duhm, 1973). The effect of 2,3-DPG on the Haldane effect under physiological conditions is shown in Figure 28.

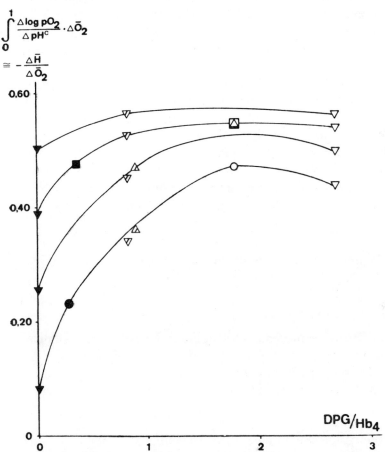

Figure 28. Effect of 2,3-DPG concentration, expressed as the molar ratio of DPG and hemoglobin tetramer, on the oxygen-linked proton binding for various values of pCO_2 at $pH^c \cong 7.20$. The four curves, drawn by eye, correspond to the following pCO_2 values: 0, 22, 34, and 80 mm Hg as read from the top. [From Arturson, Garby, Wranne, and Zaar. *Acta. Physiol. Scand.* 1974, **92**, 332. Reproduced by permission. Original sources listed therein.]

Carbon dioxide inhibits binding of 2,3-DPG through the direct effect already discussed.

Carbon Monoxide

Carbon monoxide and oxygen compete for the same sites in hemoglobin. The pioneering observations on the equilibrium of carbon monoxide with hemoglobin and its dependence upon oxygen tension were made by Douglas *et al.* (1912) and in a highly important note by J. B. S. Haldane, at the age of 19, in the same year.

The allosteric interactions are presumably very much the same as those of oxygen binding. It has been observed that protons, 2,3-DPG, and CO reduce the hemoglobin affinity of one another. There is, however, a difference between the reactions of CO and O_2 insofar as the combination of hemoglobin with CO involves greater cooperativity, and therefore its interaction energy ΔG_I exceeds that of oxygen (Roughton, 1970; see also p. 100). Furthermore, the progressive saturation of hemoglobin with CO appears to be more randomly distributed among α and β chains than that of oxygen (Ho, 1974).

Oxygen Binding and Interaction Coefficients under Physiological Conditions

Basic Considerations

From the preceding description, it is obvious that hemoglobin–ligand interactions are quite complex: Binding of any ligand influences the affinity of the hemoglobin molecule toward all others. Therefore, isothermal binding equations must take the form

$$\bar{X}_i = f_i \text{ (all } x_j) \tag{4-24}$$

where $\bar{X}_i$ is the number of moles bound per mole of hemoglobin monomer, x the activity of unbound ligand, and i and j denote oxygen, protons, carbon dioxide, 2,3-DPG, etc.

Insofar as there is as yet no comprehensive, quantitatively developed theory for ligand binding to hemoglobin, we content ourselves with a semiempirical format. Furthermore, so as to be able to invoke the laws of linked functions, we deal with a differential analog to equation (4-24), after replacing the activities by their logarithms. The alternative generalized relationship is then

$$d\bar{X}_i = \sum_{j=1}^{n} \left(\frac{\partial \bar{X}_i}{\partial \log x_j}\right)_{x_{k(k \neq j)}} d \log x_j \qquad (4\text{-}25)$$

For physiological binding of *oxygen* in the presence of protons, carbon dioxide, and 2,3-DPG, (4-25) becomes

$$d\bar{O}_2 = \left(\frac{\partial \bar{O}_2}{\partial \log pO_2}\right) d \log pO_2 + \left(\frac{\partial \bar{O}_2}{\partial pH}\right) dpH$$

$$+ \left(\frac{\partial \bar{O}_2}{\partial \log pCO_2}\right) d \log pCO_2 + \left(\frac{\partial \bar{O}_2}{\partial \log x_{DPG}}\right) d \log x_{DPG} \qquad (4\text{-}26)$$

where it is recognized that the activity of dissolved gas is equivalent to its partial pressure, and $\log x_{H^+} = -pH$. In addition, the subscripts of differentials have been dropped for simplicity.

Analogous expressions may be written for the binding of protons, carbon dioxide, and 2,3-DPG. All such relations contain one coefficient of the form $(\partial \bar{X}_i/\partial \log x_i)$ and three others of the form $(\partial \bar{X}_i/\partial \log x_j)_{j \neq i}$. The first may be called *binding coefficients* and the second *interaction coefficients*.

On the other hand, it is customary to operate in terms of interaction coefficients that differ in form from those in (4-25). The effects of protons, CO_2, and 2,3-DPG upon the oxyhemoglobin dissociation curve are instead expressed by the following differential equation *written for changes at constant* $\bar{O}_2$:

$$d \log pO_2 = \left(\frac{\partial \log pO_2}{\partial pH}\right) dpH + \left(\frac{\partial \log pO_2}{\partial \log pCO_2}\right) d \log pCO_2$$

$$+ \left(\frac{\partial \log pO_2}{\partial \log[DPG]_T}\right) d \log[DPG]_T \qquad (4\text{-}27)$$

Note that x_{DPG} has been replaced, for practical purposes and without loss of generality, by the total concentration of 2,3-DPG (free and hemoglobin-bound), $[DPG]_T$.

Equation (4-27) can also be written in terms of either $[DPG]_{free}$ or $[DPG]_{bound}$ (i.e., free or bound to hemoglobin) instead of $[DPG]_T$.

In either of the former two alternative cases, one may invoke the laws of linked functions, such that the first two interaction coefficients in (4-27) are respectively equivalent to $(\partial \bar{H}^+/\partial \bar{O}_2)_{pH}$ and $-(\partial \overline{CO}_2/\partial \bar{O}_2)_{pCO_2}$. These latter two coefficients describe *in vivo* oxygen-linked binding of protons and carbon dioxide.

Experimentally, however, the maintenance of constant $[DPG]_{free}$ or $[DPG]_{bound}$ is usually not realized; nonetheless there is evidence to the effect that $(\Delta \bar{H}^+/\Delta \bar{O}_2)_{pH,pCO_2,[DPG]_T}(\Delta \bar{O}_2 = 1.0)$ is equal, within experimental error, to

$$\int_0^1 \left(\frac{\partial \log pO_2}{\partial pH} \right)_{\bar{O}_2, pCO_2, [DPG]_T} d\bar{O}_2$$

under normal physiological conditions (Garby *et al.*, 1972; Arturson *et al.*, 1974*d*). One may, therefore, assume that the linked-functions relationships may also be applied at constant $[DPG]_T$, although this lacks rigorous theoretical and experimental justification.

The Whole Blood Oxygen Binding Curve under Standard Conditions

The binding and interaction coefficients discussed above are partial derivatives that allow the calculation of *changes* in ligand binding. Calculation of the absolute *degree* of binding under a given set of conditions requires a set of reference conditions.

The oxygen binding curve of whole blood under selected standard conditions with respect to plasma pH, pCO_2, pCO, red cell 2,3-DPG, and temperature has been reported by Arturson *et al.* (1974*a*). The standard conditions chosen were as follows: plasma pH = 7.40, $pCO_2 = 40$ mm Hg, pCO ensuring $\overline{CO} = 0.01$, $[DPG]_T = 5.0$ mmoles/liter of packed cells, and 37°C. The equilibrium data were obtained, on fresh blood drawn from apparently healthy subjects whose HbCO concentrations were below 5% of total hemoglobin, with a Radiometer DCA-1 instrument, maintaining a pCO_2 of 34 mm Hg in the oxygenation gas. In this way, the actual concentrations of effector ligands (protons, carbon dioxide, 2,3-DPG, and carbon monoxide) were quite close to those chosen as standard, and therefore the correction factors to convert from actual to standard pO_2 values (see below) were quite small.

In reality, the molar concentrations of 2,3-DPG and hemoglobin are each subject to variation as the blood is oxygenated at constant pH^{pl} and pCO_2. As may be deduced from the nomogram of Dill *et al.* (1937; reproduced in Roughton, 1964), a change from 0 to 100% saturation would effect a cellular volume decrease on the order of 1%. The accompanying change in hemoglobin oxygen affinity would hardly be measurable (see Woodson *et al.*, 1974; Sinet *et al.*, 1976).

The standard data are shown in Table V. No difference was found between male and female subjects. The values are compared with those compiled by Severinghaus (1966; see also Severinghaus *et al.*, 1972, and Roughton and Severinghaus, 1973) because his data, though lacking information on blood sample 2,3-DPG concentration, are almost certainly more reliable above 95% oxygen saturation. In this region of the curve the effect of modest variation in $[DPG]_T$ is quite small (Tyuma *et al.*, 1971).

The standard deviation of replicates was found to be about one-half the total standard deviation. This implies a fairly low degree of precision in the upper part of the curve, i.e., above 90–95% oxygen saturation. It also implies variations in factors, other than those mentioned above, that influence the oxygen affinity of whole blood. One such variable is the concentration of red cell ATP in apparently healthy subjects. ATP is an allosteric effector similar to 2,3-DPG (Rörth, 1968; Garby *et al.*, 1969; Lo and Schimmel, 1969; Udkow *et al.*, 1973; Hamasaki and Rose, 1974). The coefficient of variation of red cell ATP concentration among apparently healthy subjects is as great as 10% (Andreasson *et al.*, 1973), which would account for a few tenths of a 1-mm Hg change in pO_2. Another variable is the presence of minor hemoglobin components in the blood of healthy subjects (HbA_2, HbA_{IA}, HbA_{IB}, HbA_{IC}, and HbF). The ligand binding and interaction coefficients of these species of hemoglobin differ from those of HbA.

Recently, Tweeddale *et al.* (1976) found that the oxygen affinity of whole blood under standard conditions decreases with age: The $p(50)$ increased linearly from 27.3 mm Hg in the age group 18–39 years to 29.2 mm Hg in the age group 60–89 years. The reason for

Table V

Relation between Oxygen Tension and Oxygen Saturation of Whole Blood from Apparently Healthy Subjects under Standard Conditions[a]

$\bar{O}_2$ (%)	pO_2(mm Hg)		
	Mean	S.D.	Standard curve of Severinghaus
10	10.6	1.0	10.3
20	15.4	1.1	15.4
30	19.5	1.1	19.2
40	23.4	1.0	22.8
50	27.4	1.1	26.6
60	31.9	1.3	31.2
70	37.5	1.4	36.9
80	45.1	1.8	44.5
85	50.4	2.0	49.8
90	58.2	2.6	57.8
92	62.6	2.7	
94	68.6	3.1	
96	77.3	3.9	81.0
98	92.3	5.6	110.0

[a]From Arturson et al. (1974a). pH (plasma) = 7.40, pCO_2 = 40 mm Hg, [DPG]$_T$ = 5.0 mmol/liter of cells, HbCO = 1.0%, and temperature = 37°C.

this increase remains obscure. It is of interest to note that in the age group 18–39 years, the mean $p(50)$ value and the standard deviation were the same as those found by Arturson et al. (1974a; see Table V).

Numerical Values

The numerical values of several of the binding and interaction coefficients referred to above are well established, while others are only roughly known. Fortunately, those required for an analysis of the respiratory functions of the blood (see Chapters 5 and 6) belong to the first category.

The extensive experimental work that forms the basis for estimation of binding and interaction coefficients was performed on whole blood, erythrolysates, or concentrated hemoglobin solutions. When comparing data for whole blood with that obtained from hemoglobin solutions, it is necessary to be conscious of the difference in pH between red cells and plasma. The difference is a consequence of the impermeable, charged components in each phase and possibly also of the pump–leak cation transport system of red cells. This is discussed in more detail in Chapter 5. The correction for differences in pH may be made by analogy to

$$\left(\frac{\partial \log X}{\partial \mathrm{pH}^{\mathrm{pl}}}\right)_{\bar{O}_2} = \left(\frac{\partial \log X}{\partial \mathrm{pH}^{\mathrm{c}}}\right)_{\bar{O}_2} \left(\frac{\partial \mathrm{pH}^{\mathrm{c}}}{\partial \mathrm{pH}^{\mathrm{pl}}}\right)_{\bar{O}_2}$$

Under physiological conditions, the numerical value of $(\partial \mathrm{pH}^{\mathrm{c}}/\partial \mathrm{pH}^{\mathrm{pl}})_{\bar{O}_2}$ is in the range 0.80–0.84. It varies with pH, $\bar{O}_2$, $p\mathrm{CO}_2$, and $[\mathrm{DPG}]_T$ (see p. 131 and Tables X and XII).

Extensive experimental data have been accumulated in regard to:

(1) Oxygen binding as a function of $p\mathrm{O}_2$, pH, $p\mathrm{CO}_2$, and $[\mathrm{DPG}]_T$ in human whole blood and concentrated hemoglobin solutions (Duhm, 1971; Garby *et al.*, 1972; Siggaard-Andersen *et al.*, 1972*a*; Duhm, 1973; Arturson *et al.*, 1974*d*; Duhm and Gerlach, 1974).

(2) Proton binding of human whole blood and erythrolysates as a function of pH, $p\mathrm{CO}_2$, $[\mathrm{DPG}]_T$, and $\bar{O}_2$ (Siggaard-Andersen, 1971; Siggaard-Andersen and Salling, 1971).

(3) Carbon dioxide binding of human whole blood as a function of pH, $p\mathrm{CO}_2$, $[\mathrm{DPG}]_T$, and $\bar{O}_2$ (Bauer and Schröder, 1972; Klocke, 1973).

These data reveal the functionality of most binding and interaction coefficients. Some have already been shown here (Figures 19–25, 28). Whenever direct comparisons have been possible, the agreement has been excellent (see Arturson *et al.*, 1974*a,d*).

Arturson *et al.* (1974*a*) have tabulated their experimental data, for whole blood, of the coefficients $\Delta \log p\mathrm{O}_2/\Delta \mathrm{pH}^{\mathrm{pl}}$, $\Delta \log p\mathrm{O}_2/\Delta \log[\mathrm{DPG}]_T$, and $\Delta \log p\mathrm{O}_2/\Delta \log p\mathrm{CO}_2$ at different values of oxygen saturation, $\mathrm{pH}^{\mathrm{pl}}$, $p\mathrm{CO}_2$, and total 2,3-DPG concentration. These results are reproduced in Tables VI–VIII.

Effect of Hemoglobin Concentration

In the previous sections, numerical values were assigned to several of the binding and interaction coefficients on the basis of data obtained from either whole blood or concentrated hemoglobin

Table VI

Values for the Coefficient $-[\Delta \log pO_2/\Delta pH^{pl}]_{\bar{O}_2,pCO_2,[DPG]_T}$ [a]

pH^{pl}:					7.20				
[DPG]$_T$ (mM):		3.0			5.0			7.0	
pCO$_2$:	20	40	80	20	40	80	20	40	80
$\bar{O}_2$(%)									
10	0.34	0.26	0.18	0.36	0.28	0.21	0.37	0.30	0.25
20	0.35	0.28	0.21	0.38	0.30	0.25	0.38	0.33	0.29
30	0.35	0.29	0.23	0.39	0.32	0.27	0.39	0.35	0.32
40	0.35	0.30	0.25	0.40	0.34	0.30	0.40	0.37	0.34
50	0.34	0.31	0.27	0.41	0.35	0.32	0.41	0.39	0.36
60	0.34	0.31	0.28	0.40	0.37	0.33	0.41	0.40	0.38
70	0.33	0.31	0.29	0.39	0.36	0.34	0.41	0.40	0.39
80	0.32	0.31	0.30	0.38	0.36	0.35	0.40	0.40	0.40
90	0.30	0.30	0.29	0.36	0.35	0.35	0.40	0.39	0.39
95	0.28	0.28	0.28	0.34	0.34	0.34	0.39	0.39	0.39

pH^{pl}:					7.40				
[DPG]$_T$(mM):		3.0			5.0			7.0	
pCO$_2$:	20	40	80	20	40	80	20	40	80
$\bar{O}_2$(%)									
10	0.31	0.23	0.11	0.33	0.24	0.18	0.45	0.43	0.40
20	0.33	0.26	0.18	0.38	0.30	0.24	0.47	0.45	0.42
30	0.34	0.29	0.22	0.40	0.35	0.28	0.48	0.46	0.44
40	0.35	0.31	0.25	0.42	0.37	0.31	0.49	0.47	0.45
50	0.35	0.33	0.28	0.42	0.39	0.33	0.50	0.48	0.46
60	0.36	0.33	0.30	0.42	0.40	0.34	0.49	0.48	0.46
70	0.35	0.33	0.31	0.40	0.39	0.35	0.48	0.47	0.46
80	0.33	0.32	0.31	0.38	0.37	0.35	0.46	0.46	0.45
90	0.28	0.28	0.35	0.35	0.35	0.34	0.44	0.44	0.44
95	0.25	0.25	0.25	0.32	0.32	0.32	0.42	0.42	0.42

Table VI—continued

pH^{pl}:				7.60				
[DPG]$_T$(mM):		3.0			5.0			7.0	
pCO_2	20	40	80	20	40	80	20	40	80
$\bar{O}_2$(%)									
10	0.28	0.18	0.06	0.35	0.27	0.16	0.44	0.38	0.31
20	0.30	0.20	0.10	0.37	0.30	0.20	0.45	0.40	0.33
30	0.31	0.23	0.14	0.39	0.32	0.24	0.45	0.41	0.35
40	0.32	0.24	0.17	0.39	0.33	0.27	0.45	0.41	0.36
50	0.31	0.25	0.20	0.39	0.34	0.29	0.44	0.41	0.36
60	0.30	0.26	0.22	0.39	0.34	0.30	0.43	0.40	0.36
70	0.29	0.26	0.23	0.37	0.33	0.30	0.41	0.39	0.36
80	0.27	0.26	0.24	0.34	0.31	0.29	0.39	0.37	0.36
90	0.24	0.24	0.23	0.28	0.29	0.29	0.35	0.35	0.35
95	0.22	0.22	0.22	0.25	0.25	0.25	0.33	0.33	0.33

[a] From Arturson *et al.* (1974a).

solutions. There is, in addition to these data, a considerable body of information concerning the interactions of hemoglobin with ligands based upon experiments with dilute hemoglobin solutions. The

Table VII
Values for the Coefficient $[\Delta \log pO_2/\Delta \log[DPG]_T]_{\bar{O}_2, pH^{pl}, [DPG]_T}$ [a]

pH^{pl}:		7.20			7.40			7.60	
pCO_2:	20	40	80	20	40	80	20	40	80
$\bar{O}_2$(%)									
10	0.34	0.30	0.26	0.36	0.30	0.23	0.33	0.24	0.15
20	0.37	0.33	0.31	0.38	0.32	0.25	0.35	0.26	0.18
30	0.37	0.34	0.32	0.39	0.32	0.26	0.36	0.27	0.20
40	0.36	0.34	0.31	0.38	0.32	0.26	0.36	0.28	0.21
50	0.34	0.33	0.30	0.37	0.31	0.26	0.35	0.28	0.22
60	0.32	0.33	0.28	0.36	0.30	0.25	0.34	0.28	0.22
70	0.30	0.28	0.26	0.34	0.29	0.24	0.32	0.27	0.21
80	0.28	0.26	0.24	0.32	0.28	0.23	0.30	0.25	0.20
90	0.26	0.26	0.22	0.30	0.25	0.21	0.28	0.23	0.18
95	0.24	0.23	0.21	0.28	0.23	0.20	0.26	0.22	0.17

[a] From Arturson *et al.* (1974a).

Table VIII

Values for the Coefficient $[\Delta \log pO_2/\Delta \log pCO_2]_{\bar{O}_2, pH^{pl}, [DPG]_T}{}^a$

pH^{pl}:	7.20			7.40			7.60		
[DPG]$_T$ (mM):	3.0	5.0	7.0	3.0	5.0	7.0	3.0	5.0	7.0
$\bar{O}_2(\%)$									
10	0.08	0.07	0.05	0.18	0.14	0.09	0.22	0.17	0.10
20	0.07	0.06	0.04	0.14	0.10	0.07	0.18	0.13	0.08
30	0.06	0.05	0.04	0.12	0.09	0.05	0.15	0.11	0.07
40	0.05	0.04	0.03	0.11	0.07	0.04	0.14	0.09	0.06
50	0.05	0.04	0.03	0.10	0.06	0.03	0.13	0.08	0.05
60	0.04	0.04	0.03	0.09	0.06	0.02	0.12	0.08	0.05
70	0.04	0.03	0.02	0.08	0.05	0.02	0.11	0.07	0.04
80	0.03	0.02	0.01	0.07	0.04	0.02	0.09	0.06	0.04
90	0.02	0.02	0.01	0.05	0.03	0.01	0.07	0.05	0.03
95	0.02	0.01	0.00	0.04	0.02	0.01	0.06	0.04	0.03

[a] From Arturson *et al.* (1974a).

interpretation of such data in terms of binding and interaction coefficients is, however, complicated appreciably by the presence of dimers. Comparison of data from dilute and concentrated solutions is also complicated by the prevalence of tetramer–tetramer interactions in the latter.

Ackers *et al.* (1975) performed an extensive study of the dimerization-mediated effect of change in hemoglobin concentration upon estimation of the parameters of hemoglobin function in terms of Adair constants. Their approach was to simulate oxygen–hemoglobin equilibrium curves on the basis of a model that included dimer formation. The simulated curves were then fitted with four apparent Adair constants assuming no dimer formation. The latter were then compared with the originally assumed values. [The previously mentioned "redundancy" of Adair parameter sets (see p. 61) does not appear to have been a serious factor in this analysis.] It was found that even the small amounts of dimers present at commonly employed hemoglobin concentrations may have a devastating effect upon the reliability of fitted Adair constants. In a simulation of a typical case, the four Adair constants were estimated to be 1.06, 1.11, 0.93, and 1.01 times their true values, already at a hemoglobin concentration of 2.5 mM tetramer, while they were 2.5,

5, -1.5 (*sic*), and 1.4 times their true values at a concentration of 0.025 mM tetramer. In a 0.04 mM tetramer solution, the calculated value of $p(50)$, the oxygen tension at 50% saturation, was found to be 4 mm Hg lower than in dimer-free solution.

Several phenomena of hemoglobin function also appear to be concentration dependent in a range where the fraction of dimers should be too small to influence the results. In these cases, the explanation might be tetramer–tetramer interaction. For example, Gary-Bobo and Solomon (1968, 1971) have provided evidence for the reactions

$$n[\mathrm{Hb(NH_3^+)}_x] \rightleftharpoons [\mathrm{Hb(NH_2)}_x]_n + nx \cdot \mathrm{H}^+$$

$$n[\mathrm{Hb(COO^-)}_y] \overset{\mathrm{H_2O}}{\rightleftharpoons} [\mathrm{Hb(COOH)}_y]_n + ny \cdot \mathrm{OH}^-$$

when the hemoglobin concentration exceeds 4–5 mM tetramer. Furthermore, the 2,3-DPG affinity of both oxygenated and deoxygenated hemoglobin decreases as the concentration of hemoglobin increases (Garby and de Verdier, 1971; Klinger *et al.*, 1971; Jänig *et al.*, 1973; Udkow *et al.*, 1973; Hedlund and Lovrien, 1974; see, however, Hamasaki and Rose, 1974). Finally, the extent of oxygen-linked carbamate formation at the four terminal valines in sheep hemoglobin is considerably lower in concentrated than in dilute solutions (Baumann *et al.*, 1975).

Such data may well be related to the evidence obtained by Damaschun *et al.* (1975), from small-angle X-ray scattering in hemoglobin solutions, of structural order extending as far as 160 Å into the solvent medium at hemoglobin concentrations of 5 mM tetramer.

Carbon Monoxide

The effect of carbon monoxide on oxygen binding can be described by analogy to (4-26). At constant proton, carbon dioxide, and 2,3-DPG concentrations we have

$$d\bar{\mathrm{O}}_2 = \left(\frac{\partial \bar{\mathrm{O}}_2}{\partial \log p\mathrm{O}_2}\right)_{p\mathrm{CO}} d \log p\mathrm{O}_2 + \left(\frac{\partial \bar{\mathrm{O}}_2}{\partial \log p\mathrm{CO}}\right)_{p\mathrm{O}_2} \cdot d \log p\mathrm{CO}$$

$$(4\text{-}28)$$

The integrated form of equation (4-28) may be derived from the experimental results of Roughton and Darling (1944) and

Roughton (1970) as follows. When the simultaneous reactions of O_2 and CO are sufficient to completely saturate the hemoglobin, the following relation, known as Haldane's first law, is nearly exact over a very wide range of values for pO_2 and pCO:

$$\overline{CO}/\overline{O}_2 = M \times pCO/pO_2 \qquad (4\text{-}29)$$

where M, which depends on pH (Joels and Pugh, 1958) and 2,3-DPG concentration (Bratteby and Wadman, unpublished results), has a value of 220 to 270 in normal subjects.

Roughton (1970) and Okada *et al.* (1976) provided experimental evidence indicating that, at combinations of pO_2 and pCO *insufficient* to saturate the hemoglobin, the relative degrees of binding of the two ligands still approximate equation (4-29). It is, moreover, reasonable (Roughton, 1964) to assume that

$$\overline{CO} + \overline{O}_2 = f_0(p) \qquad (4\text{-}30)$$

where f_0 is the functional relationship between $\overline{O}_2$ and pO_2 at $pCO = 0$, and $p = pO_2 + MpCO$.

Combination of (4-29) and (4-30) yields

$$\overline{O}_2 = \frac{f_0(pO_2 + MpCO)}{1 + MpCO/pO_2} \qquad (4\text{-}31)$$

$$\overline{CO} = \frac{f_0(pO_2 + MpCO)}{1 + pO_2/MpCO} \qquad (4\text{-}32)$$

The value of M is not exactly independent of total saturation, but rather is somewhat lower at low and high values of the latter (Roughton, 1970, 1972).

Plots of (4-31) and (4-32) at pCO values of 0.04 and 0.08 mm Hg, respectively, are shown in Figure 29 together with the whole blood oxygen binding curve at standard conditions (see Table V). In these plots, the variation of M with $\overline{O}_2 + \overline{CO}$ was calculated from the $\overline{CO}$ vs. pCO relationship at $pO_2 = 0$ given by Roughton (1970), and the $\overline{O}_2$ vs. pO_2 relationship at $pCO \approx 0$ given in Table V.

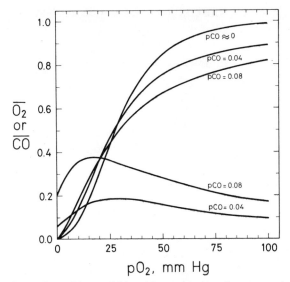

Figure 29. Saturation of hemoglobin with oxygen (top three curves) and carbon monoxide (lower two curves) in the presence of fixed pCO values (mm Hg) and otherwise standard conditions.

There are very similar effects of both pH (Joels and Pugh, 1958) and 2,3-DPG (Okada *et al.*, 1976) upon the binding curves of O_2 alone and CO alone. Therefore, it appears reasonable to assume that variations of the function f_0 with the concentrations of these effector ligands are the same as those listed in Tables VI–VIII.

Effect of Temperature

Most, if not all, of the individual reactions of ligand binding and conformational change involve a change in heat content. The equilibrium constants of the respective reactions are therefore temperature dependent according to the van't Hoff isochore:

$$\partial \ln K/\partial T = \Delta H_R/RT^2 \qquad (4\text{-}33)$$

where K is the equilibrium constant and ΔH_R the enthalpy change associated with the given reaction.

In the hemoglobin system, the determination of ΔH_R for individual reactions is complicated by the fact that the reactions are linked. For example, the binding of oxygen to hemoglobin is linked to conformational changes and to binding of other species. Thus, many experimental results give only *apparent* ΔH_R values.

An apparent equilibrium constant for oxygen–hemoglobin interaction is frequently evaluated on the basis of the Hill relationship:

$$\bar{O}_2 = Kp O_2^n/(1 + Kp O_2^n) \qquad (4\text{-}34)$$

derived on the assumption that n moles of O_2 bind, in unison, with 1 mole of hemoglobin tetramer. It follows from (4-34) that K is equal to $p(50)^{-n}$, and from (4-33) as well that

$$\left[\frac{\partial \log p O_2}{\partial(1/T)}\right]_{\bar{O}_2} = \frac{\Delta H_{O_2}}{2.3R} \qquad (4\text{-}35)$$

where ΔH_{O_2} is the enthalpy of reaction of *one* mole of oxygen (plus the enthalpies of the reactions coupled to oxygen binding).

In the present context we are interested primarily in obtaining numerical values of $[\partial \log p O_2/\partial T]$ for human whole blood as a function of $\bar{O}_2$, pCO_2, red cell pH, and 2,3-DPG concentration. This can be achieved, on a limited basis, from published data.

The association of oxygen molecules with human hemoglobin A is accompanied by evolution of heat (the reaction is *exothermic*). At pH 7.3, in the absence of 2,3-DPG and at 50% saturation with oxygen, the variation of $\log p O_2$ with $1/T$ in the range 283–303°K (10–30°C) is linear and thus yields a constant ΔH_R value, -11 kcal/mole (Benesch *et al.*, 1969). In the lower pH range where the Bohr effect is insignificant, the value is roughly 3 kcal/mole more negative, this difference being the heat of ionization of the Bohr groups (see Antonini and Brunori, 1971; Kilmartin and Rossi-Bernardi, 1973).

Binding of 2,3-DPG to deoxyhemoglobin is also exothermic; ΔH_R is between -11 and -13 kcal/mole (Benesch *et al.*, 1969; Hedlund and Lovrien, 1974). Thus, the addition of 2,3-DPG decreases the heat evolved when oxygen combines with hemoglobin. For complete oxygenation, i.e., $\Delta \bar{O}_2 = 1.0$, the net value is about -7 kcal/mol oxygen when the 2,3-DPG to hemoglobin tetramer molar ratio is 4:1 and the hemoglobin concentration is 0.06 mM.

The value of $[\partial \log p(50)/\partial T]$ is temperature dependent, since $[\partial \log p(50)/\partial(1/T)]$ is not, and the two derivatives are related by

$$\frac{\partial \log p(50)}{\partial T} = -\frac{1}{T^2} \frac{\partial \log p(50)}{\partial(1/T)} \qquad (4\text{-}36)$$

Assuming that the values of ΔH_R remain temperature independent throughout the pathophysiological range, then from equations (4-35) and (4-36) and the above-noted heats of reaction, it follows that at 37°C, $[\partial \log p(50)/\partial T] = 0.025°K^{-1}$ in the absence of 2,3-DPG and 0.016 under the stipulated excess of 2,3-DPG. In whole blood under physiological conditions, $[\partial \log p(50)/\partial T]$ is 0.024 (Astrup *et al.*, 1965), which is reasonably consistent with the other two values.

As to other factors, the pH dependence of the overall heat of oxygenation has not yet been studied in detail but is probably small in the pathophysiological pH range of, say, 6.8 to 7.8. There is, however, evidence indicating that the apparent heat of reaction of the first oxygen molecule exceeds in magnitude that of the last (Roughton, 1965; Imai and Yonetani, 1975).

Embryonic and Fetal Hemoglobins

During embryonic and fetal development, hemoglobin molecules other than HbA predominate. Though their ligand binding properties and interaction coefficients have not yet been determined with the same accuracy as those for HbA (there is no information at all for several of them), the available data allow a semiquantitative analysis.

Three different globin chains, γ, ε, and ζ, are synthesized in embryonic and fetal development in addition to α and β chains. In the smallest embryos studied, the following three hemoglobin species are most prevalent: Hb Gower 1 ($\zeta_2\varepsilon_2$), Hb Gower 2 ($\alpha_2\varepsilon_2$), and Hb Portland ($\zeta_2\gamma_2$). The primary structures of the ε and ζ chains are not yet known but that of the γ chain is (see Table II).

The ligand binding and interaction coefficients of these three particular hemoglobins have not yet been determined. However, blood from embryos with a crown–rump length of less than 35 mm and containing these hemoglobins to the extent of between 30 and

50%, the rest consisting of HbF ($\alpha_2\gamma_2$) and HbF^{acetyl} ($\alpha_2\gamma_2$ with the NH$_2$-termini of the γ chains blocked by acetate), has a high oxygen affinity [$p(50)$ between 17 and 19 mm Hg] under physiological conditions (Huehns and Farooqui, 1975). The values of the whole blood Bohr coefficient and Hill constant appear to be near normal.

Blood from fetuses with a crown–rump length of about 50 mm contains about 90% HbF. This fraction decreases continuously during gestation and is, at birth, about 75%, the remainder being HbA. As shown in Table II, the γ chains of HbF differ from the β chains in HbA in not less than 39 of the 146 residues. In spite of this large difference, however, the affinity of HbF for oxygen in the absence of 2,3-DPG and carbon dioxide is very nearly the same as that of HbA (Allen *et al.*, 1953).

The main functional difference between HbF and HbA is in their behavior toward 2,3-DPG. Both the oxy and deoxy forms of HbF bind less 2,3-DPG than the HbA forms (de Verdier and Garby, 1969) and, furthermore, the oxygen-linked binding to HbF is smaller in magnitude (Bauer *et al.*, 1968). The increase in $p(50)$ per mM of 2,3-DPG in the cells of fetal blood containing only HbF was calculated to be 0.7 mm Hg at cellular pH of 7.15, $pCO_2 \cong 40$ mm Hg, and 37°C (Versmold *et al.*, 1973; see also Bunn and Briehl, 1970), in contrast to a value of 2 mm Hg for blood containing HbA only. This phenomenon is probably explained alone by the presence, in the γ chains of HbF, of serine in the place of histidine in residue 143: the uncharged serine residue would not be expected to contribute to the binding of 2,3-DPG.

In the presence of physiological amounts of 2,3-DPG at cellular pH = 7.20 and $pCO_2 = 40$ mm Hg, deoxygenated fetal cells contain more hemoglobin carbamate than deoxygenated adult cells: 0.7 vs. 0.5 mol/mol of hemoglobin tetramer (Bauer and Schröder, 1972). The amounts of carbamino hemoglobin in oxygenated fetal and adult bloods at the same condition are each approximately 0.13 mol/mol tetramer, so that the oxygen-linked carbamino formation is larger in fetal blood. Since there is evidence, albeit in very dilute solutions, that the oxygen-linked carbamino formation in the absence of 2,3-DPG is smaller in HbF than in HbA (Bauer *et al.*,

1975), a likely explanation for the opposite result in intact cells is the diminished interaction of HbF with 2,3-DPG.

Identical values of -0.66 for the coefficient $\Delta \log pO_2/\Delta pH$ at 50% oxygen saturation and at constant base excess have been determined in erythrolysates of both adult and cord red blood cells (Versmold *et al.*, 1973). The same workers also measured the coefficient in fetal and adult whole blood and found that both have a value of about -0.50.

Bauer and Schröder (1972) found very similar values for the regression lines of $[H^+]^{pl}/[H^+]^c$ vs. pH^{pl} for fetal and adult blood in both the oxygenated and deoxygenated states. There was a small difference, however, in the change of red cell pH upon oxygenation at constant pH^{pl}: 0.038 for fetal blood and 0.047 for adult blood.

Although the data referred to above are not extensive enough to derive a complete set of binding and interaction coefficients, it appears that they may be used to describe fairly closely the oxygen binding curve of HbF and the effect thereupon of protons, carbon dioxide, and 2,3-DPG. The whole blood oxygen binding curve of red cells containing HbF only, under standard conditions, should be taken to equal that of whole blood containing HbA only in the presence of 2 mM of red cell 2,3-DPG. The proton and carbon dioxide interaction coefficients may be taken to equal those given in Tables VI and VIII, while those for 2,3-DPG may be taken as half the values given in Table VII. For blood containing both HbA and HbF, linear interpolation would presumably allow fairly accurate prediction.

The functional significance of the higher oxygen affinities of embryonic and fetal bloods has not yet been clarified. It is, however, a logical mode of ensuring adequate extraction of oxygen from maternal blood.

Hemoglobin–Ligand Kinetics in Solution

The intrinsic rates of the reversible chemical reactions between hemoglobin and its physiologically important ligands—oxygen, protons, carbon dioxide, and 2,3-DPG—have been the object of research endeavor (most fervently concerning oxygen) since the pioneering work of Hartridge and Roughton in 1923. Biochemists and molecular biologists have traditionally employed such data in tests of proposed reaction mechanisms more stringent than agreement with equilibrium data alone. Physiologists have, on the other hand, aimed at identifying rate-limiting steps in O_2 supply and CO_2 disposal, a process that, as already noted, comprises a multiplicity of reactions that proceed simultaneously with diffusion and convection. In analyzing that process, when the associated rate constants are known to exceed definable limits, a reaction may be treated as if it were infinitely fast, i.e., as if attaining equilibrium instantaneously.

Excellent reviews of oxygen–hemoglobin kinetics have been given by Gibson (1959) and Antonini and Brunori (1971).

In this section, we adopt the viewpoint of the physiologist and limit the treatment of kinetics to a discussion of empirically determined rate constants, with only incidental mention of mechanisms. This is due to our conclusion that the interpretation of hemoglobin–ligand kinetic data, rather than being any less important than the equilibrium analysis, is at a much more primitive stage of development. The reader seeking an acquaintance with sophisticated kinetic models is referred to Shulman *et al.* (1975) and Bansil *et al.* (1976).

Hemoglobin–Oxygen Interaction. The reaction between oxygen and hemoglobin is, as discussed in the foregoing sections, a complex one, inasmuch as there are four binding sites per molecule and there are apparent differences between the reactivities of the two α and two β hemes. The reactivity of the respective binding sites depends on the presence or absence of ligand at the remaining sites, i.e., binding of oxygen induces conformational changes together with release of CO_2, protons, and 2,3-DPG, all of which perturbations tend to readjust the oxygen affinity of the hemes; and, as implied by the last statement, heme reactivity to oxygen is a function of the prevailing carbon dioxide tension, pH, and 2,3-DPG concentration.

Nonetheless, most experimental measurements of the rate of change of hemoglobin oxygen saturation following perturbation from equilibrium have been analyzed in terms of a single overall reaction:

$$O_2 + Hb \underset{k_{diss}}{\overset{k_{ass}}{\rightleftharpoons}} O_2Hb \qquad (4\text{-}37)$$

where Hb represents heme *monomer*. This approach allows a satisfactory fit to the results of certain experiments, in particular, the initial phase of deoxygenation of fully saturated hemoglobin when the oxygen tension is maintained in the vicinity of zero. However, more extensive observations manifest the expected more complex behavior (two or more phases of differing relaxation time); thus kineticists have frequently adopted the sequential binding scheme of Adair (1925; see p. 61):

$$O_2 + (O_2)_{i-1} Hb \underset{k_{diss}^i}{\overset{k_{ass}^i}{\rightleftharpoons}} (O_2)_i Hb, \qquad i = 1, \ldots, 4 \qquad (4\text{-}38)$$

where Hb now represents hemoglobin *tetramer*.

A complete set of the eight rate constants in scheme (4-38) *at 37°C* has not been determined for human hemoglobin. However, Gibson *et al.* (1955) reported values at that temperature for the effective overall association constant k_{ass}, at pH = 7.1 in very dilute solution (1/1000 the erythrocyte hemoglobin concentration), as a function of hemoglobin saturation with oxygen. Values from three subjects at 0, 33, and 67% saturation ranged from 1.7 to 5.7×10^6 liters/mol/sec, with no consistent saturation dependence. Insofar as the dissociation constant was not accounted for in determining these values, there is a distinct possibility that they represent a lower limit to the actual range of association constants.

Recently, Bauer *et al.* (1973) measured the initial rate of deoxygenation of fully saturated hemoglobin (at 1/20 physiological concentration) and reported values close to 200 sec^{-1} for the effective dissociation rate constant in the physiological pH range at 37°C. That figure agrees well with most values of k_{diss} determined under similar conditions. Experiments conducted at lower temperatures (e.g., Gibson, 1970; Ilgenfritz and Schuster, 1974) indicate differences among the four k_{diss}^i (and k_{ass}^i) values of scheme (4-38), which cannot be accounted for statistically on the basis of the relative numbers of occupied binding sites per tetramer. Such results suggest that 200 sec^{-1} might prove to be a low estimate of the overall dissociation constant at 37°C.

A limited amount of data has been published on the effects of variations in the concentrations of CO_2, protons, and 2,3-DPG upon O_2–Hb reaction kinetics. Salhany (1972) demonstrated that in very dilute solutions (less than 1/3000 physiological) free of 2,3-DPG at pH 7.5 and a temperature of 23°C, the initial rate of O_2 dissociation from oxyhemoglobin was insensitive to pCO_2 variation in the range 0–75 mm Hg, whereas the initial rate of *CO* binding to deoxyhemoglobin decreased by a factor of 2 with the same variation in CO_2 tension. The k_{diss} values reported by Bauer *et al.* (1973) and referred to above were found to decrease with increasing pH (~50% per pH unit) in the physiological pH range, as previously reported by Salhany *et al.* (1970) under conditions of 1/400 physiological hemoglobin concentration and 24°C, and in the 40–85% saturation range. Modest increases in k_{diss} with increases in DPG concentration from zero to well in excess of 1 mol DPG/mol heme were also described by the latter two sets of investigators.

If the above-mentioned data at 37°C are taken to be representative of the kinetics prevailing at erythrocyte hemoglobin concentration, one can estimate the relaxation time characteristic of *in vivo* oxygen binding. Roughly speaking, the half-time for a reaction of the type denoted by scheme (4-37) is on the order of

$$\{k_{diss} + k_{ass}([O_2] + [Hb])\}^{-1}$$

Using the values of 200 sec^{-1} for k_{diss}, 5×10^6 liters/mol/sec for k_{ass}, and 1×10^{-2} M for a typical concentration of deoxygenated hemoglobin monomer (justifiably neglecting the dissolved oxygen), then the half-time may be estimated to be on the order of 0.1 msec.

Hemoglobin Interactions with CO_2, Protons, and 2,3-DPG. The kinetics of hemoglobin binding of physiological ligands other than oxygen have been accorded relatively scant attention. However, available data allow an estimate of the relaxation times associated with the equilibration of CO_2, hydrogen ions, and 2,3-DPG with hemoglobin *in vivo*.

The reaction between CO_2 and the N-terminal α-valines of hemoglobin is given by

$$CO_2 + HbNH_2 \underset{k_d}{\overset{k_a}{\rightleftharpoons}} HbNHCOOH \tag{4-39}$$

which, at physiological pH, leads instantaneously to dissociation of carbamic acid:

$$HbNHCOOH \rightleftharpoons HbNHCOO^- + H^+ \qquad (4\text{-}40)$$

Reactions (4-39) and (4-40) are further coupled to the ionization of the amino group

$$HbNH_3^+ \rightleftharpoons HbNH_2 + H^+ \qquad (4\text{-}41)$$

inasmuch as carbamino formation proceeds with the uncharged group only.

From experiments at 37°C and a range of effectively constant pH values in the physiological range, in fairly concentrated (1/7 to 1/4 physiological) deoxy-hemoglobin solutions, Forster *et al.* (1968) estimated values for k_a and k_d of 11×10^3 liters/mol/sec and 500 sec^{-1}, respectively, under the assumption of equilibration of the extremely rapid ionization reactions (4-40) and (4-41) (see the discussion of proton binding below). The corresponding half-time of reaction was on the order of 10 to 20 msec. In oxygenated hemoglobin solutions, the reaction was somewhat slower, with a half-time roughly twice as high.

The latter experiments were apparently conducted in DPG-free solution. Since 2,3-DPG decreases the hemoglobin affinity for CO_2, the kinetics of CO_2–Hb interaction under physiological conditions are somewhat different. However, if, as is believed, CO_2 and 2,3-DPG compete for the same amino sites on the β chains, the possibility remains that the intrinsic CO_2–Hb rate constants are not particularly affected by the presence of organic phosphate. On the other hand, the somewhat greater physiological hemoglobin concentration would, following the same analysis as applied to O_2–Hb kinetics, be expected to be responsible for reduced half-times.

The reactions of protons with hemoglobin fall under the general class of buffer ionization reactions, which are known to proceed at extremely high rates (Eigen and DeMaeyer, 1963). Forster *et al.* (1968) refer to unpublished observations in their laboratory, which indicate that acid neutralization by plasma proteins and hemoglobin is complete within a few milliseconds.

While the rate of binding of 2,3-DPG to hemoglobin has not been reported, that of ATP, which should not be drastically different, has. Antonini and Brunori (1970) observed that ATP–Hb interaction in dilute (1/400 physiological) hemoglobin solutions at pH 6.5 and 30°C was complete before the first observation in a rapid mixing apparatus taken 3–4 msec after mixing the two species.

The data reported in this section refer to measurements obtained in hemoglobin *solutions*. They are taken to be suggestive of the intrinsic rates of reaction in red cells, direct observation of which is precluded by simultaneous diffusion and possible membrane resistance. A discussion of rate constants determined from experiments with whole blood appears in Chapter 5.

Chapter 5

Blood as a Physicochemical System—II

Equilibria, Steady States, and Transport Kinetics of the Red Cell–Plasma Distributions

Several important properties of the blood as a transport system for oxygen, carbon dioxide, and protons are attributable to the fact that it is *a two-phase system*, i.e., a suspension of red cells in plasma, and that all three transported components are distributed between the phases.

Oxygen, carbon dioxide, and protons are passively distributed, i.e., allowed sufficient time, the plasma and red cell concentrations of each species will be consistent with interphase thermodynamic equilibrium. For the two gaseous species, this means a tendency for their respective plasma and red cell activities (i.e., partial pressures) to equalize. On the other hand, the effective impermeability of the red cell membrane to a number of charged species—most notably hemoglobin, 2,3-DPG, and plasma proteins—and the apparent pumping of both sodium and potassium between red cells and plasma are responsible for the existence of an electrical potential difference across the red cell membrane. The latter ensures that the distributions of permeable ionic species, including protons,* resemble those observed in a Gibbs–Donnan system. Thus, the proton activity tends to be appreciably greater in the erythrocyte phase under most physiological conditions.

Since the oxygen affinity of hemoglobin is determined by the erythrocyte, rather than the plasma pH value, analysis of *in vivo* blood gas transport requires a method for calculation of the *in vivo* red cell–plasma proton distribution. The latter is determined not only by the above-mentioned potential difference, but also by the reactions of hydrogen ions and, through the constraints of electroneutrality, by the distributions of all other ionic species. Furthermore, the dependence of these factors on species concentrations implies sensitivity to osmotic water shifts between the two blood phases.

Additional, vital considerations in analyzing the significance of red cell–plasma distributions are the rates of relaxation of inter- and intraphase disequilibria. The perturbations in red cell–plasma equilibrium induced by the fluxes of O_2 and CO_2 in the lungs and tissue (e.g., upset of the interphase bicarbonate ion equilibrium by rapid hydration of CO_2 and dissociation of carbonic acid in the erythrocytes) occur at estimable rates. The subsequent responses in the direction of new equilibria may be considered as effectively instantaneous if characterized by rates that are much greater or, at the opposite extreme, as insignificant if their rates are much lower.

The sections that follow comprise a discussion of these factors.

Definition of a Standard State for Measurements of Blood Composition

The circulating blood is an open system, connected to its environment, the lungs and tissues, by way of material flows. The existence of flows that differ in composition from that of the blood

---

*The permeability of protons, like those of all cations, is believed to be quite low. However, proton equilibration is effected either by that of hydroxyl ions coupled to the dissociation of water or, in the presence of CO_2, by the equilibration of CO_2 hydrolysis/carbonic acid dissociation on both sides of the erythrocyte membrane.

makes the latter composition a variable with respect to position in the circulation. Thus, in order to make comparisons among individuals with respect to the composition of the blood, it is necessary to introduce some standard or reference conditions under which compositions should be measured.

For the purpose of analyzing the respiratory functions of the blood, it is generally sufficient to consider the flows of only two components: oxygen and carbon dioxide. The flows of other components that affect the respiratory functions of the blood are, under most circumstances, so small that they may be neglected. Hence, the composition of the blood in an individual, when equilibrated with oxygen and carbon dioxide at some standard partial pressures— usually 100 and 40 mm Hg, respectively—is *effectively independent of the site* from which it was obtained. Although the composition of such blood may not be identical to that of any volume element of the blood *in vivo* in that particular individual, it represents an operationally defined standard state composition by means of which interindividual comparisons can be made.

The requirement of gas equilibrium is, however, not sufficient for a proper definition of the standard state. Besides the temperature, it is also necessary to define the time period within which the composition must be measured. This requirement is related to the fact that the system, i.e., the blood sample with its adjacent gas phase, is not in complete thermodynamic equilibrium. Two of its diffusible components, sodium and potassium, are in fact rather far from thermodynamic equilibrium and the system as a whole is running down. If, however, the glucose concentration is kept above a certain value, the rest of the system can be maintained for some hours in what may be considered a true steady state, with time-invariant intraphase concentrations of all relevant species. This time period, then, constitutes the additional requirement, and it is indeed a fortunate circumstance that it is long enough for most measurements to be possible. At the other extreme, of course, the time of equilibration must be long enough to allow relaxation of the CO_2 hydrolysis reaction in plasma, i.e., on the order of 1 min.

Under conditions in which the flows of oxygen and carbon dioxide into and out of the system *in vivo* have been constant for some time, and to the extent that one may consider the blood flow constant, the composition of the blood at any point in the circulation may also be considered time invariant. These *local* steady state distributions of components between red cells and plasma are, in general, quite different from those of the standard steady state. This distinction is an important one, as should become more evident as we proceed.

The Standard Steady State Distributions

As mentioned above, the steady state composition of the blood under standard conditions is a state of disequilibrium maintained by a continuous supply of glucose and transformation of chemical energy. This fact does not, however, exclude the possibility that one or several components in the system might be very close to thermodynamic equilibrium. This is of considerable importance, inasmuch as analysis is greatly facilitated when such conditions may be assumed to prevail.

Red Cell Water

The high permeability of the red cell membrane toward water (Forster, 1971; Naccache and Sha'afi, 1973) ensures that this component remains, under all conditions of interest, in thermodynamic equilibrium or very nearly so. Furthermore, the hydrostatic pressure in the red cells is only 2–3 mm of water in excess of that in plasma (Rand and Burton, 1964). These facts imply the following relation:

$$\mu_{H_2O}^{0,c} + RT \ln a_{H_2O}^{c} \cong \mu_{H_2O}^{0,pl} + RT \ln a_{H_2O}^{pl} \tag{5.1}$$

where $\mu_{H_2O}^{0}$ and a_{H_2O} are the standard chemical potential and activity, respectively, of water, and c and pl refer to cells and plasma, respectively.

As determined by drying erythrocytes to constant weight at 100–105°C, water occupies 0.72 liter/liter of the cells under physiological conditions (Savitz *et al.*, 1964; Funder and Wieth,

1966a). The volume of distribution of a large number of small nonelectrolytes at 37°C corresponds very closely to this value (Gary-Bobo, 1967; Gary-Bobo and Solomon, 1968). Furthermore, the amount of water in the cells determined, by osmotic shift experiments, to exhibit solute interaction equivalent to that in the suspending salt media is equal to the chemically determined total cell water (Gary-Bobo and Solomon, 1968, 1971). These observations strongly suggest that red cell water behaves as "ordinary" water toward both electrolytes and nonelectrolytes, and that it is valid to calculate the concentrations of solute species on the basis of analytically determined water. Of course, the data do not necessarily preclude the possibility that part of the water may be unavailable for ordinary solute–solvent interaction, but it would then be necessary to assume that the remaining water has such abnormal interaction that the two effects cancel, which is rather unlikely.

Unless the standard chemical potentials in equation (5.1) are different, and the above considerations make this unlikely, the water activities must be essentially the same in both phases. Measurements of solute lowering of the vapor pressure of erythrocyte fluid and plasma support this conclusion (Roepke and Baldes, 1942; Williams *et al.*, 1959).

Red Cell Ionic Composition

Table IX shows typical data on the ionic composition of normal red cells and plasma in the standard state. The values for H^+, Na^+, K^+, Cl^-, and HCO_3^- are from Funder and Wieth (1966a,b). The values of the charge concentration of impermeable species, X^-, are obtained from electroneutrality considerations.

The system in Table IX may be shown to be in osmotic equilibrium if it is assumed that: (1) the osmotic coefficients of Na^+, K^+, Cl^-, and HCO_3^- are the same in each phase (see below), and (2) the osmolarity of impermeable red cell species is 36 mOsm and that of impermeable plasma species is 2 mOsm. The value for the impermeable red cell species is in reasonable agreement with the observations of Dalmark (1975) that when, at 0°C, red cell and medium pH were equal (at 7.20), 27 mOsm of sucrose were required for osmotic

Table IX

**Ionic Compositions of Red Cell and Plasma
in Normal Oxygenated Blood at 37°C and
$pCO_2 = 40$ mm Hg[a]**

Species	Red cells	Plasma
H^+	$63 \cdot 10^{-6}$	$40 \cdot 10^{-6}$
Na^+	17	138
K^+	135	4
Mg^{2+}	1^b	1
Ca^{2+}	0.03^c	1
Cl^-	70	105
HCO_3^-	16	24
X^-	67^d	16^d

[a] Values are in milliequivalents per liter of *water*.
[b] There are about 7 meq/liter H_2O of magnesium in the
red cells, most of it complexed with 2,3-DPG and ATP
(see Berger *et al.*, 1973).
[c] Total calcium concentration (Lichtman and Weed, 1972).
An unknown but very large fraction of it is complexed.
[d] Within the red cells, X^- is predominantly the sum of
contributions of 2,3-DPG, ATP, and hemoglobin. In the
plasma, X^- is almost exclusively due to the proteins (see
Siggaard-Andersen, 1974).

equilibrium with red cells made salt permeable with nystatin treatment. It is also in fair agreement with the value calculated from the
contributions of hemoglobin, 2,3-DPG, ATP, and Mg, when one
recognizes the large osmotic coefficient of the former under
intracellular conditions (Adair, 1928; McConaghey and Maizels,
1961).

Thermodynamic Equilibria and Ion Activity Coefficients

The species Na^+, K^+, Cl^-, and HCO_3^- are permeable to the red
cell membrane. If they were passively distributed, the electrochemical potential $\tilde{\mu}$ of each would be the same in both phases, i.e.,

$$\tilde{\mu}_i^c = \tilde{\mu}_i^{pl} \tag{5-2}$$

or

$$\mu_i^{0,c} + RT \ln a_i^c + z_i F \Phi^c = \mu_i^{0,pl} + RT \ln a_i^{pl} + z_i F \Phi^{pl} \tag{5-3}$$

where F is Faraday's constant, z_i the charge of species i, and Φ electrical potential.

An examination of the possible existence of thermodynamic equilibrium for any species thus requires a knowledge of standard chemical potentials, activity coefficients, and the electrical potential difference across the membrane. There is little experimental data from which to estimate the standard chemical potentials or activity coefficients of the above four ions in erythrocyte fluid. However, available data do allow certain inferences.

Gary-Bobo and Solomon (1968) performed equilibrium dialysis experiments at 0°C in which they measured the distributions of radioactive sodium, potassium, and chloride between a 3.7 mM tetramer hemoglobin solution and NaCl/KCl solutions of varying concentration and pH (the latter controlled by phosphate buffers). The distribution ratios of sodium and potassium were always found to be the same when calculated on a weight of water basis. At salt concentrations of 150 mM, corresponding to that in red cells, the distribution ratios varied continuously between 0.98 and 1.01, as the pH was increased from 6.65 to 7.30. The isoelectric points of hemoglobin and of hemoglobin plus physiological proportions of 2,3-DPG, ATP, and Mg at the given temperature and ionic strength are not accurately known, but must certainly lie between 6.65 and 7.30 (see Winterhalter and Colosimo, 1971). Therefore, the data show that, at least at 0°C and a hemoglobin concentration of 3.7 mM tetramer, the activity coefficients of sodium, potassium, and chloride ions are very much the same as those in the corresponding salt media.

In more concentrated solutions of hemoglobin, such as in intact red cells, the hemoglobin molecules appear to interact to the extent that the net charge per hemoglobin molecule decreases as the concentration increases. Gary-Bobo and Solomon (1968, 1971) developed this idea in quantitative terms and predicted net fluxes of sodium and chloride between cells and medium due to the change in hemoglobin charge as the cells shrink and swell through osmotic gradients. The predicted fluxes were indeed observed; since no changes in activity coefficients were assumed, Gary-Bobo and Solomon argued that such changes did not occur.

Available data thus indicate that activity coefficients of univalent electrolytes in the erythrocyte fluid are quite similar to those in corresponding salt solutions. In addition, these data make it highly unlikely that the standard chemical potentials of the univalent ions are different in the two phases. In light of these considerations, equation (5-3) may be reduced to

$$\Phi^c - \Phi^{pl} = \Delta\Phi \cong (RT/z_iF)\ln(c_i^{pl}/c_i^c) \tag{5-4}$$

Insertion of the data in Table IX into the above relationship yields

$$\Delta\Phi(H^+) = \Delta\Phi(Cl^-) = \Delta\Phi(HCO_3^-) = -10\text{ mV}$$

$$\Phi(Na^+) = 53\text{ mV}, \qquad \Phi(K^+) = -83\text{ mV}$$

showing that at least two of the species must not be in thermodynamic equilibrium.

The findings that chloride ions, bicarbonate ions, and protons have consistent distributions make it highly likely that all these three ions are very close to thermodynamic equilibrium. Furthermore, measurements of the electrical potential difference across the red cell membrane have shown values consistent with this interpretation (Lassen and Steen-Knudsen, 1968; see also Lassen *et al.*, 1971). If so, sodium and potassium must be out of thermodynamic equilibrium, and the steady state concentrations of these ions in the red cells must be maintained by a continuous expenditure of energy. The mechanism(s) by which these ions are—actively—transported across the membrane is not yet known.

The electrical potential difference is due to a separation of electrical charge between the two phases. This may occur because of (1) the presence of unequally distributed, truly impermeable charged components, and/or (2) the operation of cation pump–leak systems, which render certain species effectively impermeable by ensuring their unequal distribution. The roles played by these processes in the distribution of passive ions in blood are not yet known. The case in which the sole contributions are those of truly impermeable charged components is the classical Gibbs–Donnan equilibrium (see, for example, Donnan and Guggenheim, 1932).

While this case differs fundamentally from the red cell–plasma system, there are similarities in some aspects, and so the distribution ratio of the so-called passive Cl^-, HCO_3^-, and H^+, i.e.,

$$a_{Cl^-}^c/a_{Cl^-}^{pl} = a_{HCO_3^-}^c/a_{HCO_3^-}^{pl} = a_{H^+}^{pl}/a_{H^+}^c \equiv r \qquad (5\text{-}5)$$

is often referred to as a *Donnan* distribution ratio.

Erythrocyte and Plasma Responses to Perturbations in Composition

The composition of the blood in the generally accepted standard state is listed in Table IX. The plasma and erythrocyte pH values are found to be close to 7.40 and 7.20, respectively.

Both the plasma and erythrocyte pH value respond to three perturbations typical of human physiology:

(1) addition or removal of acid or base,
(2) variations in CO_2 or O_2 tension,
(3) changes in membrane-impermeable ("nondiffusible") charges in either blood phase.

The first effect is self-explanatory. The second occurs by way of changes in either the concentration of carbonic acid or the relative proportions of deoxy- and oxyhemoglobin, which last two species differ in proton affinity. The third perturbation occurs by way of the just discussed Donnan-like distribution of diffusible ions between red cells and plasma. Because of the heats of ionization of the blood's titratable species, a change in temperature will also affect the pH value in both plasma and red cells. All such tendencies toward pH change are opposed by the blood's buffering species—most notably hemoglobin and H_2CO_3/HCO_3^-, and to lesser extents plasma protein and red cell organic phosphate.

The following is an analysis of the changes in pH that can be expected under a variety of circumstances.

Fundamental Constraints and Approach to Analysis

The resulting pH and composition of each blood phase under any particular set of conditions, e.g., specified values of pO_2, pCO_2, red cell 2,3-DPG concentration, and acid/base contents, are derivable from the known standard steady state composition through the application of appropriate physicochemical data to equations describing (1) the absence of net electrical charge in either blood phase and (2) material balance with respect to the blood's strong acid/base contents. That is, such changes as may occur between the reference and any other possible state must be consistent with (1) the preservation of each phase's electrical neutrality and (2) the fact that the changes in the nontitratable ion contents of each phase must sum to the overall change for whole blood.

Electroneutrality Conditions. According to the constraint of electroneutrality, any state assumed by the cells and the plasma must satisfy the relationship

$$\{\textstyle\sum z_i[i] = 0\}^{\text{cor pl}} \tag{5-6}$$

where z_i is the algebraic valence and $[i]$ the molar concentration of species i, and the sum is taken over all species present. The existence of a membrane potential implies a net charge imbalance in each phase. However, its magnitude is too small to detract from the validity of equation (5-6).

The electroneutrality condition may be expanded into three physiologically important terms for the plasma,

$$B^{\text{pl}} + z_{\text{Pr}}[\text{Pr}]^{\text{pl}} - [\text{HCO}_3^-]^{\text{pl}} = 0 \tag{5-7}$$

and four for the erythrocytes,

$$B^c + z_{\text{Hm}}[\text{Hm}]^c + z_{\text{DPG}}[\text{DPG}]_T - [\text{HCO}_3^-]^c = 0 \tag{5-8}$$

where Pr denotes plasma protein, Hm hemoglobin *monomer*, and $[\text{DPG}]_T$ the total cellular 2,3-DPG concentration in free and hemoglobin-bound forms. The B terms denote the charge concentrations attributable to nontitratable ionic species, i.e.,

$$\{B \equiv [\text{Na}^+] + [\text{K}^+] + 2[\text{Mg}^{2+}] + 2[\text{Ca}^{2+}] + \cdots$$
$$- [\text{Cl}^-] - 2[\text{SO}_4^{2-}] - \cdots\}^{\text{cor pl}} \tag{5-9}$$

Since we are chiefly concerned with *changes* in state, we proceed by differentiating equations (5-7) and (5-8), thereby obtaining

$$dB^{pl} + [Pr]^{pl} \, dz_{pr} - d[HCO_3^-]^{pl} = 0 \qquad (5\text{-}10)$$

$$dB^c + [Hm]^c \, dz_{Hm} + d(z_{DPG}[DPG]_T) - d[HCO_3^-]^c = 0 \qquad (5\text{-}11)$$

where the plasma protein and erythrocyte hemoglobin concentrations are assumed constant.

Plasma protein and hemoglobin charges are essentially determined by the binding/release of protons. If we restrict the analysis to isothermal changes, then this binding in the plasma is a function of pH only, expressed by the plasma nonbicarbonate buffer capacity:

$$\beta^{pl} \equiv -[Pr]^{pl} \, dz_{pr}/d\,pH^{pl} \qquad (5\text{-}12)$$

where the value of β^{pl} under physiological conditions departs only minimally from 7.7 mM/pH unit (Siggaard-Andersen, 1974).

Equation (5-10) may be rewritten as

$$dB^{pl} = \beta^{pl} \, d\,pH^{pl} + d[HCO_3^-]^{pl} \qquad (5\text{-}13)$$

It is somewhat difficult to avoid ambiguity in defining and distinguishing between hemoglobin and DPG charges. On the one hand, it is logical to consider hemoglobin molecular charge to comprise contributions from all bound ligands, DPG being no exception, and to consider changes in the charge of unbound DPG to determine the third term in equation (5-11). However, this approach presupposes knowledge of the degree of hemoglobin DPG binding as it varies under physiological and pathophysiological conditions, whereas that behavior is only approximately known at the present time.

An alternative approach, attractive because it conforms to the mode of reportage of available buffering data (see Figures 19 and 21), is to expand the sum of the second and third terms of equation (5-11) as follows:

$$d(z_{Hm}[Hm]^c + z_{DPG}[DPG]_T) = -\beta^c \, d\,pH^c + z_{DPG} \, d[DPG]_T$$

$$+ [Hm]^c \left\{ \frac{\partial z_{Hm}}{\partial \bar{O}_2} \, d\bar{O}_2 + \frac{\partial z_{Hm}}{\partial \log pCO_2} \, d \log pCO_2 \right\} \qquad (5\text{-}14)$$

where

$$\beta^c \equiv -\left([Hm]^c\frac{\partial z_{Hm}}{\partial pH^c} + [DPG]_T\frac{\partial z_{DPG}}{\partial pH^c}\right) \tag{5-15}$$

and recognition is accorded the fact that hemoglobin charge varies with pCO_2, $\bar{O}_2$, and pH^c. The additional variation of hemoglobin charge with $[DPG]_T$ can be accounted for in near-rigorous fashion by assigning z_{DPG} in equation (5-14) the value for unbound DPG calculated from the prevailing pH and free DPG pK values. This neglects changes in hemoglobin and DPG pK values that accompany the complexing of the two species; however, the approximation appears to be justified by the data of de Bruin *et al.* (1974*a*).

Siggaard-Andersen (1974) reports values of β^c at near normal $[DPG]_T$ for deoxy- and oxyhemoglobin, and at elevated $[DPG]_T$ for oxyhemoglobin, all as functions of pH^c in the physiological range, and at $pCO_2 = 0$ (see Figures 19–21).

CO_2-linked proton binding may be derived from the assumption of chemical reaction equilibrium in the carbamino binding scheme outlined in Chapter 4 [reactions (4-21)–(4-23)], i.e.

$$K_z = \frac{[HbNH_2][H^+]}{[HbNH_3^+]} \tag{5-16}$$

$$K_c = \frac{[HbNHCOO^-][H^+]}{[CO_2][HbNH_2]} \tag{5-17}$$

where $[CO_2]$ is the concentration of dissolved carbon dioxide and [HbNHCOOH] can safely be neglected. As discussed previously (see pp. 80–81), both equilibrium constants K_z and K_c are functions of $\bar{O}_2$ and $[DPG]_T$.

The number of "CO_2-labile" protons bound per monomer varies between zero and two according to

$$\frac{[HbNH_2] + 2[HbNH_3^+]}{[HbNH_2] + [HbNH_3^+] + [HbNHCOO^-]}$$

$$= \frac{1 + 2[H^+]/K_z}{1 + [H^+]/K_z + K_c[CO_2]/[H^+]} \tag{5-18}$$

Differentiation of the right-hand side of equation (5-18) with respect to $[CO_2]$ and then multiplication by $2.3[CO_2]$ leads to:

$$\left(\frac{\partial z_{Hm}}{\partial \log p CO_2}\right)_{pH^c, O_2, [DPG]_T} = -\frac{2.3(K_c[CO_2]/[H^+])(1+2[H^+]/K_z)}{(1+[H^+]/K_z + K_c[CO_2]/[H^+])^2}$$

(5-19)

Similarly, the additional buffer capacity afforded by carbamino binding may be taken to equal the difference between (1) the derivative of the right-hand side of equation (5-18) with respect to pH, and (2) the buffer capacity afforded by the same CO_2-binding amino groups in the absence of the gas. That is,

$$\beta^c = \beta^c(p CO_2 = 0)$$

$$+2.3[Hm]^c\left\{\frac{4K_c[CO_2]/K_z + [H^+]/K_z + K_c[CO_2]/[H^+]}{(1+[H^+]/K_z + K_c[CO_2]/[H^+])^2}\right.$$

$$\left.-\frac{[H^+]/K_z}{(1+[H^+]/K_z)^2}\right\}$$

(5-20)

Returning now to equation (5-11), we find that it is transformed by equation (5-14) into

$$dB^c = \beta^c\, dpH^c + d[HCO_3^-]^c - z_{DPG}[DPG]_T$$

$$-[Hm]^c\left\{\frac{\partial z_{Hm}}{\partial \bar{O}_2}\, d\bar{O}_2 + \frac{\partial z_{Hm}}{\partial \log p CO_2}\, d \log p CO_2\right\} \quad (5\text{-}21)$$

with auxiliary information provided by equations (5-19) and (5-20).

It is worthy of note that for conditions of reaction equilibrium, of the two derivatives enclosed in the brackets of relationship (5-21), the first can be identified—in modern terminology—as the Haldane coefficient, and, as discussed on pp. 64, 92, it is approximated by the Bohr coefficient, i.e.,

$$\left(\frac{\partial z_{Hm}}{\partial \bar{O}_2}\right)_{pH^c} \cong \left(\frac{\partial \log p O_2}{\partial pH^c}\right)_{\bar{O}_2}$$

(5-22)

where constancy of $p CO_2$ and $[DPG]_T$ is implied.

Similarly, the second of the two derivatives in brackets should be approximated by the negative of the slope of a plot of $\overline{CO_2}$ vs. pH^c

at constant $p\mathrm{CO_2}$ (where $\overline{\mathrm{CO_2}}$ denotes the fractional saturation of hemoglobin monomer with carbon dioxide), i.e.,

$$\left(\frac{\partial z_{\mathrm{Hm}}}{\partial \log p\mathrm{CO_2}}\right)_{\mathrm{pH^c}} \cong -\left(\frac{\partial \overline{\mathrm{CO_2}}}{\partial \mathrm{pH^c}}\right)_{p\mathrm{CO_2}} \qquad (5\text{-}23)$$

the implied constants being $\overline{\mathrm{O}}_2$ and $[\mathrm{DPG}]_T$. The above relationship is also derivable from equations (5-16) and (5-17).

Conservation of Nontitratable Ions. We now turn to the constraint of mass conservation, which governs the changes in nontitratable ionic species concentrations in each blood phase. In this regard, we introduce the whole blood B value, which is related to the respective erythrocyte and plasma values as follows:

$$B^{\mathrm{bl}} = hB^c + (1-h)B^{\mathrm{pl}} \qquad (5\text{-}24)$$

where h is the hematocrit expressed as a fraction.

Differentiation of equation (5-24) yields

$$dB^{\mathrm{bl}} = h\,dB^c + (1-h)\,dB^{\mathrm{pl}} + (B^c - B^{\mathrm{pl}})\,dh \qquad (5\text{-}25)$$

The last term accounts for erythrocyte swelling/shrinkage. The first two terms can be expanded by means of equations (5-21) and (5-13), respectively, so as to transform the above relationship into

$$dB^{\mathrm{bl}} = h\Big\{\beta^c\,d\mathrm{pH^c} - z_{\mathrm{DPG}}\,d[\mathrm{DPG}]_T + d[\mathrm{HCO_3^-}]^c$$

$$-[\mathrm{Hm}]^c\Big[\frac{\partial z_{\mathrm{Hm}}}{\partial \overline{\mathrm{O}}_2}\,d\overline{\mathrm{O}}_2 + \frac{\partial z_{\mathrm{Hm}}}{\partial \log p\mathrm{CO_2}}\,d\log p\mathrm{CO_2}\Big]\Big\}$$

$$+(1-h)\{\beta^{\mathrm{pl}}\,d\mathrm{pH^{pl}} + d[\mathrm{HCO_3^-}]^{\mathrm{pl}}\} + \{B^c - B^{\mathrm{pl}}\}\,dh \qquad (5\text{-}26)$$

The term dB^{bl} represents changes in whole blood base excess, a quantity that Siggaard-Andersen (1974) defined as the "difference in the concentration of strong base between the blood . . . and the same blood titrated to $[\mathrm{pH^{pl}}] = 7.40$ at $p\mathrm{CO_2} = 40\,\mathrm{mm\,Hg}$ and [temperature] $= 37°\mathrm{C}$," essentially complete hemoglobin oxygenation presumably being the additional condition.

The last equation, derived from the fundamental constraints of electroneutrality in each blood phase and of conservation of strong acid–base (i.e., nontitratable ions), describes the allowable changes in concentration of the blood's ionic species at constant temperature.

It is equally descriptive of the processes that occur as the blood flows through pulmonary or systemic tissue capillaries, through an artery, a vein, or membrane oxygenator, or, if contained in a test tube, as it equilibrates with a gas phase.

It is generally true of these circumstances, including the situation in the systemic capillary in a steady state, that strong acid–base is neither entering nor leaving the blood in appreciable amount, and therefore $dB^{bl} = 0$. On the other hand, the acidification of blood during exercise, the equilibration of systemic capillary blood with surrounding tissue in response to a perturbation in blood pCO_2, and simple *in vitro* titration with strong acid–base are cases in which B^{bl} is indeed a variable.

The effects of temperature change upon blood acid–base status have been omitted from the development of equation (5-26). A recent experimental study (Reeves, 1976a) has, in fact, confirmed the notion that appreciable changes in pH and pCO_2, *at constant CO_2 content*, should be anticipated as the blood flows from normothermic regions of the body to, say, hypothermic skin or hyperthermic working muscle. Interestingly though, the corresponding changes in r and h are all but negligible (Reeves, 1976b).

Applications of the Fundamental Relationships

The following are some examples of the application of equation (5-26).

Changes from One Equilibrium State to Another. We consider first situations in which all reversible chemical reactions and red cell–plasma diffusible ion distributions are equilibrated. In such circumstances equation (5-26) is modifiable by two important equilibrium relationships, which respectively connect (1) the bicarbonate, proton, and carbon dioxide concentrations in each blood phase, and (2) the cellular and plasma concentrations of individual diffusible ionic species.

The first is the Henderson–Hasselbalch reaction, which is expressible as

$$\{[HCO_3^-]10^{-pH}/[CO_2]\}_{eq}^{cor\,pl} = K_a' \qquad (5\text{-}27)$$

where "eq" denotes equilibrium conditions. As stated earlier, the term 10^{-pH} is a measure of proton *activity*.

K_a' is the overall equilibrium constant of the consecutive reactions comprising CO_2 hydration (hydrolysis) and carbonic acid dissociation:

$$CO_2 + H_2O \leftrightharpoons H_2CO_3 \leftrightharpoons HCO_3^- + H^+$$

and comprises the activity of water. The value of K_a' under physiological conditions is $10^{-6.1}$ M, subject to slight variation with pH, temperature, and ionic strength (Siggaard-Andersen, 1974).

When, at equilibrium, the *partial pressures* of CO_2 in cells and plasma equalize, the *concentrations* of physically dissolved gas differ according to the respective solubilities α_{CO_2}, defined by Henry's law:

$$\{[CO_2] = \alpha_{CO_2} pCO_2\}^{c \, or \, pl} \tag{5-28}$$

The values at 37°C for $\alpha_{CO_2}^{pl}$ and $\alpha_{CO_2}^{c}$ are 0.030 and 0.023 mM/mm Hg, respectively (Siggaard-Andersen, 1974).

The second equilibrium relationship is afforded by the value of r, which is the ratio of the ionic activities of univalent diffusible species in the two phases of the blood [see equation (5-5)]. Assuming identical bicarbonate ion activity coefficients in each phase, then

$$\frac{[HCO_3^-]^c}{[HCO_3^-]^{pl}} \frac{\rho_{H_2O}^{pl}}{\rho_{H_2O}^{c}} = \frac{10^{-pH^{pl}}}{10^{-pH^c}} = r \tag{5-29}$$

where ρ_{H_2O} is expressed in liters of water per liter of cells. [Equations (5-27)–(5-29) are internally consistent as long as the water content ratio equals that of the CO_2 solubilities.]

Review of Literature Data on Cellular/Plasma Hydrogen and Chloride Ion Distributions at Equilibrium. Table X summarizes data in the literature on the hydrogen ion distribution between red cells and plasma in normal oxygenated blood at 37–38°C and different values of plasma pH. Corresponding data for oxygenated as well as deoxygenated cord blood are reported by Bauer and Schröder (1972). Funder and Wieth (1966b) have indicated that the results are independent of whether the plasma pH is adjusted by addition of

Table X

Relation between Red Cell and Plasma pH of Normal Oxygenated Blood at 37°C

Plasma pH						pH range	$\eta\ (\mathrm{pH^{pl}}=7.40)^a$	$r\ (\mathrm{pH^{pl}}=7.40)$	Ref.
6.800	7.000	7.200	7.400	7.600	7.800				
Red cell pH									
	6.905	7.054	7.197	7.332		6.9–7.7	0.695	0.627	*b*
	6.843	6.998	7.149	7.293	7.429	7.3–7.7	0.738	0.561	*c*
6.711	6.874	7.034	7.189	7.339	7.482	6.4–8.5	0.763	0.615	*d*
	6.867	7.019	7.166	7.304		7.1–7.7	0.714	0.583	*e*
6.699	6.868	7.035	7.199	7.359	7.516	6.6–8.6	0.811	0.629	*f*
	6.863	7.020	7.174	7.321		7.0–7.7	0.752	0.594	*g*

$^a \eta = (\partial \mathrm{pH}^c / \partial \mathrm{pH}^{pl})_{O_2}$

[b] Fitzsimmons and Sendroy (1961), $r = 3.883 - 0.440 \mathrm{pH}^{pl}$.

[c] Bromberg *et al.* (1965), $r = 3.062 - 0.338 \mathrm{pH}^{pl}$.

[d] Funder and Wieth (1966*b*), $r = 3.094 - 0.335 \mathrm{pH}^{pl}$.

[e] Bauer and Schröder (1972), $r = 3.417 - 0.383 \mathrm{pH}^{pl}$.

[f] Duhm and Gerlach (1971), $r = 2.649 - 0.273 \mathrm{pH}^{pl}$.

[g] Rörth (private communication), $r = 3.095 - 0.338 \mathrm{pH}^{pl}$

acid–base or by variation of pCO_2. However, despite generally fair agreement among the different sets of data, it is noteworthy that the progressively lower r values of references f, g, and e are consistent with progressively higher pCO_2 values (see Table XI). This is indicative of an appreciable effect of carbamino formation, a reaction that makes the hemoglobin molecule more negatively charged.

Besides a possibly significant carbamino effect, highly probable sources of the discrepancies in the data listed in Table X are differences in red cell DPG concentration among different bloods. In the first place, the variation in $[DPG]_T$ among normal subjects is quite large (see p. 196). Secondly, incubation of the blood—especially at low pH values—leads to a reduction in $[DPG]_T$; this effect was in fact noted by Bauer and Schröder (1972). According to Duhm (1971; see below), a difference in red cell 2,3-DPG concentration of 0.5 mM, i.e., about 10% of the normal value or one standard deviation of the natural variation (see p. 196), is responsible for a ~ 0.01 unit red cell pH difference at fixed plasma pH.

Data on hydrogen ion activity are based on emf measurements that include liquid junction potentials that are difficult to characterize in rigorous fashion. The relative errors arising from liquid junction potentials have been studied by Salling and Siggaard-Andersen (1971), who estimate that the erythrocyte hydrogen ion activity relative to that in plasma may be overestimated by a factor of

Table XI

The Difference in Red Cell pH of Deoxygenated and Oxygenated Normal Blood, $pH^c(d-o)$, at Different Plasma pH Values and at 37°C

Plasma pH					
7.000	7.200	7.400	7.600	pCO_2(mm Hg)	Ref.[a]
ΔpH^c (d–o)					
0.058	0.062	0.067	0.074	0	(a)
0.032	0.032	0.031	0.029	36	(b)
0.030	0.038	0.048	0.062	40	(c)

[a] Regression for deoxygenated blood: (a) Duhm and Gerlach (1971), $r = 2.740 – 0.271$ pH^{pl}; (b) Rörth (private communication), $r = 3.369 – 0.369$pH^{pl}; (c) Bauer and Schröder (1972), $r = 3.175 – 0.341$ pH^{pl}.

1.03. Uncertainties of this nature have motivated measurements of the red cell–plasma chloride ion distribution as an indicator of the hydrogen ion distribution.

The chloride ion distribution has been studied by several groups of investigators (Dill *et al.*, 1937; Fitzsimons and Sendroy, 1961; Funder and Wieth, 1966*b*). In the study of Funder and Wieth, the ratio $[Cl^-]^c/[Cl^-]^{pl}$ was found to vary with pH^{pl} in much the same way as $[H^+]^{pl}/[H^+]^c$. However, the former ratio exceeded the latter by 5–10% at all plasma pH values studied. The cause of this difference is not clear, but there are several possibilities besides the liquid junction error already mentioned. Either chloride ions or hydrogen ions or both may not be in thermodynamic equilibrium. Another possibility is binding of chloride ions to hemoglobin (Rollema *et al.*, 1975). Finally, the chloride ion activity coefficients in plasma and red cells may not be identical.

In any case, the data support the contention that the hydrogen ion activity inside red cells can be measured with reasonable accuracy with appropriate emf cells, or calculated from measurements of the chloride distribution as well as plasma pH. The data also demonstrate that oxygenated red cell pH may be calculated from the plasma pH alone, provided (1) that $[DPG]_T$ is equal or close to the normal mean value, and (2) that the deviation of plasma pH from the normal value of 7.40 is a result of *acute* changes in the blood acid–base status, whether by addition of proton acceptors–donors or by changes in carbon dioxide tension.

Measurements of red cell pH in normal *deoxygenated* blood yield expectedly higher values at the same plasma pH. Available literature data for ΔpH^c $(d-o)$, the difference between erythrocyte pH values of oxy- and deoxygenated bloods at constant pH^{pl}, derived from regression lines of r vs. pH^{pl} for oxy- and deoxygenated blood samples, are listed in Table XI. The notable discrepancies among the three data sets would appear to be at least partly connected to the pCO_2 differences. As shown theoretically by Siggaard-Andersen (1974), ΔpH^c $(d-o)$ is a function of the Haldane coefficient $(\Delta z_{Hm}/\Delta \bar{O}_2)$, erythrocyte (as well as plasma) buffer capacity, and the quantity $(\Delta pH^c/\Delta pH^{pl})$. Since all three vary with pCO_2, a complex functionality of ΔpH^c $(d-o)$ with pCO_2 may be expected. It should also be noted that the assumption of a linear r vs. pH^{pl} relationship has no sound theoretical basis. Therefore, such a data-reduction method, while necessary for statistical purposes, may well distort the real situation.

Besides the plasma pH and state of oxygenation of the blood, the red cell 2,3-DPG concentration is the most important determinant of red cell pH. When 2,3-DPG (and other organic phosphate) builds up in the red cells from glucose and inorganic phosphate, the concentration of impermeable negative charge rises. Over time periods on the order of hours or possibly even days, the red cells are apparently unable to balance this negative charge by cation accumulation, but do so instead by release of chloride ions. This exchange of multivalent for monovalent ions affects osmotic balance and thereby causes the cells to shrink somewhat (Deuticke *et al.*, 1971).

The relationship between pH^c and red cell organic phosphate concentration (comprising mainly 2,3-DPG, ATP, and fructose-1,6-

Table XII

Effects of Red Cell 2,3-DPG on pH^c and $\partial pH^c/\partial pH^{pl}$ at Different Values of pH^{pl}

Regression equations for the relation between red cell pH and red cell 2,3-DPG concentration (mmol/liter H_2O) at different plasma pH values in oxygenated blood (modified from Duhm, 1971)

pH^{pl}	$(DPG)^c > 6.3$	$(DPG)^c < 6.3$
7.00	$6.94-0.0125(DPG)^c$	$6.91-0.0072(DPG)^c$
7.20	$7.12-0.0128(DPG)^c$	$7.09-0.0086(DPG)^c$
7.40	$7.30-0.0148(DPG)^c$	$7.28-0.0123(DPG)^c$
7.60	$7.46-0.0182(DPG)^c$	$7.42-0.0130(DPG)^c$
7.80	$7.64-0.0205(DPG)^c$	$7.60-0.0134(DPG)^c$

Values of $\eta = \partial pH^c/\partial pH^{pl}$ of oxygenated blood at 37°C at different red cell 2,3-DPG concentrations and plasma pH (calculated from Duhm, 1971)

$(DPG)^c/pH^{pl}$	7.00	7.20	7.40	7.60	7.80
1.0	0.89	0.88	0.87	0.86	0.85
6.0	0.86	0.84	0.82	0.80	0.78
19.0	0.70	0.67	0.63	0.60	0.56
24.0	0.59	0.56	0.53	0.50	0.45

diphosphate), at 37° and varying pH^{pl} in oxygenated blood, has been studied by Duhm (1971). Erythrocyte phosphate level was varied by incubation in the presence and absence of glucose, inosine, pyruvate, and phosphate. The data allow calculation of $pH^c - (DPG)^c$ regression lines at constant pH^{pl} values between 7.0 and 7.8, where $(DPG)^c$ is the total cellular 2,3-DPG concentration, expressed in mmol/liter H_2O, determined from the total phosphate concentration. (Corresponding values of $[DPG]_T$, i.e., in mmol/liter cells, may be derived from the data of Deuticke *et al.*, 1971.) Regression lines of the form $pH^c = a' - b'(DPG)^c$ provide good fits at 2,3-DPG concentrations between 6.3 and 30 mmol/liter red cell water. Below the value of 6.3, the slopes are much lower. Table XII lists the regression equations and derived values of η.

The experimental results and calculations discussed above appear to provide a reasonably safe basis for the calculation of pH^c from data on pH^{pl}, $[DPG]_T$, pCO_2, and $\bar{O}_2$. It should be kept in mind, however, that the data are derived from experiments in which red cells were observed within a few hours of perturbation. Funder and Wieth (1966*a,b*) have shown that under such circumstances, cation shifts do not occur to any appreciable extent, and therefore observable effects may be explained solely on the basis of changes in nondiffusible anionic charge and shifts of both anions and water.

The situation during *in vivo* changes in pH or $[DPG]_T$ may well be different. For example, in metabolic alkalosis, sodium accumulates in the erythrocytes without a corresponding loss of potassium (Funder and Wieth, 1974*a*). Furthermore, simultaneous alkalosis and treatment with digitalis may elevate red cell sodium exceedingly, while again leaving the potassium unperturbed (Funder and Wieth, 1974*b*). Thus, there are indeed circumstances in which the ionic balance of the red cell is quite abnormal. There has been no systematic study of changes in proton distribution in such instances.

As happens in response to changes in the concentration of effectively impermeable ions in the red cells, the pH^c/pH^{pl} ratio responds to changes in the concentration of impermeable ions in the plasma. Variations in the concentration of plasma proteins under physiological and pathophysiological circumstances are usually too small to significantly influence the ratio. However, the presence of citrate ions under conditions of blood storage for transfusion purposes (Funder and Wieth, 1966b) and of negative ions in radiographic contrast material (Lichtman et $al.$, 1975) may be responsible for highly significant changes.

Working Relationship for Changes in Equilibrium State. We now proceed with the transformation of equation (5-26) by means of the above-described equilibrium relationships. First, from differentiation of equation (5-27) it can be shown that

$$d[HCO_3^-]^{pl} = 2.3[HCO_3^-]^{pl}(dpH^{pl} + d \log pCO_2) \qquad (5\text{-}30)$$

In addition, from equation (5-29) we have

$$[HCO_3^-]^c = r\omega[HCO_3^-]^{pl} \qquad (5\text{-}31)$$

where $\omega \equiv \rho_{H_2O}^c / \rho_{H_2O}^{pl}$.

Finally, assuming a generally linear $r - pH^{pl}$ correlation, then

$$r = a - bpH^{pl} \qquad (5\text{-}32)$$

where a and b are functions of $[DPG]_T$ and $\bar{O}_2$ but not of pH. The above relationship implies

$$\eta \equiv \partial pH^c / \partial pH^{pl} = 1 - b/2.3r \qquad (5\text{-}33)$$

Furthermore, differentiation of equations (5-31) and (5-32), at constant $\bar{O}_2$ and $[DPG]_T$, leads to the following relation:

$$d[HCO_3^-]^c = \omega(rd[HCO_3^-]^{pl} - b[HCO_3^-]^{pl} dpH^{pl}) \qquad (5\text{-}34)$$

[It should be noted that the analysis up to this point contains the implicit assumption that variations in ω due to possible osmosis, and in a and b due to pCO_2 change, are all insignificant. The validity of this assumption may be verified by a more rigorous approach to equation (5-35) below. In a related matter, the use of constant $[DPG]_T$, rather than a constant amount of DPG *per cell*—as likely prevailed during the relevant experimental investigations—is also justified by the negligible magnitude of osmotic solvent shift.]

Equation (5-26) now can be modified through the application of equations (5-30), (5-33), and (5-34) so as to assume the following form:

$$(dB^{bl})_{\bar{O}_2,[DPG]_T} = \{h\eta\beta^c + (1-h)\beta^{pl} + 2.3(h\omega r\eta + 1 - h)$$

$$\times [HCO_3^-]^{pl}\} \, d\,pH^{pl}$$

$$+ \left\{2.3(h\omega r + 1 - h)[HCO_3^-]^{pl}\right.$$

$$\left. - h[Hm]^c \frac{\partial z_{Hm}}{\partial \log pCO_2}\right\} d \log pCO_2$$

$$+ \{B^c - B^{pl}\} \, dh \tag{5-35}$$

Equation (5-35) leads directly to expressions for:

(1) The slope of the *in vitro* strong acid–base titration curve of whole blood determined at constant carbon dioxide tension:

$$\left(\frac{\partial B^{bl}}{\partial pH^{pl}}\right)_{\bar{O}_2,[DPG]_T,pCO_2} = h\eta\beta^c + (1-h)\beta^{pl}$$

$$+ 2.3(h\omega r\eta + 1 - h)[HCO_3^-]^{pl} \tag{5-36}$$

$$+ (B^c - B^{pl})\left(\frac{\partial h}{\partial pH^{pl}}\right)_{\bar{O}_2,[DPG]_T,pCO_2}$$

(2) The slope of the *in vitro* CO_2 equilibration curve of whole blood:

$$\left(\frac{\partial \log pCO_2}{\partial pH^{pl}}\right)_{\bar{O}_2,[DPG]_T,B^{bl}}$$

$$= \frac{h\eta\beta^c + (1-h)\beta^{pl} + 2.3(h\omega r\eta + 1 - h)[HCO_3^-]^{pl} + (B^c - B^{pl})\phi}{2.3(h\omega r + 1 - h)[HCO_3^-]^{pl} - h[Hm]^c(\partial z_{Hm}/\partial \log pCO_2)} \tag{5-37}$$

where $\phi = (\partial h/\partial pH^{pl})_{\bar{O}_2,[DPG]_T,B^{bl}}$.

We consider first the second of the above two slopes. In oxygenated normal whole blood of hematocrit 0.44, $pCO_2 = 40$, and $pH^{pl} = 7.40$, and on the basis of Bauer and Schröder's (1972) data for (1) K_c and K_z (*see p.* 138), (2) pH^c (see Table X), and (3) $\alpha^c_{CO_2}$ (0.026 mM/mm Hg), the first three terms in the numerator of equation (5-37) are 21.3, 4.3, and 38.6 mM/pH unit, respectively. From a theoretical analysis of the cellular/plasma–diffusible ion distribution accounting for cellular osmotic balance, Siggaard-Andersen (1974) estimated a value for ϕ of -0.054 (pH unit)$^{-1}$. Furthermore, on the basis of the same author's models of plasma and erythrocyte fluid, $(B^c - B^{pl})$ can be assigned a value of 52 meq/liter. Thus we estimate that, under normal conditions,

$$(B^c - B^{pl})\phi = -2.8 \text{ mM/pH unit}$$

Finally, the two terms in the denominator of equation (5-37) are, respectively, 41.7 and 1.3 mM.

The slope of the CO_2 equilibration curve is thus calculated to be -1.43. If one neglects the contributions from swelling–shrinkage and carbamino buffering [i.e., by letting $\beta^c = \beta^c (pCO_2 = 0)$, discarding the second term in the denominator of (5-37), and applying the r vs. pH^{pl} regression at $pCO_2 = 0$ of Duhm and Gerlach (1971), see Table X], the resulting value is -1.58. Surprisingly, it is the latter value that better agrees with the experimental value of -1.57 reported by Siggaard-Andersen (1974) for $pCO_2 = 40$ mm Hg.

Turning to the slope of the acid–base titration curve, if one assumes that the $(\partial h/\partial pH^{pl})$ terms in equations (5-36) and (5-37) are equal, then the value of what may be described as the whole blood buffer capacity at constant pCO_2 is calculated to be 61.4 mM/pH unit. If one again neglects volumetric and carbamino affects, the value is 67.1 mM/pH unit, which is nearly identical to the value of 67.2 mM/pH unit that can be obtained from the interpolated experimental data depicted in Figure 10 of Siggaard-Andersen (1974).

Simplification of the Basic Relationships. The previous analysis can be simplified by discarding in equation (5-26) and its successors those terms attributable to CO_2-linked hemoglobin proton binding and osmotically driven volumetric change. Moreover, we may assume the general applicability of the r vs. pH^{pl} data of Duhm and Gerlach (1971) and Duhm (1971), which were registered in the absence of CO_2. These approximations are believed justified by: (1) the relatively small extent of carbamino buffering (which can be. shown to be true also of *deoxygenated* blood) as derived from equations (5-19) and (5-20); (2) the similarly small effect of erythrocyte shrinkage–swelling; and (3) the relatively insignificant difference among both r and η values derived from the data obtained at various pCO_2 levels. Furthermore, the errors introduced by neglect of carbamino buffering and the effect of CO_2 upon r tend to offset each other; and use of the data of Duhm and Gerlach (1971) and Duhm (1971) provides a self-consistent correlation of r with pH^{pl}, $\bar{O}_2$, and $[DPG]_T$.

Equation (5-26) now can be rewritten in its reduced form:

$$dB^{bl} \cong h\{\beta^c \, dpH^c - z_{DPG} \, d[DPG]_T + d[HCO_3^-]^c$$

$$- [Hm]^c (\partial z_{Hm}/\partial \bar{O}_2) \, d\bar{O}_2\}$$

$$+ (1-h)\{\beta^{pl} \, dpH^{pl} + d[HCO_3^-]^c\} \tag{5-38}$$

Constraint once again to constant DPG concentration and oxygen saturation, and application of equations (5-30), (5-33), and (5-34), further reduce the above to

$$(dB^{bl})_{\bar{O}_2,[DPG]_T,} \cong \{h(\beta^c \eta - \omega b[HCO_3^-]^{pl}) + (1-h)\beta^{pl}\} \, dpH^{pl}$$

$$+ \{h\omega r + 1 - h\} \, d[HCO_3^-]^{pl} \tag{5-39}$$

In Vitro versus in Vivo CO_2 Equilibrations Curves. The previously discussed *in vitro* CO_2 equilibration curve is often plotted in $HCO_3^{-pl} - pH^{pl}$ coordinates. From equation (5-39), the theoretical slope of such a curve is approximated by

$$\left(\frac{\partial [HCO_3^-]^{pl}}{\partial pH^{pl}}\right)_{\bar{O}_2,[DPG]_T,B^{bl}}$$

$$= -\frac{h(\beta^c \eta - \omega b[HCO_3^-]^{pl}) + (1-h)\beta^{pl}}{h\omega r + 1 - h} \tag{5-40}$$

For oxygenated blood of hematocrit 0.44 and pCO_2 of 40 mm Hg, the calculated slope is -31.8 mM/pH unit. This agrees quite well with the values of -31.9 and -29.1 mM/pH unit predicted by Lloyd and Michel (1966) and by Siggaard-Andersen (1974), respectively, on the basis of somewhat different data sets and theoretical approaches. The actual value consistent with the experimental value of $\partial \log pCO_2/\partial pH^{pl}$ and equation (5-30) is reported by Siggaard-Andersen (1974) to be -29.0.

Strikingly different $[HCO_3^-]^{pl} - pH^{pl}$ relationships are obtained from measurements on blood samples taken from subjects as they breathe gas of progressively altered carbon dioxide tension. The reason is that in such studies B^{bl} *is a variable* rather than a constant. This is a consequence of equilibration of systemic capillary blood with surrounding tissue (Shaw and Messer, 1932), as clarified below.

Following a perturbation of whole body pCO_2 values, the bicarbonate ion concentrations in the blood and interstitial fluid (ISF) attain new sets of values, determined largely by the available nonbicarbonate buffer capacities. Since the latter value is much greater in the blood, the immediate change in bicarbonate concentration is much greater in the erythrocytes and plasma than in ISF. However, since bicarbonate ions can penetrate the capillary wall in exchange for other anions, e.g., Cl^-, the $[HCO_3^-]$ values in the blood and ISF approach a new Donnan-like equilibrium. The net result of this "Hamburger shift" between blood and ISF is that the blood base excess changes and in a direction opposed to that in pCO_2, which in turn has the effect of amplifying the blood pH change. Thus, during *in vivo* CO_2 equilibration, the buffer capacity of the blood appears to be diminished, because the blood's buffers must in effect control ISF pH as well.

A theoretical analysis of the equilibration of blood and ISF, based again on the constraints of electroneutrality in each phase and conservation of total base, can be developed by straightforward analogy to equations (5-13) and (5-24), assuming that ISF–plasma proton activity and bicarbonate concentration ratios satisfy the following relationship:

$$[HCO_3^-]^{ISF}/[HCO_3^-]^{pl} = 10^{-pH^{pl}}/10^{-pH^{ISF}} = r' \qquad (5\text{-}41)$$

The slope of the *in vivo* CO_2 equilibration curve is thus theoretically approximated by

$$\left(\frac{\partial[HCO_3^-]^{pl}}{\partial pH^{pl}}\right)_{(B^{bl}+B^{ISF}),\, \bar{O}_2, [DPG]_T}$$
$$= -\frac{h(\beta^c\eta - \omega b[HCO_3^-]^{pl}) + (1-h)\beta^{pl} + \theta\beta^{ISF}}{h\omega r + 1 - h + \theta r'} \qquad (5\text{-}42)$$

where $\theta = V^{ISF}/V^{bl}$, and V denotes volume.

An analogous relationship is derived, with a different theoretical approach by Dell and Winters (1970). For normal man, they suggest that $\beta^{ISF} = 1.8$ mm/pH unit and $r' = 1.1$, while V^{Bl} and V^{ISF} are, respectively, 0.075 and 0.187 liters/kg body weight, or $\theta = 2.5$. On the basis of these additional data and equation (5-42), one predicts a value of -8.2 mm/pH unit for the slope of the *in vivo* CO_2 equilibration curve, whereas Dell and Winters report that experimental results indicate a value of -12.7 mm/pH unit.

The discrepancy between theoretical and experimental values is not surprising, given the appreciable uncertainty regarding ISF parameters and approximations introduced by the treatment of the three fluid phases in terms of average compositions. Furthermore, prolonged exposure of tissue to altered CO_2 tensions eventually stimulates additional channels of pH regulation. Within hours a similar exchange of acid–base and bicarbonate occurs between the (blood + ISF) and the highly buffered intracellular fluid. Over still longer periods both the kidneys and bone respond, the latter through the slow equilibration of alkali carbonate with surrounding tissue. Comprehensive discussions of the mechanisms of pH control are presented by Davenport (1974), Siggaard-Andersen (1974), and Woodbury (1974).

Calculated Whole Blood Equilibria. Before we proceed to application of the electroneutrality/base conservation relationships to the analysis of *in vivo* transport, let us first review how the available reaction equilibrium and electrolyte distribution data may be applied.

First of all, the relationship between oxygen tension and hemoglobin saturation is illustrated in Figure 30 for: (1) standard conditons with respect to pH^{pl} (7.40), pCO_2 (40 mm Hg), $[DPG]_T$ (5.0 mm), and temperature (37°C), and (2)–(5) otherwise identical conditions except for the indicated change of one of these variables. The standard curve is that listed in Table V; that at elevated temperature was calculated using the correction (see p. 103)

$$pO_2(T, \bar{O}_2) = pO_2(37°C, \bar{O}_2) \cdot 10^{0.024(T-37)}$$

while all three other curves were derived from the standard data by application of the interaction coefficients listed in Tables VI–VIII.

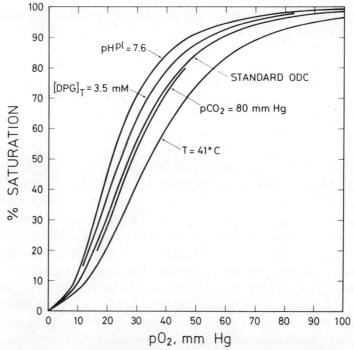

Figure 30. Oxygen dissociation curves of hemoglobin A. All curves at standard conditions of temperature, 37°C; $pH^{pl} = 7.40$; $pCO_2 = 40$ mm Hg; and $[DPG]_T = 5.0$ mM, except as indicated otherwise.

The equilibrium value of $\overline{CO_2}$, the average number (≤ 1) of moles of CO_2 bound per mole heme monomer at 37°C, may be estimated as a function of pCO_2, pH^c, $\bar{O}_2$, and $[DPG]_T$ as follows:

The amount bound to fully oxygenated hemoglobin at the stated pCO_2 and pH^c is calculated on the basis of equilibrium of reactions (4-21), (4-22), and (4.23), i.e.,

$$\overline{CO_2}(\bar{O}_2 = 1.0) = \frac{K_z K_c [CO_2]^c}{K_z K_c [CO_2]^c + K_z [H^+]^c + ([H^+]^c)^2} \quad (5\text{-}43)$$

where the values of K_z and K_c are 1.79×10^{-8} and 1.13×10^{-5} mol/liter, respectively, as reported by Bauer and Schröder (1972) for normal erythrocyte 2,3-DPG concentration. This value of $\overline{CO_2}$ is assumed to approximate the true value, whatever the value of

$[DPG]_T$, insofar as the effect of 2,3-DPG upon CO_2 binding to *oxy*hemoglobin is relatively small (see p. 81).

The desired value is then obtained by the following formula of linked functions based on assumption

$$\overline{CO_2} - \overline{CO_2}\,(\bar{O}_2 = 1.0) = \int_{1.0}^{\bar{O}_2} (\partial\overline{CO_2}/\partial\bar{O}_2)_{pCO_2}\, d\bar{O}_2$$
$$\cong \int_{\bar{O}_2}^{1.0} (\partial \log pO_2 / \partial \log pCO_2)_{\bar{O}_2}\, d\bar{O}_2$$

$$(5\text{-}44)$$

where the interaction coefficient $\partial \log pO_2 / \partial \log pCO_2$ may be obtained as a function of $[DPG]_T$ from Table VIII.

We are now in a position to calculate the equilibrium composition of blood under all physiological and pathophysiological conditions. Let us first look at the values derived when pH^{pl} is treated as an independent variable. (We in fact consider the latter and pH^c to be *derived* quantities insofar as their values depend on the blood's base excess, cellular 2,3-DPG concentration, and the prevailing gas tensions. The following section approaches the problem on that basis.)

Figure 31 comprises the carbon dioxide equilibration curves of oxygenated and deoxygenated whole blood at $pH^{pl} = 7.40$ and normal $[DPG]_T$, temperature, and hematocrit. Also included are the individual components of the total amount of absorbed gas,* with the concentrations of erythrocyte bicarbonate and carbamate having been derived from the appropriate values of pH^c (and pH^c calculated from the r vs. pH^{pl} data of Duhm and Gerlach, 1971; see Tables X and XI). The figure manifests the relatively small contributions of physically dissolved and hemoglobin-bound gas, as well as the relation between the magnitudes of cellular and plasma bicarbonate resulting from (1) the greater *amount* of plasma, (2) the greater concentration of *solvent* water in the plasma (0.94 vs. 0.72 kg/liter in the cells), and (3) an r value well below unity.

*Recently published data of Gros *et al.* (1976) have confirmed the generally assumed negligibility of *plasma* carbamate. Under normal arterial conditions, the estimated amount was about one-half that of dissolved CO_2 in plasma. While correspondingly greater values are to be expected in, for example, hypercapnia and/or alkalosis, the contribution of plasma carbamate to the arteriovenous CO_2 *difference* is estimated to remain negligible.

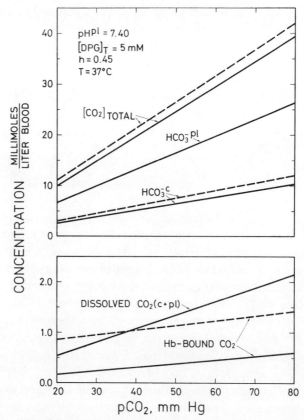

Figure 31. Carbon dioxide dissociation curves of normal oxygenated (solid lines) and deoxygenated (broken lines) human whole blood. $T = 37°C$, $pH^{pl} = 7.40$, $[DPG]_T = 5$ mM, $h = 0.45$.

Figure 32 explores the effect of varying $[DPG]_T$ at $pCO_2 = 40$ and otherwise the same conditions as in the preceding figure. Added are the erythrocyte pH values in oxygenated and deoxygenated blood. Because of the appreciable decreases in the latter values as $[DPG]_T$ increases, the total carbon dioxide follows the same trend. This is a result of diminishing erythrocyte bicarbonate and carbamate concentrations. In deoxygenated blood, the effect of $[DPG]_T$ upon carbamate formation is magnified directly by the competition of DPG and CO_2 for the same hemoglobin sites (see p.80).

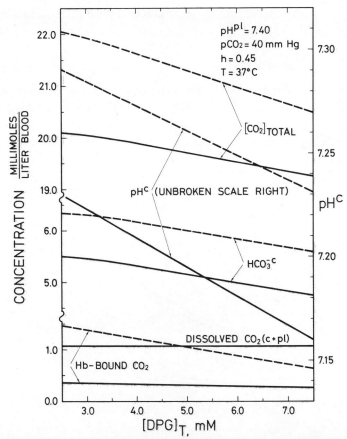

Figure 32. Effect of variation in erythrocyte 2,3-DPG concentration upon red cell pH in, and carbon dioxide absorption by, oxygenated (solid lines) and deoxygenated (broken lines) human whole blood. $T = 37°C$, $pH^{pl} = 7.40$, $pCO_2 = 40$ mm Hg, $h = 0.45$.

Figure 33, finally, illustrates the response to variation of pH^{pl}. There is an expectedly profound effect upon the concentrations of all forms of reacted CO_2.

Working Relationships for the Analysis of Steady-State in Vivo Transport.   We now turn to the two types of change in blood state that are of primary interest in the remaining chapters of this book:

(1) Variations in the overall character of the circulating blood, which remain effective for periods that are long by comparison with the time of circulation, and

(2) The cyclical changes undergone by the blood as it circulates.

By the first sort of perturbation we mean a change in blood base excess, arterial gas tension, or $[DPG]_T$. By the second we mean the continuous adjustments of pH, pCO_2, pO_2, $\bar{O}_2$, etc., that result from the exchange of oxygen and carbon dioxide in lungs and tissue.

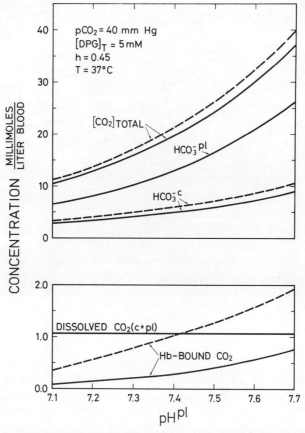

Figure 33. Effect of variation in plasma pH upon carbon dioxide absorption by oxygenated (solid lines) and deoxygenated (broken lines) human whole blood. $T = 37°C$, $pCO_2 = 40$ mm Hg, $[DPG]_T = 5$ mM, $h = 0.45$.

Analysis of Changes in the Composition of Arterial Blood. To illustrate the first group of changes, we consider the blood about to enter the systemic capillaries, having traversed the arterial system. This particular condition is selected so that we may retain the previous assumption of blood equilibration without introducing appreciable approximation. To determine the values for pH^c and pH^{pl} that must theoretically prevail at a given set of values for h, pO_2, pCO_2, $[DPG]_T$, and B^{bl}, we start by integrating equation (5-38) between limits defined by the standard steady state (I) and the state we seek to determine (II), i.e.,

$$\Delta B^{bl} = h \left\{ \int_{I}^{II} \beta^c \, dpH^c - \int_{I}^{II} z_{DPG} \, d[DPG]_T + \Delta[HCO_3^-]^c \right.$$

$$\left. - [Hm]^c \int_{I}^{II} (\partial z_{Hm}/\partial \bar{O}_2) \, d\bar{O}_2 \right\}$$

$$+ (1-h)\{\beta^{pl}\Delta pH^{pl} + \Delta[HCO_3^-]^{pl}\} \tag{5-45}$$

where the *delta* quantities signify differences between values of the respective terms at these two conditions.

In the standard state, $\bar{O}_2 = 1.00$, $pCO_2 = 40$ mm Hg, $[DPG]_T = 5.0$ mM, and $pH^{pl} = 7.40$; from the data of Duhm and Gerlach (1971), listed in Table X (see also Table IX), $pH^c = 7.198$; plasma and cellular bicarbonate concentrations are calculated, on the basis of equation (5-27), to be 23.9 and 11.5 mM, respectively.

The prevailing values of $\bar{O}_2$, pH^c, and pH^{pl} must satisfy equation (5-45). These three variables are themselves related by available data describing oxygen–hemoglobin equilibrium (see Tables VI–VIII) and the relationship between r and pH^{pl} (Duhm and Gerlach, 1971; Duhm, 1971; see Tables X–XII). The latter data are for normal $[DPG]_T$ at $\bar{O}_2 = 0$, and a wide range of $[DPG]_T$ at $\bar{O}_2 = 1.0$. We assume that r for normal 2,3-DPG content at intermediate saturations may be estimated by linear interpolation, and that the desaturation correction is the same at all $[DPG]_T$ values. The oxygen–hemoglobin equilibrium data of Arturson *et al.* (1974a) are given over ranges of values for pH^{pl}, pCO_2, and $[DPG]_T$, from which the oxygen tension at any value of $\bar{O}_2$ and set of the latter three variables encountered under physiological and pathophysiological conditions can be derived easily by interpolation or minimal extrapolation.

Given the above-described equilibrium data and the prevailing values of pO_2, pCO_2, and 2,3-DPG concentration, it follows that a guess of pH^{pl} leads successively to values for $\bar{O}_2$ and pH^c. The complete set of properties can be substituted into equation (5-45), which then provides a test for the correctness of the assumed plasma pH. In order to perform the latter operation, it is first necessary to develop a format for evaluation of the three integrals in the equation.

Consider first the integrated charge difference associated with a change in $[DPG]_T$. As discussed elsewhere (see pp. 90–96), $[DPG]_T$ adjustments are brought about by perturbations in the erythrocyte glycolytic system that are mainly induced by changes in the time-averaged values of pH^c and $\bar{O}_2$. Depending on the actual nature of the phosphate transfer across the erythrocyte membrane, i.e., upon the value of n in the exchange of 1 molecule of $(H_n PO_4)^{n-3}$ for $3-n$ molecules of Cl^- (assuming Cl^- to be the ion thereby mobilized), the buildup–breakdown of 2,3-DPG is inherently coupled with some specific change in B^{bl}. Although a limited amount of data on this exchange is available (see, e.g., Rapoport and Guest, 1939), it is not obvious what the value of n should be, nor whether it is constant. We therefore make the assumption that the two terms in equation (5-45) due to a change in $[DPG]_T$ and associated change in B^{bl} offset one another, so that we need only concern ourselves with changes in the blood's base excess brought about by other means (e.g., exercise or the ingestion of acid–base).

The above line of reasoning does not rule out the possibility of a 2,3-DPG-induced change in the remainder of the blood's composition. On the contrary, because of the dependence of r upon $[DPG]_T$ (Table XII), an increase in the latter at, say, constant pCO_2 in oxygenated blood lowers the value of r and therefore is responsible for a *decrease* in pH^c simultaneous with an *increase* in pH^{pl}.

With regard to the integrated charge differences due to changes in pH^c and $\bar{O}_2$, the necessary values of β^c are presented in Figure 21. Values for the differential Haldane coefficient, as a function of pH^c, pCO_2, $[DPG]_T$, and $\bar{O}_2$, may be estimated on the basis of equation

(5-22) from data for $(\partial \log pO_2/\partial pH^{Pl})_{\bar{O}_2}$ (see Table VI), by division of the value for the latter partial derivative by the value of η.

One may consider the changes of pH^c and $\bar{O}_2$ as if they proceeded serially, and thus evaluate the first integral with $\bar{O}_2$ constant at 1.00, and the integrated Haldane effect with pH^c constant at its value in state II.

Figure 34 illustrates the application of equation (5-45) to the determination of equilibrium blood composition. All curves are drawn for $[DPG]_T = 5.0$ mM, $pCO_2 = 40$ mm Hg, $pO_2 = 100$ mm Hg, $h = 0.45$, and $T = 37°C$. What is varied independently is the base excess, ΔB^{bl}. The dependent variables are then the cellular and plasma pH values, as well as all the other quantities plotted in Figures 30–33. The solid curves portray the relationships between the two pH values, at a given value of ΔB^{bl}, as demanded by equation (5-45). For each of these curves, only one point corresponds to a condition of cellular/plasma proton (or, for that matter, bicarbonate ion) equilibrium. The broken line is the locus of all such equilibrium conditions, as derived from r vs. pH^{pl} data. Thus, the points of intersection yield the equilibrium blood pH values that,

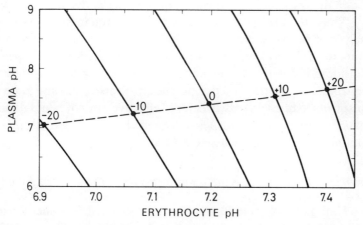

Figure 34. Graphical determination of equilibrium red cell and plasma pH values as functions of whole blood base excess ΔB^{bl} in oxygenated whole blood. $T = 37°C$, $h = 0.45$, $[DPG]_T = 5.0$ mM, $pCO_2 = 40$ mm Hg. Broken line depicts the pH^c–pH^{pl} (Donnan) equilibrium relationship; solid lines are loci of pH values that satisfy equation (5-45) for the indicated values of base excess; ● denotes equilibrium condition at indicated base excess (mmol/liter whole blood).

theoretically, must prevail at the assigned values of blood base excess. Similarly obtained results comprising, in addition, variable $[DPG]_T$, pCO_2, pO_2, and h are contained in Chapter 8.

Analysis of Changes Undergone by the Blood as It Circulates. The validity of equation (5-45) is not diminished by the possible non-equilibrium of any or all of the reversible processes involved, i.e., ligand binding to hemoglobin, carbon dioxide hydrolysis, or relaxation of diffusible ion μ gradients between cells and plasma. However, in the application of that equation to the changes undergone by the circulating blood during and after the uptake and release of oxygen and carbon dioxide, it is necessary to consider the actual *rates* of these processes before proceeding to invoke chemical equilibrium relationships such as linked functions, the Hasselbalch–Henderson equation, or correlations of r vs. pH^{pl}. In particular, the existence of effective equilibrium *locally within the capillaries* is contingent upon there being sufficient time for relaxation; the characteristic relaxation time must be small by comparison with the time period characteristic of the transport-induced perturbation. Similarly, the same relaxation time governs the rate of residual equilibration in the course of flow through the arteries and veins.

Thus, as a prelude to the deployment of equation (5-45) in the analysis of *in vivo* transport dynamics, it is important to arrive at an estimate of the *in vivo* kinetics of chemical reactions and species translocations. With this in mind, we revert to a brief review of available data on the kinetics of these processes, making note of conspicuous differences between the effective rates of hemoglobin–ligand reactions in cell suspensions and those determined in free solution, which were discussed in Chapter 4.

Review of Data on the Kinetics of Relaxation Processes in Blood

Hemoglobin–Ligand Binding in Cell Suspensions. As noted in the earlier section on solution kinetics Gibson and co-workers (1955) reported values on the order of 5×10^6 liters/mol/sec for k_{ass}, the effective association constant in oxygen binding to hemoglobin at pH 7.1, 37°C, and very low hemoglobin concentration. The typical time for 50% completion of reaction was less than 10 msec. This is in rather strong contrast with the same authors' observation of half-times on the order of 50 msec for the reaction of oxygen in human red cell *suspensions* at the same temperature, and over a range of pH values. Somewhat shorter reaction times were measured by Staub *et al.* (1961), who also found a continuous increase in association rate constant with saturation level. Bauer *et al.* (1973) determined values for k_{diss}, the overall dissociation constant for the same interaction, that were an order of magnitude below the corresponding values measured in free solution.

The most frequently suggested reason for discrepancies between kinetic constants determined in homogeneous solution and cell suspensions is the existence of concentration gradients within the interior of the erythrocytes, i.e., diffusional limitation. Another debated possibility is the finite permeability of the erythrocyte membrane to oxygen (see Forster *et al.*, 1957; for a critical review of early theoretical and experimental investigations of these factors, see Roughton, 1959). The experimental evidence is not all conclusive. Sirs (1967, 1974), for example, determined, in experiments conducted near room temperature, nearly identical values in solutions and cell suspensions for the rate constant characteristic of the release of the first oxygen molecule from fully saturated hemoglobin. Since there is little doubt that the experiments conducted in the rapid mixing apparatus using free solution were free of significant diffusional resistance, the results of Sirs may be construed to be indicative of a similar absence in cell suspensions as well. Still, it can be argued that by operating at subphysiological temperature, and focusing upon what is generally believed to be the slowest of the four oxygen dissociations, the extent of diffusional limitation is minimized.

The controversy regarding interpretation of experimental results is aggravated somewhat by discrepancies among the kinetic data reported by various investigators. Several explanations have been advanced in this regard, among them the differences in experimental technique and the importance of unstirred layers of plasma on the erythrocyte surfaces, the thickness of which depends upon the flowrate through the rapid mixing apparatus. A critical discussion of these factors is presented by Mochizuki (1970).

Data on the kinetics of reaction in intact cells between hemoglobin and its three physiologically important effector ligands are, as one might expect, rather sparse. The exception is carbon dioxide binding, for which Kernohan and Roughton (1968) determined essentially the same association rate constant at 25°C in solutions and cell suspensions (both oxygenated and deoxygenated). Similarly, Forster *et al.* (1968) found reasonable agreement between the association constant they obtained at 37°C in solution and one calculated on the basis of earlier experimental results with blood, as reported by Constantine *et al.* (1965).

Klocke (1973) deduced a half-time of 140 msec for the release of carbamate CO_2, from a study of the complex kinetics of oxygenation-linked release of carbon dioxide from previously reduced erythrocytes. Klocke pointed out that the observed half-time is large compared with the values suggested by the results of Kernohan and Roughton (1968) and Forster and co-workers (1968). It might therefore be of interest to measure the rate of release of CO_2 from hemoglobin *solutions* under comparable conditions.

CO_2 Hydration/Dehydration in Solution and Cell Suspensions. The free solution kinetics of the noncatalyzed hydration (hydrolysis) of carbon dioxide and dehydration of carbonic acid at 37°C have been reinvestigated recently by Garg and Maren (1972), who also review previous literature on this subject. The overall reaction scheme is, as noted earlier, written rigorously as

$$CO_2 + H_2O \underset{k_{-1}}{\overset{k_1}{\rightleftharpoons}} H_2CO_3 \rightleftharpoons HCO_3^- + H^+$$

The second step is so extremely rapid (Eigen and DeMaeyer, 1963) that bicarbonate, protons, and carbonic acid may be assumed, in the physiological context, to exist in a continual state of equilibrium. Furthermore, since the pK of carbonic acid dissociation, p$K_{H_2CO_3}$, is below 4, [H_2CO_3] is always negligible by comparison with [HCO_3^-] in the physiological pH range. As such, the overall reaction is often represented by

$$CO_2 + H_2O \underset{k_b}{\overset{k_1}{\rightleftharpoons}} HCO_3^- + H^+$$

where k_b is equal to $k_{-1} \times 10^{pK_{H_2CO_3}}$ The net rate of reaction is, accordingly, either

$$k_1[CO_2] - k_{-1}[H_2CO_3] \qquad \text{or} \qquad k_1[CO_2] - k_b[HCO_3^-][H^+]$$

where k_1 incorporates the activity of water.

Garg and Maren (1972) report values of 0.145 and 49.6 $\sec^{-1}$, respectively, for k_1 and k_{-1}, in general agreement with earlier reports. These constants imply a half-time on the scale of 10 sec, which far exceeds the ~ 1 sec residence time of the blood in most capillaries. The uncatalyzed reaction in plasma was recently identified as the source for the slow phase of whole blood pH and CO_2 equilibration in the experiments and analysis of Forster and Crandall (1975), thus confirming the astute deductions of Roughton (1935).

The conversion of CO_2 into protons and bicarbonate as the blood traverses the systemic capillaries, and the reverse process in the lungs, is made possible by the presence of carbonic anhydrase in the erythrocytes, an enzymic protein that catalyzes the hydration–dehydration reaction. Estimates of the accelerative factor at 37°C are generally on the order of 10^4. Values derived recently from relaxation experiments with blood suspensions are 16,000 (Klocke, 1973) and 5000 (Holland and Forster, 1975). The values in hemolysates and cell suspensions are essentially the same (Kernohan and Roughton, 1968). Thus, it is safe to say that the equilibration of erythrocyte protons, carbon dioxide, and bicarbonate ions is all but complete within a few milliseconds.

The Hamburger Shift. The presence of carbonic anhydrase in the erythrocytes and the high permeability of the red cell membrane to CO_2 alone ensure that a significant portion of the CO_2 that enters the blood from tissue is nearly instantaneously converted to HCO_3^- and H^+, and that the reverse occurs with similar alacrity in the lungs. Moreover, the role of carbonic anhydrase is greatly expanded by means of the rapid exchange of bicarbonate and chloride ions across the erythrocyte membrane (the "Hamburger shift"). The latter process in whole blood is characterized by a half-time of approximately 100 msec (Luckner, 1939).

The Operating Relationship. The rapid cellular/plasma equilibrations of carbon dioxide and bicarbonate ions, plus the effectively instantaneous equilibrations of CO_2 and H_2CO_3 in the cells and of H_2CO_3, HCO_3^-, and H^+ in each phase, do *not* constitute a means for the effective catalysis of plasma CO_2–HCO_3^-–H^+ equilibration. Nor is one furnished by the additional transmembrane transport of either hydroxyl ion or undissociated carbonic acid, as the fluxes of both species must be negligibly small [see Crandall *et al.* (1971) on OH^-, and Booth (1938) on H_2CO_3].

In Chapter 6, it is noted that, in regard to capillary blood, it is generally fair to assume the effectively instantaneous equilibration of hemoglobin–ligand interactions as well as erythrocyte CO_2 hydration–dehydration. On the other hand, the longer times required for the relaxation of cellular/plasma HCO_3^- gradients and of the plasma CO_2 hydration reaction necessitate allowance for finite kinetic rates.

In light of (1) the presumed constancy of both B^{bl} and $[DPG]_T$, and (2) the discussion in the preceding paragraphs, equation (5-45) may be subdivided into two separate but coupled relationships, one for the cells and one for plasma, as follows:

$$h\,\delta B^c = h\left\{\beta^c\,\delta pH^c + \delta[HCO_3^-]^c - [Hm]^c \frac{\partial z_{Hm}}{\partial \bar{O}_2}\,\delta\bar{O}_2\right\}$$

$$= -(1-h)\,\delta B^{pl} = -(1-h)\{\beta^{pl}\,\delta pH^{pl} + \delta[HCO_3^-]^{pl}\} \qquad (5\text{-}46)$$

where the δ implies a difference in the values of the pertinent blood property evaluated at successive locations along a vessel; the cellular bicarbonate and oxyhemoglobin concentrations and Haldane coefficient are evaluated from reaction equilibrium relationships; and the δB terms are due to the exchange of chloride between the two blood phases. It is further implied that the displacement between discrete locations is sufficiently small to justify the use of constant values for both β^c and $\partial z_{Hm}/\partial \bar{O}_2$.

For applications to the arteries and veins, in which the residual disequilibria in the aftermaths of lung and tissue perfusion are relaxed, equations (5-46) may be simplified further by the assumption of interphase bicarbonate equilibrium at all locations. This is because in the relevant time scale, i.e., that associated with the equilibration of plasma CO_2 hydrolysis, the Hamburger shift is in effect instantaneous.

Chapter 6

The Dynamics of Oxygen, Carbon Dioxide, and Proton Transport under Normal Conditions

In this chapter we develop a quantitative evaluation of the factors that govern the blood's performance of its respiratory functions. Toward that goal, we advance a relatively simple model of the *in vivo* transport system, a set of phenomenological and conservation relationships descriptive of its steady-state behavior, and the results of numerical analysis of these relations.

We choose to approach the problem by assuming, perhaps arbitrarily, that the total system is geared to the ensurance of oxygen supply to metabolizing tissue, and that the performance of that function requires the provision of capillary blood oxygen tensions sufficient to overcome diffusional loss in tissue. It is thus implied that the need to supply oxygen, rather than the need to carry CO_2 or to moderate the fluctuations in pH, determines the changes in blood flow, hematocrit, oxyhemoglobin dissociation curve, etc., that take place in response to the normal as well as pathophysiological perturbations in system properties considered in this and the final chapter of this book. Nonetheless, the carriages of O_2, CO_2, and protons are treated with comparable levels of rigor, and so the performance of the latter two functions are indeed examined in appreciable detail.

The principal results of this theoretical investigation are sets of values for the blood characteristics that are calculated to guarantee representative oxygen demands. In the process of generating such data, we derive profiles of oxygen tensions in tissue and of species concentrations in the circulating blood.

Following the development of our model of the *in vivo* transport system and analysis of its behavior in the steady state, we apply it to the simulation of gas exchange in normal individuals at rest and progressive degrees of physical activity. In Chapter 8, we consider the particular compensatory mechanisms the body may deploy to ensure proper O_2 supply under a variety of physicochemically characterized pathological conditions.

The Model System

Geometric Considerations

A theoretical evaluation of the blood's functioning as a supplier of oxygen necessitates the assumption of a capillary–tissue model. In such a framework it is possible to estimate the actual demands placed upon the blood. An analysis of the physics of diffusion and reaction of oxygen in tissue reveals the pO_2 requirements placed upon the blood, while the coupling of those processes to the simultaneous changes in the flowing blood allows a simulation of the *in vivo* gas exchange process.

Since the pioneering work of Krogh (1918–1919*b*), a rather large number of theoretical analyses of capillary–tissue oxygen transport, and in a few instances of carbon dioxide transport as well, have appeared in the published literature. These are reviewed by Reneau *et al.* (1967), Middleman (1972), Leonard and Bay Jørgensen (1974), and Guillez (1976). Almost without exception, such analyses have been aimed at the calculation of tissue pO_2 profiles, using capillary oxygen tensions that were either assumed in advance or determined simultaneously on the basis of rather simplified representations of blood chemistry. Only recently has that chemistry been included in appreciable detail, but in the contexts of pulmonary (Wagner and West, 1972; Hill *et al.*, 1973*b*; Hlastala, 1973) and placental (Hill *et al.*, 1973*a*) rather than capillary–tissue gas exchange.

The general lack of attention to the vagaries of blood chemistry is doubtless attributable to two primary factors: (1) the emphasis upon tissue oxygen tensions, and (2) the late discovery of 2,3-DPG's profound effect upon oxygen–hemoglobin equilibrium, together with findings of correlations between red cell DPG content and degrees of abnormality of other gas transport parameters (see Chapter 8).

Nearly all theoretical models stem from that of Krogh (1918–1919*b*), who in light of morphological studies of skeletal muscle revealing regularly spaced and parallel capillaries (Krogh, 1918–1919*a*) supposed that tissue pO_2 could be predicted by assuming

> ... each capillary to supply oxygen independently of all others to a cylinder of tissue surrounding it. In a transverse section such a cylinder is represented by an area which can be taken as circular and the average area belonging to each capillary can be calculated from a counting of the number of capillaries in a transverse section by division of its total area with the number found.

Thus, the capillary–tissue pair of Krogh is illustrated in cross section as shown in Figure 35.

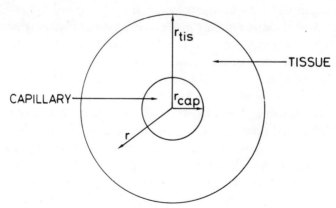

Figure 35. Krogh's (1918–1919*a*) capillary–tissue pair in cross section.

The difference between the oxygen tensions at the capillary–tissue interface and at any radius r, as derived by Krogh's mathematician Erlang, is given by

$$p\,O_2^{bl} - p\,O_2^t(r) = \frac{m}{P_{O_2}^t}\left\{\frac{r_{tis}^2}{2}\ln\frac{r}{r_{cap}} - \left(\frac{r^2 - r_{cap}^2}{4}\right)\right\} \qquad (6\text{-}1)$$

where m is the *zero-order* O_2 consumption rate and $P_{O_2}^t$ the physical permeability of oxygen in tissue, i.e., the product of O_2 solubility and diffusivity. ($P_{O_2}^t$ is also known as the "Krogh diffusion constant" of oxygen.)

As we discussed in Chapter 3, equation (6-1) is the solution to the steady-state continuity equation written in cylindrical coordinates, which governs the simultaneous diffusion and irreversible reaction of oxygen under circumstances in which the angular and axial components of diffusion are negligible, i.e.,

$$\frac{1}{r}\frac{d}{dr}\left(r\frac{dp\,O_2^t}{dr}\right) = \frac{m}{P_{O_2}^t} \qquad (6\text{-}2)$$

The associated boundary conditions are

$$p\,O_2^t(r_{cap}) = p\,O_2^{bl}, \qquad \frac{dp\,O_2^t}{dr}(r_{tis}) = 0$$

which respectively imply the absence of an interfacial diffusional resistance and the vanishing of the O_2 flux at the radial extremity of tissue supplied by the individual capillary.

Each of the assumptions made to this point imposes what may be shown to be generally second- or higher-order approximations in the calculation of requisite blood oxygen tensions. One would not expect from equation (6-1) the capability to anticipate precisely, for example, the onset of anoxia in nonuniformly perfused tissue (see Bourdeau-Martini *et al.*, 1974). Still, one finds that this rather straightforward relationship is quite reasonable as a tool for comparison of the gross effects of changes in flowrate, hematocrit, hemoglobin oxygen affinity, etc. The mathematical assumptions and approximations are examined by Meldon (in preparation).

A representative "Krogh cylinder" of tissue, *of constant radius* and supplied by a single microvessel, has often been presumed in order to estimate tissue pO_2 profiles (e.g., Kety, 1957; Tenney, 1974). This approach is mathematically convenient and derives partial support from studies of transverse sections of mammalian skeletal muscle (e.g., Hammersen, 1968; Plyley and Groom, 1975), which show a regularity of capillary spacing consistent with Krogh's early observations. Nonetheless, the question of the constancy of effective tissue radius remains unresolved after investigations in smaller mammals. Eriksson and Myrhage (1972) reported a 40% greater capillary density at the *venous* end of *cat tenuissimus* muscle microvasculature, while Myrhage and Hudlická (1976) found the reverse trend, i.e., 30% greater capillarization at the *arterial* end of the *rat extensor hallucis proprius* muscle microcirculation.

In view of the appreciable complexity found even in skeletal muscle capillary networks, and the greater irregularity of arrange-ment in other tissues (Krogh, 1918–1919b), the approach we choose is simply to evaluate the *maximum* volume of tissue that can be supplied by an individual capillary. That is, then, the theoretical case in which the zones supplied by adjacent capillaries do not impinge upon one another—let us presume though that they do in fact just meet tangentially—and their radial extremity is now defined not only by the absence of an oxygen *flux*, but also by an oxygen *tension* of *zero*. Thus, the local radius of the supply zone is allowed to vary (Figure 36) with blood oxygen tension, through the functionality one obtains by setting $r = r_{tis}$ and $pO_2^t(r) = 0$ in equation (6-1). The result is

$$pO_2^{bl} = \frac{mr_{cap}^2}{4P_{O_2}^t}\left\{1+\frac{r_{tis}^2}{r_{cap}^2}\left(\ln\frac{r_{tis}^2}{r_{cap}^2}-1\right)\right\} \qquad (6\text{-}3)$$

This equation is plotted in Figure 37.

Given values for the intrinsic tissue metabolic rate m, tissue O_2 permeability constant $P_{O_2}^t$, and capillary radius r_{cap}, we now have a relationship between the local blood oxygen tension pO_2^{bl} and the radius of tissue, r_{tis}, which is supplied by the individual capillary with oxygen. Rigorously speaking, pO_2^t could only reach zero at finite radii in the hypothetical case of true zero-order oxygen consump-tion. However, there is evidence that the critical pO_2 of the mitochondrion is well below 1 mm Hg [see, for example, Schindler,

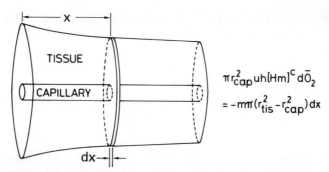

Figure 36. Cylindrical disk showing balance between tissue consumption and oxyhemoglobin flow.

1964, cited in Kessler, 1974; Stahrlinger and Lübbers, 1973; and Clark *et al.*, 1976; other investigators, among them Chance *et al.* (1965), have reported values on the order of one mm Hg]. This allows calculation of the maximum rate of oxygen supply in the above manner with little reduction of accuracy.

Our goal, as originally stated, was to evaluate the oxygen supply capability of blood that is described by a particular set of compositional characteristics (hemoglobin and 2,3-DPG concentrations, acid–base status, etc.). To do so, *we calculate the rate at which it must flow in order that the representative capillary may accommodate a specified total volume of tissue.*

Among the inherent consequences of our approach are that the tissue radius decreases along the capillary in reflection of the falling blood pO_2, as is implied in Figure 37. Furthermore, because of this effect, the shape of the tissue zone of supply departs from that of a "Krogh cylinder" in the direction of what one might anticipate with *countercurrent* blood flow in neighboring capillaries that are in a parallel, regularly spaced array. Because of the steepness of the oxyhemoglobin dissociation curve for a good portion of the range of blood pO_2 values between artery and vein, the decreases in pO_2^{bl} and therefore r_{tis} are in fact small except near the capillary's entrance.

The major difference between the constant and variable radius approaches—where the former is carried out under the assumption that the flowrate is that necessary to avoid anoxia at the *venous* end—is that when the required volumes of tissue (per capillary) are the same in both, the variable radius framework generates consistently lower pO_2^{bl} values, blood flows, and tissue pO_2 values. The average tissue oxygen tensions calculated with the chosen model are generally between 5 and 10 mm Hg. This range is considerably below that of 20–35 mm Hg revealed by *in vivo* pO_2 histograms determined with microelectrodes (as reviewed by Kessler, 1974). On the other hand, Coburn and co-workers (Coburn and Mayers, 1971; Coburn, 1973) have applied the spectrophotometric technique of Millikan (1937) for measurement of muscle myoglobin saturation, and Haldane's first law (see p. 100) to the determination of average muscle pO_2, and found values consistently in the 1–10 mm Hg range. The striking discrepancy between results derived from these two approaches has not been resolved. In any event, the chosen model is forced to conform with blood flowrates in the physiological range by selecting the required average radius of oxygenated tissue per capillary so that venous pO_2 values are in the range observed *in vivo*.

Analysis of Plasma and Red Cell Compositional Profiles

While on the one hand, the flux of oxygen to tissue depends upon blood gas tension, the latter tension varies along the capillary as a result of that very flux. Thus the changes in blood and tissue from one point along the capillary to another are coupled to each other, and therefore, in order to determine the degree of tissue oxygenation, it is necessary to determine the blood oxygen tension profile simultaneously.

The fluxes of oxygen and carbon dioxide between blood and tissue induce changes in the blood's concentrations of carbon dioxide and free protons. Since the latter two species are effectors of oxygen–hemoglobin equilibrium, the determination of blood oxygen tension profiles requires estimation of local pCO_2 and pH. The analysis that follows, therefore, comprises a simulation of the simultaneous changes of hemoglobin O_2 saturation, pO_2, and pH in the circulating blood.

It is possible to estimate the composition of the two blood phases everywhere along the simplified blood loop illustrated in Figure 38

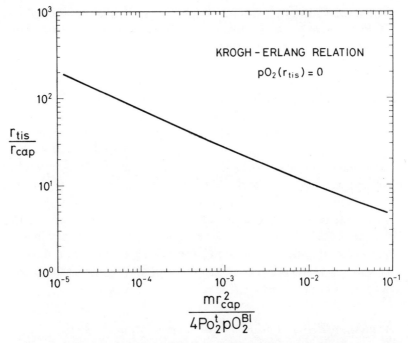

Figure 37. Relationship between the two dimensionless groups, r_{tis}/r_{cap} and $mr^2_{cap}/4P^t_{O_2}pO^{bl}_2$, implicit in equation (6-3), the Krogh–Erlang relationship when the oxygen tension at the tissue's radial extremity is equal to zero.

by solving a set of equations describing the physics of transport and chemical reaction. To make such an analysis tractable, it is necessary to disregard temporal variations attributable to respiration, the possibly continuous or sporadic opening and closing of capillaries, pulsation of the heart, turbulence in the arteries, etc. The analysis that follows leads then to a picture of the gas transport system in the steady state, i.e., in which the compositional properties vary with position but not with time.

Capillary Blood Relationships. The generalized relationships for species conservation in the systemic capillaries are derived with the following assumptions:

1. Within each phase, concentrations may be regarded as uniform radially.

2. Axial diffusion is negligible.
3. The blood's linear velocity as well as hematocrit and the capillary diameter are all constant.

The appropriate equations are then

$$u\frac{d[i]^c}{dx} = -(r_{sv}J_i^{c-pl} + \rho_i^c) \tag{6-4}$$

for the red cells, and

$$u\frac{d[i]^{pl}}{dx} = \left(\frac{h}{1-h}\right)r_{sv}J_i^{c-pl} + \frac{2J_i^{t-pl}}{r_{cap}(1-h)} - \rho_i^{pl} \tag{6-5}$$

for the plasma, where:

$[i]$ = molar concentration (mol/cm^3)

x = distance from entrance of capillary (cm)

ρ_i = rate of depletion by chemical reaction within the blood (mol/cm^3/sec)

r_{sv} = ratio of erythrocyte surface area to volume (cm^{-1})

J_i^{c-pl} = transmembrane flux from erythrocyte to plasma (mol/cm^2/sec)

J_i^{t-pl} = flux from tissue to plasma (mol/cm^2/sec)

i denotes the pertinent chemical species

Oxygen. The equations for physically dissolved oxygen in cells and plasma and for hemoglobin-bound gas in the cells (of which the concentration equals $[Hm]^c \cdot \bar{O}_2$) may be combined so as to eliminate the chemical reaction and membrane transport terms. With the justifiable neglect of gradients in concentration of physically dissolved gas, the result is

$$\frac{d\bar{O}_2}{dx} = \frac{2J_{O_2}^{t-pl}}{uhr_{cap}[Hm]^c} \tag{6-6}$$

The flux of oxygen (negative as written) is equal to the amount consumed per unit time in the surrounding cylindrical disk of tissue divided by the interfacial area, i.e.,

$$J_{O_2}^{t-pl} = -\frac{m}{2r_{cap}}(r_{tis}^2 - r_{cap}^2) \tag{6-7}$$

The last two relationships may be combined to give

$$\frac{d\bar{O}_2}{dx} = -\frac{m}{uh[Hm]^c}\left(\frac{r_{tis}^2}{r_{cap}^2} - 1\right) \tag{6-8}$$

Equation (6-8) expresses the balance between tissue oxygen consumption and oxyhemoglobin flows into and out of the cylindrical disk illustrated in Figure 36.

The time constants associated with O_2 equilibration in hemoglobin solutions and whole blood were discussed in the sections on kinetics of Chapters 4 and 5. On the basis of an analysis of the various steps in capillary–tissue exchange, Lawson and Forster (1967) showed that, in general, the overall process of oxygen–hemoglobin interaction within the blood is intrinsically so rapid that little accuracy is lost if one considers pO_2^{bl} to be not only radially uniform, but also equilibrated with the local hemoglobin saturation. *Thus, pO_2^{bl} may be calculated at each axial location from the prevailing values of $\bar{O}_2$, pH^c, pCO_2, $[DPG]_T$, and temperature, on the basis of available equilibrium data.* Since $[DPG]_T$ and—at least at rest—the temperature may be considered constant along the capillary, one need in fact only determine the local values of pH^c and pCO_2.

Carbon Dioxide. If one neglects the axial diffusion of CO_2 in tissue as was done in regard to O_2, then the rate at which carbon dioxide enters the blood at any point may be equated with that of oxygen's entry into tissue multiplied by the respiratory quotient q_R, i.e., $J_{CO_2}^{t-pl}$ may be set equal to the product $-q_R J_{O_2}^{t-pl}$. That the resulting blood pCO_2 is uniform at any axial location may safely be assumed in light of recent experimental confirmation (Silverman *et al.*, 1976) that erythrocytes are highly permeable to the gas.

Physically dissolved gas reacts to form appreciable amounts of bicarbonate and hemoglobin carbamate. The former reaction proceeds for the most part in the cells, after which the bicarbonate distributes between the two blood phases. On the basis of equations (6-4) and (6-5) applied to these species, the gradient in total carbon dioxide concentration may be expressed as

$$\frac{d}{dx}\left\{\left(\alpha_{CO_2}^c + \frac{1-h}{h}\alpha_{CO_2}^{pl}\right)pCO_2 + [HCO_3^-]^c + [Hm]^c\overline{CO_2}\right.$$

$$\left. + \frac{1-h}{h}[HCO_3^-]^{pl}\right\} = \frac{2J_{CO_2}^{t-pl}}{ur_{cap}h} \tag{6-9}$$

where it has been noted that the effectively uniform pCO_2 at any x is associated with cellular and plasma $[CO_2]$ values that are proportional to the respective solubility coefficients.

Since the catalyzed hydrolysis of CO_2 within the cells is intrinsically an even more rapid process than oxygen–hemoglobin interaction (see Chapter 5), it too may be treated as if equilibrated locally. Thus, from equation (5-27), we may write

$$[HCO_3^-]^c = K_a' \alpha_{CO_2}^c pCO_2 / 10^{-pH^c} \tag{6-10}$$

Moreover, in light of the associated time constant (see Chapters 4 and 5), the carbamino reaction may be taken to be in equilibrium as well without appreciable error. Thus the value of $\overline{CO_2}$ may be calculated, as previously described (see p. 138), from the prevailing values of pH^c, pCO_2, $\overline{O}_2$, and $[DPG]_T$.

In addition to equation (6-9), a second differential equation descriptive of carbon dioxide species is provided by expansion of equation (6-5) for bicarbonate ion, i.e.,

$$u \frac{d[HCO_3^-]^{pl}}{dx} = \frac{r_{sv}h}{1-h} J_{HCO_3^-}^{c-pl} + k_1 \alpha_{CO_2}^{pl} pCO_2 - \frac{k_{-1} 10^{-pH^{pl}}[HCO_3^-]^{pl}}{K_{H_2CO_3}} \tag{6-11}$$

(see p. 148).

The transmembrane flux of HCO_3^-, which is balanced by a simultaneous flux of Cl^-, may be described by the semiempirical formula

$$J_{HCO_3^-}^{c-pl} = P_{HCO_3^-}([HCO_3^-]^c - \omega r[HCO_3^-]^{pl}) \tag{6-12}$$

where $P_{HCO_3^-}$ is an effective permeability constant. The terms ω and r are the equilibrium distribution coefficients of water and diffusible monovalent ions as defined in Chapter 5. The value of ω may be assumed constant at 0.77, while r should be taken to vary with $\overline{O}_2$, $[DPG]_T$, and pH^c, rather than pH^{pl}, since cellular and plasma protons are generally not equilibrated *in vivo*, whereas the charge on the hemoglobin molecule is a function of *cellular* pH.

Equation (6-12), rather than the oft-deployed Goldman equation (1943), is applied here in view of its prior usage (Klocke, 1973) in the determination of the effective bicarbonate permeability from experiments performed under near-physiological conditions. Since the flux of bicarbonate ion is coupled to that of chloride, the assigned value of $P_{HCO_3^-}$ [3×10^{-4} cm/sec at 37°C, as adapted from the experimental data of Klocke (1973, 1976)] is only valid at normal chloride concentrations.

Protons.   Rather than apply equations (6-4) and (6-5) to the proton concentrations in each blood phase, one may employ the electroneutrality–base conservation relationships derived in Chapter 5. This is because the changes in pH^c and pH^{pl} imply changes in the concentrations of electrical charge due to hemoglobin, 2,3-DPG, bicarbonate ion, and plasma protein, which must satisfy equations (5-46). The changes in B^c and B^{pl} are simply those arising from the HCO_3^-/Cl^- shift, i.e., the amount by which the B value of either phase changes is algebraically identical to the amount of bicarbonate ion that enters it, per unit volume, via the red cell membrane.

Initial Conditions in the Systemic Capillaries.   The mathematical relationships derived up to this point govern the *changes* in blood composition along the systemic capillaries. What remains to be done before it is possible to calculate the *absolute* concentrations at any coordinate value is to determine the conditions at the arterial end of the microcirculation. It is generally assumed that the blood entering the systemic capillaries is equilibrated at the "arterial" pressures of oxygen and carbon dioxide, i.e., at those in the blood leaving the lung, the latter being equal to (or nearly the same as) those in the alveoli. However, the noncatalyzed hydration–dehydration of CO_2 requires a period on the order of 1 min in order to attain near-equilibrium, and even at rest the blood spends on the order of only 1 sec in the lungs and 20 sec in the arterial system. As such, the CO_2, protons, and bicarbonate ions in the plasma entering the systemic capillaries must be disequilibrated to a degree.

The consequence of the slow formation of CO_2 from plasma bicarbonate (which, as discussed in Chapter 5, is nevertheless mitigated by the HCO_3^-/Cl^- shift) is that appreciably less CO_2 can be released during the time of lung passage than would be in the event that the blood—entering the lungs with the same venous composition, and exposed to the same alveolar gas phase—remained in the alveoli for a longer period of time. Just how far from equilibrium the reaction is displaced, and the significance of this factor, may be estimated by including within the model the changes undergone by the blood in the arteries, veins, and lungs. A schematic diagram of the circulatory loop chosen for this purpose is included in Figure 38.

In a steady-state analysis of this system, the conditions assumed at any one point in the circulation need be identical with those derived for the same point following one full cycle. Thus a matching process is required, and this might at first appear to be a rather onerous task. However, analysis reveals that a solution may be obtained with little trial and error.

In traversing the pulmonary capillaries under normal conditions, the blood *gas tensions* do indeed equilibrate fairly rapidly with those in the alveoli. Small alveolar/arterial pCO_2 gradients may exist with healthy lungs (Hlastala, 1973), while substantial gradients in pO_2 should be expected in cases of alveolar–capillary membrane diffusion impairment (Rahn and Farhi, 1964). Nonetheless, it appears reasonable to assume that the blood leaving the lungs is at least equilibrated *internally, except* in regard to plasma CO_2 hydrolysis and the ratio of the proton activities in the two blood phases. That this is likely to be the case was established by the simulations of Hill *et al.* (1973*b*), who also indicate that the interphase disequilibrium of bicarbonate ions is quickly dissipated in the arteries.

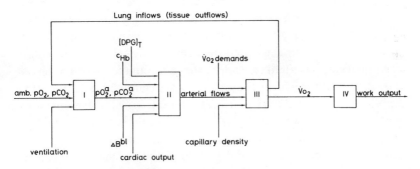

Figure 38. A schematic diagram of the gas transport system. Box I translates the pulmonary ventilation, ambient air, and pulmonary blood into alveolar gas tensions. Box II represents the complex transfer function yielding arterial flow of physically dissolved and chemically bound O_2 and CO_2. Box III translates arterial supply of oxygen, and tissue morphology and metabolic requirements into oxygen consumption (and carbon dioxide production). Box IV translates oxygen consumption into work.

One may therefore proceed with the supposition that the mixed blood leaving the lungs is partially equilibrated as just described and, somewhat arbitrarily, fix the associated values of pO_2 and pCO_2 (e.g., 90 and 40 mm Hg, respectively, under normal resting conditions). *The detailed composition of each blood phase at the entrance to the arterial system is then completely determined by the further supposition of a value for the prevailing erythrocyte pH.* That is, a guess of pH^c, together with the given values of $[DPG]_T$, pO_2, and pCO_2:

1. Allows the calculation of equilibrium values for $\bar{O}_2$, $\overline{CO_2}$, and $[HCO_3^-]^c$, as well as r.
2. The latter two values determine $[HCO_3^-]^{pl}$.
3. The value of pH^{pl} is that necessary to satisfy overall electroneutrality equation (5-45) at the given blood base excess.

The corresponding initial conditions in the systemic capillaries may then be determined by analysis of the chemical changes undergone by the blood in the arterial system.

Time Courses of Chemical Relaxation in the Arterial and Venous Systems. Just as the transport processes within the microcirculation are modeled by those occurring in a representative capillary, the chemical relaxation of the blood in the arterial and venous systems is, for simplicity, simulated by single flows. These are taken to be described by intraphase compositions that, for a given element of blood, vary with the time elapsed since its entry into that portion of the circulation. Thus the equations already derived for the purpose of simulating the changes undergone by systemic capillary blood may again be applied in the case of the arteries and veins, after simply substituting d/dt for $u\,d/dx$, and setting the gas fluxes into and out of the blood at zero. It should be noted, though, that appreciable gas exchange across periarteriolar walls in the hamster cheek pouch has, in fact, been measured by Duling and Berne (1971). The significance of this phenomenon in man remains to be determined.

Changes Undergone in the Pulmonary Capillaries. An appropriate starting point in the simulated blood "loop" is the entrance to the arterial system, where, as described above, the conditions are determined by the assumption of a value for pH^c. From these conditions and the time spent in the arterial system, numerical analysis yields an estimate of the composition of blood entering the systemic capillaries. This leads successively to the changes occurring in the peripheral circulation and then in the veins. To close the loop, the changes undergone by the blood as result of gas exchange in the lungs may be calculated and checked against the composition assumed at the start.

The correctness of the pH^c value assumed to prevail at the entrance to the arterial system may be examined by substitution of the implied changes in blood electrolyte concentrations undergone in the lungs into equations (5-46), together with effective values for both the erythrocyte nonbicarbonate buffer capacity and Haldane coefficient.

Determination of Systemic Capillary Blood Flowrate

We now have the complete set of mathematical relationships necessary to simulate our model system: equation (6-3), which relates blood pO_2 to the radius of oxygenated tissue; equation (6-8), which relates the consumption of oxygen by tissue to the change in blood O_2 content; the oxygen–hemoglobin equilibrium data, as a function of pCO_2, pH, $[DPG]_T$, and temperature, provided in Chapter 4; a set of auxiliary relationships that allow the simultaneous determination of local pH and pCO_2 values; and a method for handling the nonequilibrium conditions at the entrance to the systemic capillaries.

We may now employ the model to investigate any number of situations. The constants of a particular steady state, i.e., the parameters that may be assigned fixed values prior to numerical simulation, are the blood's hematocrit, temperature, base excess, 2,3-DPG concentration, postlung gas tensions, its flowrate through the microcirculation, and residence times in the arterial and venous systems; systemic capillary dimensions; and tissue oxygen permeability and consumption rate. The primary result is the volume of tissue oxygenated by the blood flowing through the model capillary.

We are interested in the set of parameters that ensure a given value of that volume of tissue. Though, in principle, any one of the above-mentioned parameters may be selected as the unknown quantity, we have chosen the systemic capillary blood flowrate as the quantity that must vary in order to arrive at the desired O_2 supply. In fact, as long as there is a sufficiently high arterial O_2 tension, the flowrate is the *only* parameter that can *always* ensure the desired extent of oxygenated tissue. The flowrate is, furthermore, a measure of the energy expenditure of the heart.

Our scheme, then, is to vary systemic capillary blood flowrate, along with the initial arterial erythrocyte pH until (1) the calculated volume of metabolizing tissue agrees with that desired, and (2) the value of pH^c assumed at the start of an iteration is consistent with the resulting changes undergone in the lungs. The authors were able to obtain convergence within ten iterations by means of an *ad hoc* recursion procedure. The latter procedure, and the numerical technique employed are described by Meldon (in preparation).

Simulation of Gas Transport at Rest

Base Case

In order to simulate the exchange of oxygen and carbon dioxide in healthy individuals under resting conditions, we have chosen to use the set of parameters listed in Table XIII, as selected from available literature. The additional data needed to calculate the binding of oxygen, carbon dioxide and protons to hemoglobin, and cellular/plasma Donnan distributions have already been discussed in Chapters 4 and 5. The so-called standard values are typical of those quoted for normal human beings. Capillary radii may vary between 3 and 5 μm; interestingly, though, r_{tis} calculated from equation (6-3) is rather insensitive to such variation, as may be inferred from Figure 37. Capillary length L may vary anywhere from 100 to 1000 μm or more; changing L leads simply to proportional changes in required blood velocity.

The profiles drawn in Figures 39a and 39b were obtained by numerical analysis when the average radius of oxygenated tissue was required to be 150 μm. That demand led to a capillary blood velocity of 667 μm/sec, or a capillary residence time of 750 msec. The

Table XIII
Parameter Values Employed in Simulation of Gas Exchange at Rest

Quantity	Value	Comment and/or reference
m	3×10^{-9} mol/cm^3/sec (0.4 ml/100 g/min)	Whole body average, from data assembled by Lightfoot (1974)
$P^t_{O_2}$	2.2×10^{-14} mol/cm/sec/mm Hg	Kawashiro *et al.* (1975)
β^{pl}	7.7×10^{-3} equiv/liter/pH unit	Siggaard-Andersen (1974)
$\alpha^{pl}_{CO_2}$	3.0×10^{-5} mol/liter/mm Hg	Siggaard-Andersen (1974)
$\alpha^c_{CO_2}$	2.3×10^{-5} mol/liter/mm Hg	Siggaard-Andersen (1974)
ω	0.77	Siggaard-Andersen (1974)
$P_{HCO_3^-}$	3×10^{-4} cm/sec	Adapted from data of Klocke (1973, 1976)
r_{sv}	1.84×10^4 cm^{-1}	Paganelli and Solomon (1957)
k_1	0.145 sec^{-1}	Garg and Maren (1972)
k_{-1}	49.5 sec^{-1}	Garg and Maren (1972)
p$K_{H_2CO_3}$	3.6	p$K_{H_2CO_3}$ − log $(K_1/K_{-1}) = 6.1$
Temperature	37.0°C	Standard value
[Hm]^c	2×10^{-2} mol/liter	Standard value
h	0.45	Standard value
[DPG]$_T$	5×10^{-3} mol/liter	Standard value
q_R	0.8	Standard value
L	5×10^{-2} cm	Standard value
r_{cap}	4×10^{-4} cm	Standard value
ΔB^{bl}	0	Standard value
Arterial pO_2	90 mm Hg	Standard value
Arterial pCO_2	40 mm Hg	Standard value
Arterial residence time	20 sec	Standard value
Venous residence time	40 sec	Standard value

calculated venous conditions indicated in the figures are: blood pO_2, 35 mm Hg; pCO_2, 49 mm Hg; hemoglobin O_2 saturation, 63%; plasma pH, 7.35; erythrocyte pH, 7.18. Such conditions correspond to a somewhat greater degree of oxygen extraction than is generally reported for the whole body at rest, or somewhat less extraction than in resting or lightly exercising skeletal muscle.

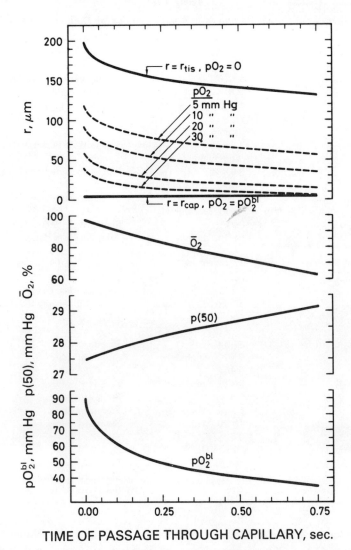

Figure 39(a). Results of simulation of oxygen–carbon dioxide exchange under resting conditions: Profiles within the systemic capillary of blood oxygen tension, $p(50)$, hemoglobin O_2 saturation, and of tissue radii corresponding to the tissue's extremities (solid line and curve) and loci of constant pO_2 (broken curves).

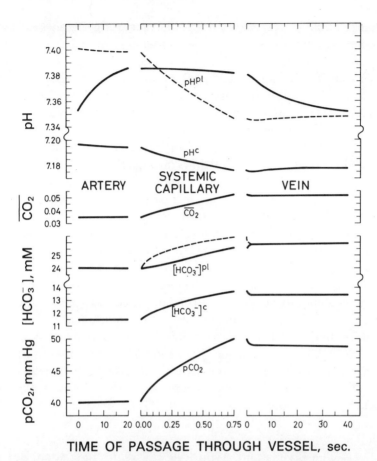

Figure 39(b). Results of simulation of oxygen–carbon dioxide exchange under resting conditions: Profiles within the arterial, systemic capillary, and venous systems of pCO_2, erythrocyte and plasma bicarbonate concentrations, moles of carbon dioxide bound per mole hemoglobin monomer, and erythrocyte and plasma pH (all solid curves). Broken curves denote hypothetical plasma bicarbonate concentration and pH in equilibrium with the respective erythrocyte values.

The tissue radius was found to vary between 197 and 132 μm. More than half of that change occurs within the first one-fifth of the capillary, while only one-fifteenth of the change occurs in the last fifth. This can be seen to be a consequence of the rapidly changing blood oxygen tension near the arterial end of the capillary and slowly changing pO_2 near the venous end. The decreasing rate of change of blood pO_2 is itself due to the increasing steepness of the oxyhemoglobin dissociation curve, as well as to the relatively lower rates of O_2 extraction as pO_2 decreases. The small effect of longitudinal tissue O_2 diffusion would be felt most near the arterial end, and tend to lessen the gradients along x. The rates of change of *all* species concentrations decrease along the capillary because of the decreasing fluxes between capillary and tissue.

Because of the increase in carbon dioxide tension and decrease in erythrocyte pH as the blood flows through the capillary, there is a small but appreciable shift in the oxyhemoglobin dissociation curve, which is characterized by an increase in $p(50)$ from 27.4 to 29.1 mm Hg. The change in erythrocyte pH is as little as 0.02 unit, despite the release of approximately 4 mmol of protons per liter of cells by the hydrolysis of CO_2 and dissociation of carbonic acid, and another $\frac{1}{2}$ mmol of protons by the dissociation of hemoglobin carbamic acid. This is because ~ 3.5 mmol of hydrogen ions are bound to hemoglobin by virtue of the Haldane effect ($\Delta \bar{H}^+/\Delta \bar{O}_2$), and all but a minute fraction of the remaining protons are buffered by the hemoglobin, 2,3-DPG, and other titratable components of erythrocyte fluid. The even smaller change in pH^{pl} within the capillary, 0.004 unit, is due to the very slight extent of plasma CO_2 hydrolysis.

Several interesting consequences of the finite rates of plasma CO_2 hydrolysis and HCO_3^-/Cl^- shift are also brought out in the figures:

(1) The plasma and erythrocyte pH values only attain near-equilibrium with one another at the end of the veins, where pH^{pl} is calculated to be within 0.004 unit of the theoretical value in equilibrium with the prevailing erythrocyte pH. The same difference attains a value of 0.042 unit in the blood leaving the lungs, and 0.035 unit at the end of the systemic microcirculation.

(2) The change in erythrocyte pH within the veins is only from 7.176 to 7.178, whereas the change in plasma pH is from 7.381 to 7.355. Thus, despite the nonequilibrium at the end of the capillary, it is possible to derive an excellent estimate of the value of end-capillary pH^c by sampling of venous blood. As long as the time elapsed between sampling and pH measurement is at least $\frac{1}{2}$ min, the

error incurred by calculating that pH^c value on the basis of equilibrium with the measured pH^{pl} will be less than experimental error. The same is true as regards the sampling of arterial blood in order to investigate erythrocyte pH at the exit of the lungs.

(3) The carbon dioxide tension increases within the arteries from 40.0 to 40.2 mm Hg, and decreases within the veins from 50.0 to 48.7 mm Hg. Both the greater time spent in the veins and neglect of the residual, interphase bicarbonate disequilibrium at the entry to the arteries (see below) are responsible for there being a greater pCO_2 change in the veins. The changes in blood oxygen tension in response to those in pCO_2 and pH^c within the arteries and veins are all but negligible.

(4) The plasma bicarbonate concentration lags behind that in the erythrocytes. During the first 100 msec into the capillary, $[HCO_3^-]^{pl}$ increases by only 0.1 mM, while $[HCO_3^-]^c$ increases by six times that amount. By the end of the capillary, $[HCO_3^-]^{pl}$ has nevertheless increased from 24.0 to 25.6 mM, but is still 0.8 mM below the value in equilibrium with $[HCO_3^-]^c$. This disequilibrium is relaxed well within the first second of flow through the veins (the time required is exaggerated in the figure); since red cell CO_2 hydrolysis responds effectively instantaneously to the transfer of bicarbonate from cells to plasma, there is a simultaneous drop in pCO_2 and cellular pH. It should be pointed out that the capillary bicarbonate disequilibrium is likely to be less than that calculated here, since Klocke (1976) reported difficulty in determining $P_{HCO_3^-}$ with precision, and indicated that the actual value may be several times that applied here. In any event, the transport of oxygen to tissue is rather insensitive to variations in $P_{HCO_3^-}$ in our model, as was the elimination of CO_2 in the lungs according to the model of Klocke (1976).

The interphase bicarbonate disequilibrium at the end of the pulmonary capillaries, disregarded here for mathematical convenience, must be responsible for mirror-image effects in the entrance region of the veins.

Of the various forms of absorbed carbon dioxide, bicarbonate accounts for 82% of the amount taken up in the systemic capillary, dissolved gas 11%, and hemoglobin carbamate the remaining 7%.

The latter fraction is well below the values frequently quoted until quite recently. That is because prior estimates were based upon measurements of carbamino binding to purified oxygenated and deoxygenated hemoglobin solutions, whereas the *in vivo* effect is compromised by both the competition of CO_2 and 2,3-DPG for hemoglobin binding sites and the saturation dependence of oxygen-linked CO_2 binding (see pp. 79–85). At subnormal 2,3-DPG concentrations or blood oxygen tensions, and at above normal pH values, the relative contribution of carbamate may well be greater, but is not estimated to exceed 15% (see p. 214).

The significance, at rest, of the changes within the systemic capillaries due to the allosteric interactions of O_2, CO_2, and protons with hemoglobin was examined by simulation of the following situation:

1. The oxyhemoglobin dissociation curve was fixed at that determined by arterial pO_2 and pH, so that $p(50)$ was 27.4 mm Hg everywhere along the capillary.
2. Consistent with (1), the coefficients $\partial \bar{CO}_2 / \partial \bar{O}_2$ and $\partial \bar{H}^+ / \partial \bar{O}_2$, i.e., oxygen-linked CO_2 and proton binding (the latter being the Haldane effect), were eliminated; CO_2 binding was determined by the association constants for *oxy*hemoglobin; similarly, the erythrocyte buffer capacity β^c and the equilibrium Donnan distribution coefficient r were chosen to be those for oxygenated blood.

The more significant calculated results were as follows:

1. Because of the fixed position of the dissociation curve, the required blood flowrate was 8% higher than previously calculated. The effect was mitigated somewhat by a fall in venous pO_2 from the previous 35.3 to 34.7 mm Hg.
2. Red cell pH decreased along the capillary to 7.13 as opposed to 7.18.

In interpreting the first result, one should realize that *constancy* of the dissociation curve *per se* is not the key factor. Had the curve been fixed at that determined by normal *venous* conditions [with

$p(50) = 29.1$ mm Hg], the required flowrate would have been correspondingly *lower*. With regard to further simulation though, it is clear that for resting conditions relatively little error would be introduced by the assumption of a constant effective dissociation curve. As to the pH effect, the slowness of the plasma CO_2 hydrolysis again ensures minimal pH^{pl} variation along the capillary, and therefore the potential significance of a larger drop of pH^c is unclear.

A Simplifying Approximation

As noted in the preceding section, although the plasma pH is found to change appreciably in both the arteries and veins as the plasma CO_2 hydration reaction equilibrates, the simultaneous (and oppositely directed) adjustments in erythrocyte pH are very small. In fact, for the purpose of relating pO_2 to hemoglobin oxygen saturation, we are primarily interested in the estimation of pH^c. Thus, it would seem sufficient to approach the same problem by simply assuming that the blood entering the capillaries is in overall reaction equilibrium at the gas tensions previously stipulated to prevail at the exit from the lungs. Indeed, when this is done, one finds that the capillary blood pH^c profile and the blood flowrate necessary for tissue oxygenation differ imperceptibly from their original estimates. The only notable differences are, of course, that the plasma pH at the capillary entrance is an equilibrium value of 7.398 instead of the previous value of 7.385, and the corresponding end-capillary plasma pH is 7.394 instead of 7.381. The time-averaged erythrocyte pH calculated by means of the more rigorous "loop" simulation is essentially the same as calculated in the simplified scheme by arithmetic averaging of the pH^c values calculated at the entrance and exit of the capillaries, a fact worthy of note in regard to the coupling of $[DPG]_T$ and pH^c (see p. 216). In light of these results, the extensive calculations of simulated pathophysiological conditions for Chapter 8 were performed using this simplified approach. [The same approximation was used to calculate the results of Meldon and Garby (1975), while the complete circulatory loop was the basis of those of Meldon and Garby (1976).]

Oxygen Transport in Exercise

There are several important changes in the fundamental characteristics of the gas transport system that occur during exercise. In fact, each subsystem—the lungs, the heart and circulation, the blood, and the tissues—responds in a fashion that accommodates the profound increase in oxygen demand evoked by an increasing level of physical performance. Pulmonary ventilation and cardiac output each increase linearly with oxygen uptake up to near-maximal consumption rates (Wasserman and Whipp, 1975), while blood flow is redistributed so that an increasing fraction is directed to muscle (Wade and Bishop, 1962). Blood oxygen affinity decreases as a result of both lactic acidosis and hyperthermia (Thompson *et al.*, 1974). Finally, the recruitment of capillaries reduces the distance over which oxygen must diffuse in tissue (Landis and Pappenheimer, 1963).

A rigorous analysis of the changes in blood gas transport properties during exercise is complicated appreciably by the thermal changes associated with changing levels of activity. This appears to be particularly true with respect to the reequilibration of blood flowing between the lungs and warmer, heavily active muscle (Reeves, 1976*a*). We shall therefore consider only the basic features of capillary–tissue O_2 transport in exercise, and in the framework of an even further simplified mathematical approach.

Let us consider the importance of three particular factors in O_2 supply to working muscle: capillary density, blood O_2 affinity, and the heretofore neglected phenomenon of myoglobin-facilitated O_2 diffusion in tissue. To do so, we retain the original approach of calculating the volume of tissue that can be oxygenated by a single capillary by means of the Krogh–Erlang relation in the form of equation (6-3). For simplicity though, rather than determine the position of the oxyhemoglobin dissociation curve as it varies along a capillary because of increases in pCO_2 and proton concentration, we make the approximation of invoking the Hill equation (see p. 102):

$$\bar{O}_2 = \frac{\{pO_2^{bl}/p(50)\}^n}{1+\{pO_2^{bl}/p(50)\}^n} \qquad (6\text{-}13)$$

where, under normal conditions, $p(50)$ is 27.4 mm Hg and n is 2.95, as may be derived from the standard dissociation curve of Arturson *et al.* (Table V) between saturation levels of 20 and 90%.

A simple relationship between blood flowrate and the average radial extent of tissue oxygenated by an isolated capillary—or, looked at differently, between the average capillary density (supposing, as we have, that the capillaries are arranged so that their zones of supply just fill space) and the minimum required flowrate— may be derived by returning to equation (6-8).

To begin with, equation (6-8) may be rearranged and written in integrated form as

$$I \equiv \int_{\bar{O}_2^v}^{\bar{O}_2^a} \frac{d\bar{O}_2}{(r_{\mathrm{tis}}/r_{\mathrm{cap}})^2 - 1} = \frac{mL}{uh[\mathrm{Hm}]^c} \qquad (6\text{-}14)$$

The integral I between any set of venous (v) and arterial (a) saturation values, may be calculated by numerical quadrature (e.g., using Simpson's rule) in a straightforward manner, since $(r_{\mathrm{cap}}/r_{\mathrm{tis}})^2$ is related to $\bar{O}_2$ by means of equations (6-3) and (6-13).

The connection between equation (6-14) and the desired relationship between flowrate and average radius of oxygenated tissue, $\tilde{r}_{\mathrm{tis}}$, may not be obvious at this point. However, the latter quantity is defined by another integrated form of equation (6-8):

$$uh[\mathrm{Hm}]^c r_{\mathrm{cap}}^2 (\bar{O}_2^a - \bar{O}_2^v) = mL(\tilde{r}_{\mathrm{tis}}^2 - r_{\mathrm{cap}}^2) \qquad (6\text{-}15)$$

Furthermore, the blood flowrate Q per unit volume of tissue is, by definition, expressed by

$$Q = ur_{\mathrm{cap}}^2 / L\tilde{r}_{\mathrm{tis}}^2 \qquad (6\text{-}16)$$

Since in general $\tilde{r}_{\mathrm{tis}}^2 \gg r_{\mathrm{cap}}^2$, equation (6-15) may be combined with (6-14) to yield

$$I = (r_{\mathrm{cap}}/\tilde{r}_{\mathrm{tis}})^2 (\bar{O}_2^a - \bar{O}_2^v) \qquad (6\text{-}17)$$

and with (6-16) to yield

$$Q = (m/h[\mathrm{Hm}]^c)/(\bar{O}_2^a - \bar{O}_2^v) \qquad (6\text{-}18)$$

Thus, for any set of arterial and venous saturations, and values for m, h, $[\mathrm{Hm}]^c$, and r_{cap}: (1) the integral I may be evaluated and related to $\tilde{r}_{tis}$ via equation (6-17); (2) Q may be obtained from equation (6-18); and (3), by assuming a range of venous conditions, the $\tilde{r}_{tis}$–Q relationship is thereby derived. Interestingly, the results are independent of capillary length L.

Figure 40 shows the calculated relationship, at four different levels of metabolic activity, between blood flowrate Q and both the

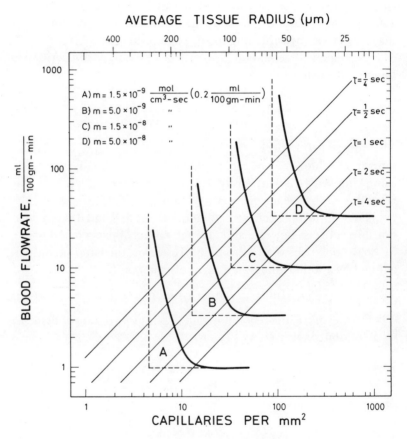

Figure 40. Theoretical values of required blood flowrate per unit mass of muscle tissue vs. capillary density (or average radius of tissue oxygenated by a representative vessel), at metabolic rates corresponding to (A) rest and (B) lightly, (C) moderately, and (D) heavily working muscle. Vertical broken lines denote high-flow, minimum capillarization asymptotes. Horizontal broken lines denote high O_2 extraction, minimum flowrate asymptotes. Forty-five-degree lines are loci of constant blood residence time in the microcirculation.

average radius of oxygenated tissue $\tilde{r}_{tis}$ and the corresponding capillary density, assumed equal to $1/\pi\tilde{r}_{tis}^2$. The four metabolic rates correspond to resting plus lightly, moderately, and heavily exercising muscle (no corrections having as yet been made for changes in oxygen–hemoglobin interaction parameters during physical activity). Besides the theoretical curves, lines of constant capillary residence time τ are also included. Since the latter quantity is equal to L/u, the equation of such lines is $Q = r_{cap}^2/\tau\tilde{r}_{tis}^2$ [see equation (6-18)].

Finally, for each consumption rate in Figure 40, there are drawn asymptotes denoting the respective minimum possible capillary densities (vertical broken lines) and blood flowrates (horizontal broken lines). The minimum capillary density is defined by the r_{tis} value at arterial blood pO_2, i.e., if the blood flowrate is infinite, the blood oxygen tension may theoretically be maintained throughout the capillary at its arterial value. At the other extreme, the minimum blood flowrate is approached as the capillary density is allowed to increase without bound. In the limit, the venous blood pO_2 approaches zero, and therefore, by setting $\bar{O}_2^v$ in equation (6-18) equal to zero, the asymptotic value of Q may be obtained. These asymptotes are essentially independent of the chosen model for capillary–tissue geometry.

Inspection of Figure 40 reveals that increases in not only cardiac output, but also in capillarization, are *required* for increasing physical activity. Furthermore, the latter increases may be so large (without exceeding the anatomical limit in skeletal muscle of some 300 capillaries/mm^2) as to allow a *reduction* in venous blood pO_2 with exercise and therefore a relatively smaller increase in blood flow than in O_2 consumption. For example, with a constant capillary residence time of 1 sec, it is apparent that the 33-fold increase in m between rest and heavy exercise may be accommodated by a 20-fold increase in flow. Indeed, as reported by Thompson *et al.* (1974; see also Asmussen, 1965), femoral venous blood oxygen tension decreases from ~ 26 mm Hg at rest to ~ 20 mm Hg in exercise.

An additional factor that tends to diminish the required increase in cardiac output concomitant with exercise is the rightward shift of the oxyhemoglobin dissociation curve. This is induced by the rise in temperature and decrease in base excess, the latter by virtue of the diffusion of lactic acid from muscle. Because of the shift of the curve, more oxygen is delivered per hemoglobin molecule when operating between the same arterial and venous O_2 tensions. Furthermore, a rightward shift of the steep portion of the curve means that a greater drop in pO_2 through the capillary allows the same average effective tension (as may be deduced from Figure 41).

Thompson *et al.* (1974) report the following average parameters for femoral venous blood in long-term heavy exercise: $pH^{pl} =$ 7.27, $T = 40.7°C$, $pCO_2 = 54.1$ mm Hg. If we assume a standard erythrocyte 2,3-DPG concentration of 5 mM (rather than the value

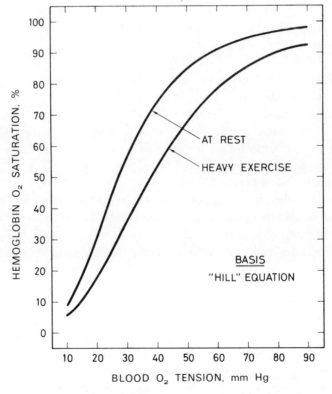

Figure 41. Oxyhemoglobin dissociation curves under standard resting conditions and during heavy exercise, as approximated by equation (6-13). Hill constant n equals 2.95 at rest and 2.7 in exercise. $p(50)$ values are 27.4 and 38 mm Hg, respectively. See text for further discussion.

of 4 mм measured by Thompson *et al.*), then the $p(50)$ value at the reported venous conditions is 38 mm Hg, in agreement with that determined by the investigators. Furthermore, the Hill constant n becomes 2.7 (as opposed to 2.95 under standard conditions), as derived from the respective oxygen tensions at 20 and 90% saturation values, obtained from the equilibrium data of Chapter 4.

If we apply these latter $p(50)$ and n values to the calculation of O_2 supply in heavily exercising muscle, then with a capillary density of, say, 160 vessels/mm^2 ($\tilde{r}_{tis} \approx 45 \ \mu$m) the required blood flowrate is found to be 49 ml/100 g/min, as opposed to 82 with the standard dissociation curve. Part of the explanation for this difference is that the rightward-shifted curve allows a venous blood pO_2 of 26.5 mm Hg, whereas the standard curve requires a value of 31 mm Hg, i.e., the average effectively capillary pO_2 is the same in each instance, despite the difference in venous values, because of the differing positions and shapes of the two dissociation curves (see Figure 41).

Facilitated Gas Transport in Tissue

Oxygen–Myoglobin

One last factor in *muscle* tissue O_2 supply, which we have neglected up to this point, is the *steady-state* carriage of O_2 by myoglobin. The notion that this heme protein can serve such a role—similar to that of hemoglobin discussed by Kreuzer (1970)— besides being a transient source of O_2 during periods of insufficient blood supply, was first suggested by Wittenberg (1959). This view has recently been strengthened by the experiments of Wittenberg *et al.* (1975) and Kreuzer *et al.* (1976). In the first of these two studies, the steady-state uptake of oxygen by bundles of pigeon breast muscle fibers *in vitro* was shown to be severely compromised by the abolition of myoglobin O_2 binding, which is normally of 1:1 stoichiometry, through a number of reagents that do not impair tissue metabolism of oxygen. Similarly, Kreuzer *et al.* (1976) found that the O_2 flux in muscle slabs sliced from chicken gizzards was significantly reduced by carbon monoxide, an agent for blockage of myoglobin O_2 binding. Such results tend to confirm an appreciable mobility of myoglobin in intact muscle, in contrast to an earlier suggestion (Goldfischer, 1967) that the protein is bound to the myofibrils.

Besides protein mobility, an additional requirement for myoglobin-facilitated O_2 diffusion is the existence of a gradient in the saturation of the protein with oxygen. Since the $p(50)$ of myoglobin is approximately 3.4 mm Hg in active muscle (as estimated from the data of Boulton and Holly, 1975; see also Rossi-Fanelli and Antonini, 1958), saturation is nearly complete at blood pO_2 values, whereas desaturation at the tissue's radial extremity requires oxygen tensions approaching zero, as are most likely to occur in heavy exercise.

The diffusion of oxymyoglobin simultaneous with oxygen has the effect of increasing the effective diffusivity of the gas. As a result, a greater amount of tissue may be oxygenated at the same blood gas tensions, as may be inferred from Figure 37. The numerical factor by which the O_2 permeability is effectively multiplied, when the tissue pO_2 reaches zero at the radial extremity, is (see Wyman, 1966; Murray, 1974) given by

$$P_{O_2}^t = P_{O_2}^t([Mb] = 0)\left\{1 + \frac{D_{Mb}[Mb]S_{Mb}^{bl}}{pO_2^{bl}P_{O_2}^t([Mb] = 0)}\right\} \qquad (6\text{-}19)$$

where Mb denotes myoglobin, and D_{Mb}, $[Mb]$, and S_{Mb}^{bl} are, respectively, its diffusivity, total concentration in oxygenated and deoxygenated forms, and saturation with oxygen at blood O_2 tension; i.e., $S_{Mb}^{bl} = pO_2^{bl}/pO_2^{bl} + 3.4$, assuming effective equilibrium.

The *physical* permeability of O_2 in tissue, $P_{O_2}^t([Mb] = 0)$, is the product of its diffusivity and physical solubility, while $[Mb]S_{Mb}^{bl}$ is the concentration of oxymyoglobin at the capillary–tissue interface. As such, the permeability enhancement factor, i.e., the term in the brackets of equation (6-19), is equal to $1 + (D_{Mb}/D_{O_2})([O_2Mb]/[O_2])$. The first of the latter two factors is certainly well below unity, since the diffusivity of oxygen is on the order of 10^{-5} cm²/sec while that of myoglobin is not likely to exceed 10^{-6} cm²/sec. However, since the oxymyoglobin *concentration* can be in the range 0.1–0.5 mM, while that of physically dissolved gas at the capillary–tissue interface is generally lower by a factor of ten, the net effect may indeed be appreciable.

Let us assume a myoglobin concentration of 0.5 mM (Biörck, 1949, quoted in Wittenberg, 1970), and a diffusivity of 2.5×10^{-7} cm^2/sec, as determined by Moll (1968) in muscle *homogenate* (any other combination of [Mb] and D_{Mb} such that their product is unchanged will give the same result). The oxygen permeability enhancement factor that one then calculates from equation (6-19) varies between 1.06 and 1.42 as blood pO_2 is made to decrease from an arterial value of 90 to a possible venous value as low as 10 mm Hg.

The increased effective $P_{O_2}^t$ values may be interpreted as allowing proportionally lower blood pO_2 values without jeopardizing tissue oxygenation [see equation (6-3) and Figure 37). To estimate the possible physiological consequence of this in O_2 to supply to working muscle, we have applied the analysis developed in the preceding section, with the modification implied by equation (6-19) (Meldon, 1976). Assuming the above-quoted values of myoglobin diffusivity and concentration, as well as the capillary density of 160 per mm^2 and rightward-shifted oxyhemoglobin dissociation curve discussed in the preceding section, one finds that *heavy* exercise may now be promoted with a venous oxygen tension of 19 rather than 26.5 mm Hg. Because of the appreciable amount of oxygen that is released by the hemoglobin between 26.5 and 19 mm Hg, the required blood flowrate decreases from 49 to 40.6 ml/100 g/min.

If the capillary density is instead 150/mm^2, then in the absence of myoglobin (or if it is immobile) a venous pO_2 of 31 mm Hg is required, along with a Q of 57.4 ml/100 g/min. With myoglobin, there is again about a 20% decrease in Q to 45.9, together with a decrease in venous pO_2 to 24 mm Hg. Moreover, if D_{Mb} is actually twice as great, i.e., 5×10^{-7} cm^2/sec as estimated by Wyman (1966), then there are further decreases in required venous pO_2 and flowrate to 16 mm Hg and 38.4 ml/100 g/min, respectively. The actual relief of cardiac output demands is a function of how much more O_2 is released by the hemoglobin as the required level of blood oxygen tension decreases.

In summary, the important determinants of the significance of myoglobin-facilitated O_2 transport are (1) the protein's diffusivity and concentration, (2) the radial gradient in its saturation with oxygen, and (3) the steepness of the oxyhemoglobin dissociation curve in the prevailing range of venous pO_2 values. The last aspect is especially intriguing in that it calls to mind a special sort of "teamwork" between the two oxygen-binding heme proteins.

Carbon Dioxide–Bicarbonate

A phenomenon resembling myoglobin-mediated O_2 transport in muscle is the carriage of carbon dioxide in tissue in the form of bicarbonate ion. The strongest evidence in favor of this hypothesis was presented recently by Kawashiro and Scheid (1976), who report that the effective Krogh diffusion constant for CO_2 in rat skeletal muscle tissue *in vitro* varies with the partial pressure of the gas according to the empirical formula

$$P^t_{CO_2} = 29\{1 + 1.7 \, e^{-0.027pCO_2}\}\frac{\text{mol}}{\text{cm-sec-mm Hg}} \times 10^{-14} \quad (6\text{-}20)$$

where pCO_2 is expressed in mm Hg.

The greater effective CO_2 permeability at lower gas tensions is consistent with a greater portion of the net flux of the gas deriving from bicarbonate diffusion. This is a rather more complex phenomenon than that of oxygen–myoglobin interaction, insofar as the flux of bicarbonate ion is coupled to that of a counterion and limited, in the absence of a catalyst like carbonic anhydrase, by the kinetics of CO_2 hydration–dehydration. In any event, the consequence of an enhanced CO_2 permeability, if indeed there is one *in vivo*, must be a smaller pCO_2 gradient between tissue and blood (Kawashiro and Scheid, 1976). However, since the gradients are estimated to be on the order of 0.1 mm Hg at rest and no more than 2 mm Hg in exercise, the physiological significance is not clear.

An interesting sidelight to this story involves three of this century's preeminent respiratory physiologists: August Krogh, A. V. Hill, and F. J. W. Roughton. Hill first noted in 1928 that the ratio of the tissue CO_2 and O_2 permeabilities reported by Krogh (1918–1919a) was rather in excess of what one might have anticipated on theoretical grounds: "It seems rather curious that the larger molecule should diffuse faster." He therefore suggested the possibility of facilitated transport: "... if the bicarbonate ion is able to diffuse, the diffusion of total carbon dioxide may be more rapid than that of free carbon dioxide at the same gradient of pressure." Notably, though, Hill treated Krogh's CO_2 permeability with reservation, since it arose from a single experimental determination. Krogh himself commented that the value "may possibly be too high."

Later, Roughton (1935), who had recently discovered carbonic anhydrase, reasoned that a lack of the enzyme in tissue would be a blessing in that it would preclude the conversion of appreciable amounts of CO_2 into an ionic species that could only slowly permeate cell membranes: "... in its absence the CO_2 is able to diffuse away rapidly without loitering appreciably by the wayside in the form of bicarbonate ions." This, however, neglects what *now* appears to be possibly appreciable enhancement of *intracellular* CO_2 transport. Hill, in turn, in his 1965 memoirs, disowned his original conclusion on grounds similar to those of Roughton (though apparently influenced by a rather high estimate of the ratio of CO_2 and O_2 solubilities in tissue), adding the comment that the ambiguously high CO_2 permeability in frog muscle "... is probably due to CO_2 penetrating the boundary membrane of the muscle fibers rather quicker than O_2."

Chapter 7

Some Physiological Control Systems

It is typical of living organisms that their different parts interact functionally. Much of modern physiology—systems physiology—is preoccupied with both the formal and quantitative aspects of such interactions, which may be of several different kinds. The very simplest are trivial in the sense that they are direct results of mass transfer or reaction stoichiometry. For example, the increase in arterial pO_2 observed after an increase in alveolar pO_2 is required by the permeability of the alveolar–capillary membrane to oxygen, and the decrease in red cell pH upon oxygenation is a direct consequence of the simultaneous binding of O_2/release of protons by hemoglobin. Much more complex interactions stem from feedback mechanisms, and these are invariably interpreted as serving some specific function, e.g., the maintenance of blood pH or tissue pO_2 within certain ranges. In describing such cases, the variables kept constant are often said to be *controlled,* and the same word is also used to describe situations in which a complete set of variables is changed in concert so as to maintain a certain function.

Use of the word *control* in regard to cause-and-effect phenomena in living organisms requires comment. Engineers have long been concerned with systems in which it is required that a particular quantity be held at a certain level or vary in a certain fashion with the value of a given input. There is no problem identifying the particular property controlled in an engineer's device—it was built with that purpose in mind. However, such identification in living systems raises a fundamental difficulty: Since purpose remains an elusive concept in biology, the word control has, in fact, no meaning there other than that normally assigned to it in the context of cause and effect. Application of engineering control theory to biology tends to imply that somehow there *is* logic in assigning purpose to phenomena in living systems. This apparent contradiction needs elaboration.

The problem is perhaps best elucidated by an example. Suppose that we establish the functional relationship between steady-state concentrations of hemoglobin and of plasma erythropoietin stimulating factors (ESF) through experiments wherein the latter are controlled by the investigator, e.g., by continuous infusion at different rates in animals whose endogeneous production has been inhibited. Let us presume that the observed relationship is such that the steady-state hemoglobin levels monotonically increase with plasma ESF level. We might then say that the hemoglobin level is determined by the ESF level. Suppose further that we again seek to establish the same functional relationship, but this time by means of experiments wherein the *hemoglobin* levels are controlled by the investigator, e.g., by continuous infusion of red cells at different rates in animals whose bone marrow has been inhibited. We now find that the hemoglobin and ESF levels are *negatively* correlated. The striking discrepancy between the two observed relationships leads us to conclude that we have studied two different subsystems.

Finally, in a third experiment the animals are left to "control themselves," and we find but one pair of ESF and hemoglobin levels. This pair is, incidentally, identical with that at the intersection of the two functional relationships. We might then arrive at the working hypothesis or model shown in Figure 42, where the transfer functions housed in the boxes are the respective relationships established by the first two experiments.

The following question may now be posed: Is the hemoglobin level "controlled" by the ESF level or vice versa? One answer is that

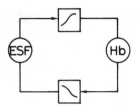

Figure 42

the uniqueness of the steady-state levels found in the third experiment implies a mutuality of cause and effect inherent to the combination of the two transfer functions, and that use of the words *control* and *regulation* is neither here nor there. This answer, while technically correct, is not very satisfying. In order to characterize the system further and, in particular, to find the biophysical and biochemical mechanisms underlying the transfer functions, it indeed makes sense to enquire as to the purpose of the system. Preliminary considerations would suggest that it is not the purpose of the hemoglobin level to *control* the ESF level, but rather that it is much more reasonable to assume the opposite and that the system must somehow be involved with blood respiratory function. The working model might therefore look like Figure 43, where the hemoglobin concentration is thought to be a factor in a new variable, say the oxygen release capacity of the blood, *ORC*, i.e., the number of moles of O_2 that are bound (or released) per mm Hg O_2 tension.

This line of reasoning immediately suggests critical experiments, since an additional factor in the ORC is the hemoglobin O_2 affinity, which might therefore influence the ESF level in predictable

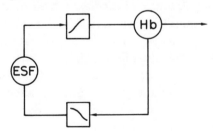

Figure 43

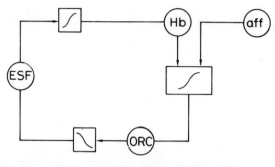

Figure 44

fashion. Thus we may tentatively replace the hemoglobin concentration as the "controlled" variable by the ORC and redo the model as shown in Figure 44, where the new transfer function describes just how the ORC varies with hemoglobin level and O_2 affinity. Experiments confirm this model (see p. 201), which inclines us to believe that the system works to "control" the ORC.

The story may now repeat itself in regard to, say, the effect of varying blood flow. It thus happens that during the course of scientific study of a physiological system, different "purposes" appear and fade as that system's inner workings become more clearly defined. In such fashion, engineering control theory, comprising powerful data reduction techniques, has found widespread application in physiology, and its heuristic value cannot be doubted.

The Controlled Gas Transport System

In Chapter 6, the complete gas transport system was analyzed in terms of the dependence of tissue O_2 consumption upon the parameters of lung output (arterial pO_2 and pCO_2), the circulation (cardiac output/local blood flow), the blood (hemoglobin and 2,3-DPG concentrations, hemoglobin affinity for ligands), and tissue geometry and intrinsic metabolic rate (see Figure 38). A procedure was developed for evaluating the effects of changes in individual parameters upon the system's output. Individual parameters were treated as if they were independent of one another, with the exception of blood flowrate, which was varied so as to ensure a fixed tissue oxygen consumption.

In this chapter, we discuss in a qualitative and introductory way a most important property of the system that has been neglected up till now. Each subsystem—the lungs, the circulation, the blood, and tissues—receives inputs, and at least one input to each is an output from another subsystem. This makes the complete system operate in a "controlled" fashion as just described and, according to one's imagination, it is possible to identify a number of variables that can be said to be controlled.

One representation of the complete system, that of Figure 38 amended so that the inputs whose sources were previously unaccounted for (red cell 2,3-DPG, hemoglobin concentration, cardiac output, ventilation, and tissue capillarization) are now control loop outputs, is shown in Figure 45. It is constructed on the basis of the following generally accepted interactions:

(1) The input to lung respiratory function, here subsumed under the term ventilation, arises in special regions of nerve tissue which sense the chemical composition (and flow?) of the blood; the rate and depth of respiratory muscular movement are thus adjusted by nerve impulse.

(2) The determinants of blood flow or cardiac output comprise several types of input—locally induced metabolic changes affect local blood vessels so as to induce changes in the flow through them, and chemical events in specific tissue elements of the brain and peripheral nervous system affect the circulation either systematically or locally through nervous impulses.

(3) Capillarization, which determines tissue diffusional distances, is mediated by locally induced chemical events.

The input–output relationships of the respiratory, circulatory, and tissue subsystems are fields of classical physiology. Both their qualitative and quantitative aspects have been subject to intense study during past decades. A critical and comprehensive treatment of them is beyond the scope of the present endeavor. However, insofar as two key parameters of the control system, the hemoglobin and red cell 2,3-DPG concentrations, are properties of the blood itself, their input–output relationships are considered below. An elaborate discussion of these relationships would be expected to

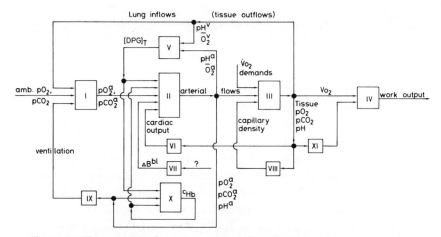

Figure 45. The previously drawn input–output flow diagram of the transport system (Fig. 38) as amended by a number of feedback loops. Box V translates arterial and venous pH and $\bar{O}_2$ values into red cell 2,3-DPG concentration. Box VI contains the transfer function relating the physicochemical events in the tissues to cardiac output/local blood flow. Box VII is the complex functionality determining blood base excess (see Chapter 5). Box VIII represents the translation of tissue events into a change in capillarization. Box IX translates arterial blood composition into ventilatory responses. Box X is the transfer function of the ESF system. Box XI is a proposed (see p. 227) transfer function for the relation of tissue pH to the thermodynamic efficiency of energy transduction.

contain both a description of mechanism and quantitative evaluation of the efficiency of control. We defer the latter to Chapter 8 and thus confine the discussion of this chapter to some basic physiological facts regarding red cell 2,3-DPG and whole blood hemoglobin concentrations.

The Red Cell 2,3-DPG Concentration

2,3-Diphosphoglycerate is an intermediate in glycolysis, the metabolic process whereby glucose is converted anaerobically into pyruvate and lactate. The main functions of this process in red cells are (1) production of adenosinetriphosphate (ATP) for transport and synthetic work; (2) production of reduced nicotinamide adenine nucleotides (NADH and NADPH) for reduction of methemoglobin and oxidized glutathion; and (3) production of

2,3-DPG, which serves as an allosteric effector of the reactions of hemoglobin with O_2, CO_2, and protons.

The glycolytic system is highly organized in the sense that it contains many feedback control loops. It is also an open system inasmuch as not only its initial reactant and final products, but also several important regulator compounds are permeable in the red cell membrane. The concentration of 2,3-DPG is thus moderated by factors associated with the remainder of the gas transport system. As such, it is only within that broader framework that its control can satisfactorily be discussed.

The red cell glycolytic system has been studied extensively in recent decades. A comprehensive and critical review was written by Rapoport (1968). A more recent review, dealing principally with the system's control features, is that of Jacobasch *et al.* (1974). Still another, dealing mainly with 2,3-DPG, was published by Duhm and Gerlach (1974).

2,3-DPG and the Red Cell Glycolytic System

The main features of glycolysis and phosphoglycerate metabolism in red cells are shown in Figure 46. The pentose phosphate pathway (PPP), connecting ribose-6-P with F-6-P and glyceraldehyde-3-P, is outlined in Figure 47 and discussed in more detail in the section dealing with control of the system's oxidation–reduction potential (p. 204).

The physiological significance of the 2,3-DPG shunt pathway and 2,3-DPG concentration in tissue cells in general is not well established, but it is clear that the pathway offers a means for the regulation of cellular ATP content. The phosphoglycerate kinase (PGK) reaction yields one high-energy bond in ATP, whereas the chemical energy of the acylphosphate group in 1,3-DPG is irreversibly dissipated when the 2,3-DPG bypass route is taken.

2,3-DPG inhibits the kinase reactions involving phosphofructokinase (PFK) and pyruvate kinase (PK), and may thereby serve to control the overall rate of glycolysis. It also functions as a ubiquitous cofactor in the phosphoglycerate mutase (PGM) reaction. In contrast to tissue cells in general, the red cell 2,3-DPG concentration

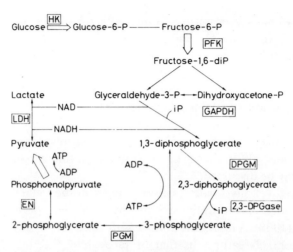

Figure 46. Outline of the red cell glycolytic system. Reactions shown with heavy arrows are, under physiological conditions, far from thermodynamic equilibrium. Enzymes are shown within boxes: HK, hexokinase; PFK, phosphofructokinase; GAPDH, glyceraldehyde phosphate dehydrogenase; DPGM, diphosphoglycerate mutase; PGK, phosphoglycerate kinase; 2,3-DPGase, 2,3-diphosphoglycerate phosphatase; PGM, phosphoglycerate mutase; EN, enolase; PK, pyruvate kinase; LDH, lactic acid dehydrogenase.

exceeds by two orders of magnitude that needed for maximal velocity of the PGM reaction. The function of this very high concentration in many mammalian erythrocytes, including those of man, appears to be fully explained by the allosteric interaction of 2,3-DPG with hemoglobin and thus its effect on these cells' oxygen transport function.

The concentration of 2,3-DPG is determined by its formation and degradation in the two reactions catalyzed by diphosphoglycerate mutase (DPGM) and 2,3-diphosphoglycerate phosphatase (2,3-DPGase), as shown in Figure 46. The rate of formation of 2,3-DPG is determined primarily by the concentration of its immediate precursor, 1,3-DPG, since the apparent K_m value of the mutase for 1,3-DPG is ~0.5 μM, which exceeds the physiological concentration

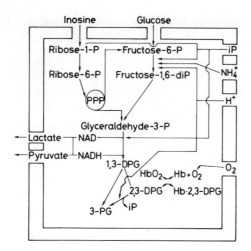

Figure 47. A diagrammatic illustration of the effect of some permeable components on red cell glycolysis.

of 1,3-DPG. The rate is further determined by the concentration of 2,3-DPG itself, since DPGM is very strongly product inhibited (K_i is approximately 1 μM). The maximal activity of DPGM in human erythrocytes at 37°C is 250–400 μmol/ml/hr. However, interactions among the metabolites under normal physiological conditions— with 2,3-DPG levels about 10,000 times those of 1,3-DPG—force the enzyme to work at an extremely low fraction of its capacity, less than 1 μmol/ml/hr.

The concentration of 1,3-DPG is governed by several of the enzymic steps of the glycolytic process:

(1) The PFK reaction is the principal controller of the overall glycolytic rate; its activity is influenced by the concentrations of several species—ATP, ADP, protons, ammonium ions, and inorganic phosphate (see Figure 47).

(2) Glyceraldehyde-3-phosphate dehydrogenase (GADPH) catalyzes the oxidation of glyceraldehyde-3-phosphate to 1,3-DPG

with NAD as a hydrogen acceptor; this step might well control the formation of 1,3-DPG under conditions of high pH and low NAD/NADH ratio; inorganic phosphate promotes the reaction.

(3) The PGK reaction operates close to its thermodynamic equilibrium under physiological conditions; as such, changes in the concentrations of any remaining reactant and/or product (ATP, ADP, and 3-phosphoglycerate) rapidly change the concentration of 1,3-DPG.

(4) PK catalyzes the conversion of phosphoenolpyruvate to pyruvate and, since the enolase (EN) and phosphoglycerate mutase (PGM) reactions are close to their respective thermodynamic equilibria, a change in the PK step affects the concentration of 1,3-DPG via back reaction.

The rate of degradation of 2,3-DPG is controlled by 2,3-DPG phosphatase (2,3-DPGase), which has the lowest capacity of any enzyme connected with erythrocyte glycolysis, about 0.1 μmol/ml/hr at 37°C. The optimal pH of the reaction is $\sim$6.5, so a decrease in pH from the normal value of 7.2 activates the enzyme, while an increase causes inhibition, as does an increase in sulfate ion concentration. The apparent K_m of 2,3-DPGase for 2,3-DPG at pH 7.2 is as low as 1 μM, and therefore an appreciable change in degradation rate at constant pH can result only from a change in the enzyme's activity. It may be activated by a number of ions, among them chloride and inorganic phosphate. Of potential interest is the stimulation by phosphoglycolate: 60 μM of this ion, which can exist in red cells at such a concentration, enhance the activity of 2,3-DPGase 1500 times.

The degree of participation of the 2,3-DPG shunt pathway in the overall glycolytic process has been variously estimated to be from 10 to 25% under normal conditions with high pO_2. Thus, the flow of "half-glucose" molecules through the shunt under such conditions is between 0.2 and 0.5 μmol/ml/hr, or some 5–10% of the 2,3-DPG pool per hour. Under other conditions, the shunt flow may be much higher. Red cells depleted of 2,3-DPG accumulate 0.4–0.8 μmol/ml/hr of it during the initial hours following reinjection (Valeri and Hirsch, 1969; Beutler and Wood, 1969).

Effects of External Signals. The red cell 2,3-DPG concentration is subject to external control, inasmuch as the red cell membrane is permeable to several species that affect the functional state of glycolysis. An outline of these interactions is shown in Figure 47.

At fixed concentrations of pyruvate and lactate, the rate of dehydrogenation of glyceraldehyde-3-P to 1,3-DPG is fixed by its coupling to the NAD/NADH system. On the other hand, the blood's concentrations of both pyruvate and lactate, and therefore the erythrocyte glycolytic rate, depend on—and presumably can be set by—factors external to the red cells. This fact has been successfully exploited in *in vitro* systems, in conjunction with the addition of inosine and inorganic phosphate, so as to obtain blood with very high levels of 2,3-DPG. However, its significance *in vivo* has not yet been clarified.

Inosine, which is freely permeable in the red cell membrane, increases the overall glycolytic rate and thereby the concentration of 2,3-DPG. There is a large capacity of purine nucleoside phosphorylase, $\sim 1000\ \mu mol/ml/hr$, to convert inosine to hypoxanthine and ribose-1-phosphate. The ribose moiety enters the glycolytic pathway by way of the pentose phosphate pathway (see Figure 47), thus bypassing the hexokinase or hexokinase-plus-PFK steps. The physiological significance of this mechanism for red cell 2,3-DPG control also remains to be elucidated.

Changes in glucose concentration within the physiological and pathophysiological range do not affect red cell glycolysis, because the K_m of hexokinase for glucose, $\sim 50\ \mu M$, is far below these concentrations. The glycolytic rate and 2,3-DPG concentration are, however, profoundly effected by phosphate ions, which reduce ATP inhibition of PFK and thereby increase the enzyme's affinity for fructose-6-phosphate. Phosphate ions may also mitigate glucose-6-phosphate inhibition of hexokinase, as well as stimulate the flux via GADPH, at least under conditions where the NAD concentration is maintained at a reasonable level. The low 2,3-DPG level in experimentally induced hypophosphatemia is due to the last mechanism (see further p. 240).

Ammonium ions act as cofactors of PFK, at least partly by annulling ATP inhibition. An increase in erythrocyte 2,3-DPG concentration follows *in vitro* incubation of whole blood with ammonium at concentrations comparable to those observed clinically, e.g., in liver cirrhosis (see p. 240).

Protons have several effects upon red cell glycolysis. An increase in proton activity inhibits both the hexokinase and, more importantly, the PFK step, the latter through sensitization of the enzyme to ATP inhibition. On the other hand, protons increase the activity of 2,3-DPGase. At present, a quantitative rationalization of these effects is not possible. It is, however, a matter of fact that most clinical situations with acidosis, respiratory or metabolic, are accompanied by low erythrocyte 2,3-DPG levels, and the converse is found in alkalosis. The data are discussed in detail in Chapter 8.

Oxygen affects the glycolytic system by releasing hemoglobin-bound 2,3-DPG. This increases the inhibition of hexokinase and PFK and decreases the flow of reactants through all steps (Rapoport *et al.*, 1976). Oxygen also affects the system by causing the release of hemoglobin-bound protons. Experimental data on which to base a firm conclusion as to the relative importance of these two mechanisms are still lacking. The available data are discussed in more detail in Chapter 8.

Variations in Red Cell 2,3-DPG Concentration under Physiological Conditions

The red cell 2,3-DPG concentration, $[DPG]_T$, averages ~ 4.5 mmol/liter of packed cells in apparently healthy male subjects and ~ 5.0 mmol/liter in apparently healthy females. There is appreciable scatter among such subjects, the coefficient of variation being $\sim 10\%$ (Hjelm, 1969; Andreasson *et al.*, 1973; Arturson *et al.*, 1974*a,b*), but no variation with age (Tweeddale *et al.*, 1976). The day-to-day variation within normal subjects has not yet been studied.

There is a rather marked change in $[DPG]_T$ with time of day, presumably in relation to physical activity (Böning *et al.*, 1975*a*). Thus, the value is quite constant from about noon until midnight, but decreases continuously thereafter to a value 10% lower between 7 and 8 AM. Apparently, the diurnal variation is not related to one of plasma inorganic phosphate, or plasma or red cell pH.

An inverse relationship is found between $[DPG]_T$ and the whole blood hemoglobin concentration, c_{Hb} (grams per liter of whole blood). That the correlation is rather strong is brought out by the fact that the coefficient of variation of $[DPG]_T$ levels at a given c_{Hb} level is considerably below 10%. Because of this, the mean values of $[DPG]_T$ from different groups of subjects are related to the distributions of hemoglobin levels within them.

In males with 120–150 g/liter of hemoglobin, the regression of values determined by Hjelm (1969) was

$$[DPG]_T = 13.5 - 0.064c_{Hb}$$

while in females with 110–145 g/liter of hemoglobin, it was

$$[DPG]_T = 11.1 - 0.052c_{Hb}$$

where, as before, the 2,3-DPG concentration is expressed in millimoles per liter of packed cells. Later studies, employing other methods for 2,3-DPG determination, indicate somewhat higher values, but essentially the same variation with sex and hemoglobin level.

The reason for the correlation of $[DPG]_T$ with c_{Hb} in the latter's normal range is not fully understood, but of considerable interest is the fact that it continues to hold at lower hemoglobin levels. Thus, subjects with anemia generally have abnormally high erythrocyte 2,3-DPG concentrations (see Chapter 8). If the correlation is indeed continuous, then subjects at the lower end of the "normal" hemoglobin range may well be considered to have reacted as anemic subjects, which illustrates the difficulty of defining the "normal" range of a continuous variable.

The mechanism underlying the $[DPG]_T$–c_{Hb} relationship in anemic subjects is discussed in detail in Chapter 8, but one factor of importance is worth mentioning here. There is a strong, positive correlation, in a variety of experimental and clinical conditions, between steady-state plasma pH level in the range 7.0–7.7 and $[DPG]_T$ in the range 1–8 mM (see Table XV and pp. 215–219). For subjects with hypoproliferative anemia, the linear regression has a slope of ~ 15 mM per plasma pH unit. Almost certainly this relationship is due largely to the above-described pH dependence of the red cell glycolytic system.

Moreover, subjects with anemia have, on the average, a higher plasma pH than normal (see pp. 222–223). In the hemoglobin range 40–170 g/liter, the pH increases by between 0.006 and 0.010 pH units per decrease of 10 g/liter of hemoglobin. Estimation of that ratio over the normal range of hemoglobin concentration is uncertain. It appears, though, to be somewhat smaller than the overall average. That is consistent with the fact that if we use the average $\Delta pH/\Delta c_{Hb}$ value to predict the $[DPG]_T-c_{Hb}$ correlation in the normal c_{Hb} range, we obtain a value that exceeds what is observed.

The difference in average 2,3-DPG level between sexes, 0.3–0.5 mM, is consistent with the observation that the arterial plasma pH of normal female subjects exceeds that of normal men by between 0.01 and 0.02 pH unit (Siggaard-Andersen, 1974).

During pregnancy, there is a steady increase in $[DPG]_T$. At term it is about 30% higher than normal (Rörth and Bille-Brahe, 1971). Concomitant with this increase is a progressively increasing alkalosis due to hyperventilation. The value of $[\Delta DPG]_T/\Delta pH^{pl}$ is ~ 20 mM per pH unit.

Red cell 2,3-DPG levels show a characteristic variation during the first year of human life (Delivoria-Papadopoulos *et al.*, 1971; Versmold *et al.*, 1973). During the first 2 to 3 days of life, the concentration is very similar to that prevailing during adulthood. Between days 3 and 5, there is an abrupt 20–25% increase in concentration, which is maintained through most of the first year. The value then decreases over the next year or so to the normal adult value. The large increase seen between days 3 and 5, and maintained until about day 9, cannot be attributed to a change in red cell pH (Versmold *et al.*, 1973). It may, however, result from changes in phosphate metabolism mediated by increases in plasma and erythrocyte inorganic phosphate content. Card and Brain (1973) have shown that the high plasma inorganic phosphate levels found in normal children are associated with increased red cell organic phosphate concentrations and decreased whole blood oxygen affinity. The implication may well be that the plasma inorganic phosphate provides a mechanism for shutting down erythrocyte production at this stage of life. The increased $[DPG]_T$ level would tend to inhibit the production of ESF (see below).

Physical training has been claimed to increase the $[DPG]_T$ level, but the evidence is inconclusive (see Böning *et al.*, 1975*b*).

The Whole Blood Hemoglobin Concentration

General Aspects

The whole blood hemoglobin concentration c_{Hb} is the essential determinant of blood O_2 transport function and, through the buffer capacity, of its CO_2 transport function as well. It is therefore not surprising that c_{Hb} is a regulated quantity. The relevant control system has been investigated extensively enough that its workings can be described in some detail.

The amount of circulating hemoglobin at any time, $N(t)$ (i.e., c_{Hb} times blood volume), is related to its respective production and destruction rates P and D by

$$N(t) = \int_0^t P\,dt - \int_0^t D\,dt + N(0)$$

where t denotes time.

Under steady-state conditions, i.e., when $dN/dt = 0$, the destruction rate D may be conveniently expressed in terms of the mean life span of circulating red blood cells $\bar{T}$ as

$$D = N/\bar{T}$$

Under steady-state physiological conditions, $\bar{T}$ is on the order of 100 days, $D = P = 0.01N$, and the system operates with very slow turnover.

There is no known feedback mechanism by which the body regulates its hemoglobin concentration through the destruction rate. Mean cell life span is difficult to determine with precision, but there is no evidence that it is causally related to N. On the other hand, the production rate is controlled by a well-known negative feedback system in which c_{Hb} is an important transfer function parameter.

The Erythropoietin System

Erythropoiesis stimulating factors (abbreviated ESF or erythropoietin) are found in the plasma and urine in a variety of conditions characterized by increased red cell production. Furthermore, ESF production increases after phlebotomy and decreases after red cell transfusion. These findings support the contention that c_{Hb} is determined by ESF.

Erythropoiesis stimulating factors have been particularly resistant to efforts at their chemical characterization as distinct molecular species. At least one, though, is a glycoprotein some 30% of which is carbohydrate, and of that 30% about 10% is sialic acid. The chemistry has been reviewed by Lowy (1970).

The *target* in bone marrow is an early precursor cell referred to as a *committed* or *unipotent stem cell*. Increased erythropoiesis after injection of ESF is clearly due to an increasing number of maturing cells, but probably as well to a shortening of the intermitotic intervals among precursor cells. Rifkind *et al.* (1974) have recently reviewed this subject extensively.

Subjects with *polycythemia vera* have high hemoglobin levels, but low concentrations of ESF in their urine. This indicates the presence of inhibitors in the system, perhaps at the level of the target organ. High concentrations of hemoglobin are found in a number of conditions with neoplasma in which there also is increased ESF production. There is no evidence for general hypoxia in such cases, and thus no obvious explanation for the high c_{Hb} level.

Subjects with arterial hypoxemia, i.e., with low arterial pO_2, almost invariably have hemoglobin levels above the normal range. This suggests that c_{Hb} is monitored by a system sensitive to oxygen tension.

Subjects with increased oxygen consumption, e.g., those with thyreotoxicosis, have normal hemoglobin levels, but increased cardiac output. This may be taken to suggest that the monitoring system is located on the arterial side of the circulation.

Subjects with a high blood O_2 affinity due to high-affinity hemoglobins have elevated c_{Hb} levels. The relationship is such that c_{Hb} increases with decreasing ORC (Bellingham, 1972, 1974; see further pp. 235–236). Similarly, subjects with a low blood O_2 affinity due to low-affinity hemoglobins have subnormal c_{Hb} as long as their oxygen binding curve is not shifted so far as to compromise O_2 uptake in the lung. Also in the same vein, changes in pH that affect blood O_2 affinity are associated with changes in ESF output (Miller *et al.*, 1973). Such observations suggest that the monitoring system consumes oxygen, and that its output varies inversely with that consumption.

Subjects with generally impaired blood flow tend to have normal hemoglobin levels. This would seem to be of definite functional importance since in their case an increased c_{Hb}—and consequent increase in blood viscosity—would be distinctly disadvantageous. This imposes an interesting constraint upon the pO_2 monitoring system: it must either be placed in a region where there is efficient autoregulation of blood flow, or it must be perfused by blood vessels subject to so-called *plasma skimming*. The latter phenomenon occurs in blood vessels that depart at a large angle from the mother vessel; the hematocrit in the daughter vessel varies inversely with blood flow, and therefore the flow of hemoglobin through it is effectively independent of the volumetric flowrate through the larger vessel.

Such insights notwithstanding, the essential nature of the erythropoietin system remains regrettably not well known. A schematic diagram based on present evidence is shown in Figure 48. The kidney appears to be the production site of either an erythropoietin-activating agent or erythropoietin itself. Release of this factor from the kidney is demonstrably insensitive to changes in blood flow, which is consistent with the above line of reasoning.

Variations under Physiological Conditions

The blood hemoglobin concentrations of apparently healthy men and women living at sea level average 150 and 130 g/liter, respectively. The distribution of values in samples selected for health is very nearly Gaussian (Garby, 1970), with a coefficient of variation between 5 and 7%. The mechanism behind this fairly large variation has not been studied in detail. Garby *et al.* (1967) found that inter- and intraindividual variations in apparently healthy females constitute about 60 and 35%, respectively, of the total variation. It is nearly certain that most of the short-term intrain-

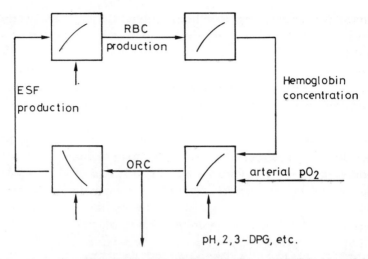

Figure 48. A schematic representation of the system for control of the hemoglobin concentration. ORC is the oxygen release capacity of the blood, i.e., the number of moles of oxygen that can be taken up or released per liter of blood when the partial pressure of oxygen varies between fixed limits.

dividual variation is due to plasma volume fluctuation incidental to blood respiratory function.

The physiological and clinical significance of the c_{Hb} differences between the sexes and between normal subjects of the same sex is not known. However, other blood properties involved in gas transport function are significantly correlated with c_{Hb}. As mentioned previously, red blood cells from normal males contain on the average 0.3–0.5 mm less 2,3-DPG than those of normal females. Moreover, in normal subjects of like sex, $[DPG]_T$ and c_{Hb} levels are inversely related. Finally, as also mentioned previously, the arterial pH of female subjects is slightly higher than that of males. The cause-and-effect relationships here remain to be clarified; current hypotheses are detailed in the discussion of anemia (Chapter 8).

Protection against Oxidation of Hemoglobin

The structure and function of the hemoglobin molecule are critically dependent upon the state of oxidation of certain atoms and groups of atoms, among them heme iron and several –SH groups. The red cell membrane is permeable to a number of species bearing oxidation–reduction equivalents, e.g., pyruvate and lactate. Consequently, the stability of the oxidation state of critical groups depends upon a continuously functioning metabolic system that acts—in erythrocytes and other cells—as a "buffer" with respect to oxidation–reduction equivalents. Although in erythrocytes this system does not appear to function in the sense of a feedback system, it is natural to deal with it here in connection with glycolysis. A number of rather comprehensive and critical reviews of this subject have recently been published (Keitt, 1972; Jaffé, 1974; Lionetti, 1974; Hsieh and Jaffé, 1975).

The Heme Groups

In deoxyhemoglobin, the porphyrin rings plus bound iron are electrically neutral. By convention, the electrons in the complex are "divided" among the atoms, with iron usually assigned the oxidation number 2+. As mentioned previously (p. 66), binding of an O_2 molecule to iron is associated with the transfer of electron density from the iron atom to the oxygen molecule. The bond is not truly ionic, but rather a result of strong π-electron donation from Fe^{2+} to the oxygen molecule, and synergistic σ-donation from one oxygen atom to iron. The deoxygenated iron–porphyrin complex has, however, a tendency to lose an electron much more completely and permanently than the oxygenated form. In doing so, its charge becomes more positive, and the iron may then be assigned the oxidation number 3+. The iron in this state cannot donate electrons to dioxygen from its low-energy d orbitals as readily as can Fe^{2+}, and its sixth coordination position is instead occupied by either water or hydroxyl ion, the relative proportions of which depend on medium pH. This form of hemoglobin is commonly referred to as either *methemoglobin* or *ferrihemoglobin*.

The tendency toward oxidation of hemoglobin iron is offset by a system in red cells that ensures a sufficient electron pressure to maintain the ratio of hemoglobin: methemoglobin (or Fe^{2+}:Fe^{3+}) at about 100:1. Under steady-state physiological conditions, between 0.5 and 3% of the hemoglobin molecules are oxidized to methemoglobin per day, and the rate of reduction is the same. The autooxidation rate is proportional to the concentration of *deoxy*hemoglobin, inasmuch as *oxy*hemoglobin is that much more resistant to oxidation. Methemoglobin formation may be much greater under certain pathological conditions and, since the capacity for reduction is limited, an increased rate of oxidation is generally accompanied by an increased methemoglobin level.

There are at least four biochemical mechanisms, or pathways, for the reduction of methemoglobin to hemoglobin in normal erythrocytes. The glycolytic system is the source of electrons for each. As shown in Figure 46, reduced nicotinamide adenine dinucleotide (NADH) is generated by the conversion of glyceraldehyde-3-P to 1,3-DPG. Although the formation of NADH in this step is coupled to the reduction of pyruvate to lactate, pyruvate can also diffuse out of the red cells and thus retain its electrons for other purposes. Another potential electron donor is reduced nicotinamide adenine dinucleotide phosphate (NADPH), which is formed in the pentose phosphate pathway (PPP). The relation of the PPP to the remainder of the glycolytic system is shown in Figure 49 (for further details, see Lionetti, 1974).

The rate of NADH formation through the glyceraldehyde-3-P→1,3-DPG step is between 2 and 3 mmol/liter of cells/hr. Since there are 20 mmol of heme/liter of cells, as much as 15% of them can

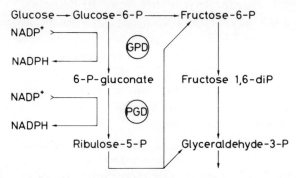

Figure 49. An outline of the relation between the pentose phosphate shunt and the glycolytic system. GPD, glucose-6-phosphate dehydrogenase. PGD, 6-phosphogluconate dehydrogenase.

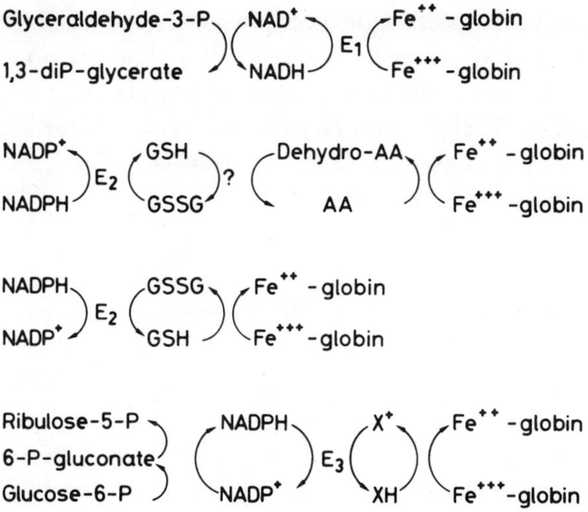

Figure 50. Metabolic pathways in human erythrocytes by which methemoglobin can be reduced to hemoglobin. E_1, NADH-methemoglobin reductase; E_2, oxidized glutation reductase; E_3, NADPH-dehydrogenase (methemoglobin reductase); AA, ascorbic acid (after Jaffé, 1974).

in principle be reduced by this mechanism hourly. This theoretical maximum far exceeds the rate required under physiological conditions, but the actual process is limited by the size of the pyruvate outflux relative to that of lactate.

Similarly, some 10% of the glucose molecules consumed under physiological conditions pass through the PPP. Thus the rate of NADPH formation is about 0.2 mmol/liter of cells/hr, which also exceeds the rate required for normal methemoglobin reduction.

The reduced coenzymes afford considerable chemical potential for the reduction of methemoglobin iron by a variety of mechanisms, as shown in Figure 50. Under physiological conditions, most of the electrons appear to derive from NADH, which can pass them on to cytochrome b_5 in a reaction catalyzed by cytochrome b_5 reductase. Apparently, reduced cytochrome b_5 can pass the electrons on further to iron atoms without catalysis. NADPH can reduce oxidized glutathion by way of a glutathion reductase, and the reduced glutathion can then reduce methemoglobin directly. In still another pathway, reduced glutathion promotes the conversion of dehyd-roascorbic acid to ascorbic acid. Finally, there is an NADPH-dependent methemoglobin reductase that can be very active in the presence of artificial electron carriers such as methylene blue. These last three pathways are not, however, believed to be of significance under physiological conditions.

The –SH Groups

Most proteins contain free sulfhydryl groups, and proper function is usually contingent upon their remaining free. Hemoglobin contains six –SH groups per tetramer, two in each β chain, and one in each α chain. Of these, only the F9β residues are titratable, and they are situated quite close to the heme groups. When such –SH groups are oxidized, the bonds joining heme and globin are weakened to the extent of possible cleavage. Loss of heme makes globin much more prone to denaturation.

Hemoglobin, enzymes, and red cell membrane proteins are all protected from sulfhydryl oxidation by a specific glutathion (GSSG) reductase, which receives electrons from NADPH. Reduced glutathion acts as an oxidation–reduction buffer by reacting with oxidants and thus sparing the more important protein –SH groups. The reaction of reduced glutathion with organic peroxides, e.g., fatty acids, is catalyzed by an enzyme, GSH peroxidase, which also catalyzes the breakdown of hydrogen peroxide.

Disturbances of the Respiratory Functions of Blood

The functions of the integrated gas transport system are to ensure that O_2 supply to tissue be in accord with metabolic demand, and that absorption of the CO_2 thereby produced serve to maintain tissue pCO_2 and pH within given ranges. Any perturbation of a system property that works against the fulfillment of these requirements may be regarded as a disturbance of transport system function.

Several key transport system parameters are properties of the blood (see Figure 45), among them the concentration of hemoglobin and the various determinants of its affinity toward O_2, CO_2, and protons. A deviation of any of these parameters from normal may be regarded as a disturbance of *blood* respiratory function.

The first to describe disturbances of blood respiratory function in terms of its altered oxygen affinity was K. A. Hasselbalch, who studied the blood from eight patients in 1917. There is an interesting background to his investigation, as is brought out by the following passage from a paper by Astrup (1969):

> Hasselbalch's studies were initiated by reports from Barcroft's laboratory where Peters had found a straight-lined correlation between the negative logarithm of the binding constant K in Hill's equation and the pH of a blood sample, and this fact was then used in Barcroft's laboratory to calculate the pH of a

blood sample by determining the K-value from corresponding oxygen saturation and oxygen tension values. Peters and Barcroft then supposed that the position of the oxyhemoglobin dissociation curve was constant. To Hasselbalch it seemed awkward to determine the pH of the blood in this way, and he writes: "Ich vermute, dass künftig jedermann, der die Reaktion des Blutes bestimmen will, die CO_2-Bindung und nicht die O_2-Bindung desselben dafür verwertet wird." And as he did not believe that the straight line in Peters–Barcroft's curve had a constant position, he investigated 6 normal persons, but "zu meiner Uberraschung" found lines very similar to the Peters–Barcroft curve. However, Hasselbalch was not a man who gave up a fight when he was convinced that his opinion on a subject was the right one. He began to study patients. In 3 of 8 patients, the position of the dissociation curve was normal, but the other cases had abnormal positions. One of the patients had pernicious anemia, with a hemoglobin concentration 25% of the normal value, and here he found a displacement of the curve to the right. In a patient with uremia, Hasselbalch found the curve displaced to the left, T_{50} was changed to approximately 23 mm Hg. More pronounced changes were found in blood from a patient with diabetic coma and from a patient with gout. The T_{50} values were approximately 22 and 21 mm Hg, respectively.

There is often no problem in identifying clinical conditions of very severe discrepancy between tissue demand and gas transport capacity. However, in the vast majority of clinical conditions in which a disturbance in gas transport function is suspected on the basis of indirect observation and educated guesswork, corroborative proof is not obtained. The difficulty is that there are no simple measurements by which abnormal tissue metabolism, due to inadequate oxygen delivery or carbon dioxide removal, can be quantitated. This does not preclude the description of a subject with, say, chronic pulmonary emphysema and arterial pO_2 of 40 mm Hg, in terms of hypoxia. It implies, however, that since there is no simple way of measuring the degree of tissue hypoxia, there is also no definite way of knowing which symptoms and signs relate directly to tissue hypoxia and to what degree, and which relate to the effort of the body to compensate for the primary disturbance or accompanying abnormalities.

One way to come to grips with this situation is to define tissue hypoxia in terms of readily observable quantities known to be closely associated with the performance of the gas transport system. One might, for instance, agree to consider deviations from normal values of cardiac output, arterial pO_2, or hemoglobin concentration as quantitative measures of tissue hypoxia. Such reasoning underlies the definition and evaluation of various types of hypoxia encountered in clinical medicine: stagnant hypoxia due to impaired blood flow, hypoxic and anemic hypoxia due, respectively, to decreases in arterial pO_2 and hemoglobin concentration. Although such conventions have the advantage of clear definition and observability, they are not likely to be of much general value. There are two main problems. The first is the complexity of the relations between the different subsystem outputs, i.e., cardiac output, arterial pO_2, hemoglobin concentration, etc., and the total output of the gas transport system. Because of this, the effect of a perturbation of one subsystem output upon overall performance is not easily predicted. The second, more serious problem is that the operation of compensatory feedback loops makes it very difficult if not impossible to maintain that an observed abnormality in one or more subsystem outputs must be associated with a corresponding abnormality of total performance.

At this stage, we may well question the logic of dealing with readily observable quantities only, while continuing to define hypoxia in terms of what actually occurs in the tissues. This question is clearly of importance and actually concerns whether or not present knowledge in physiology can be profitably applied to clinical medicine. Its answer appears, though, to be affirmative to the extent that the two main obstacles mentioned above can be overcome. A practical solution is to simulate a model of the real system along the lines of that which we have developed and detailed in Chapters 3 and 6. Such a model translates available information into a description of the relationship between tissue metabolism and total gas transport system function. To the extent that what is derived from it is representative of what occurs *in vivo*, the model may be employed to derive quantitative information on the contributions of *measurable* subsystem outputs to the overall function of serving the tissues.

The results of simulations of abnormal conditions are presented here, as in Figure 40, in the form of plots of the flow of blood necessary to ensure the required supply of oxygen to tissue *versus* the values of other key parameters. The choice of blood flow as an indicator of disturbed gas transport function, albeit arbitrarily made, is attractive in that the circulation is the paramount energy consumer of the total system of gas transport. Except as otherwise noted, the metabolic rate and average radius of tissue supplied by the representative capillary are identical to those assumed in Chapter 6 for normal resting conditions. The same is true of the hematocrit, blood base excess, and arterial gas tensions, etc., except when an abnormality of one or more of these parameters is the disturbance in question.

While factors such as the whole blood hemoglobin and erythrocyte 2,3-DPG levels, base excess, and arterial gas tensions may in principle vary independently, the greater number of combinations are eliminated in the true-life system through constraints imposed by feedback systems of the like described in Chapter 7. Bearing this in mind, we take frequent account of the coupling between variables observed in a large number of clinical and experimental situations.

For purposes of exposition, it is necessary to classify the disturbances of the respiratory functions of the blood. While perhaps the most logical means of doing so would derive from a systems analysis of the integrated entity shown in Figure 45, our choice is a compromise that places the disturbances due to abnormalities of acid–base balance, erythron function, and lung function in a more clinical perspective. Because of our analytical approach, disturbances of circulatory function are not discussed in a separate section. However, the figures indicating calculated changes in cardiac output (local blood flow) needed to compensate for a disturbance in one or another subsystem may equally well be interpreted as implying the possible responses of the latter subsystems to a disturbance of the cardiovascular system.

Abnormal Acid–Base Balance

General Discussion and Results

Disturbances in the acid–base balance of the blood are generally followed by changes in its gas transport function. The mechanisms underlying these alterations were detailed in the previous chapters and may be summarized as follows: Perturbations in plasma hydrogen ion activity are accompanied by similar changes in the erythrocytes. The changes in red cell pH modify hemoglobin oxygen affinity through the Bohr effect and also induce changes in red cell 2,3-DPG concentration, $[DPG]_T$. The latter in turn (1) directly affect hemoglobin oxygen affinity and (2) cause a readjustment of the ratio of the cellular and plasma proton activities and thereby an additional, indirect effect on O_2 affinity. Furthermore, both the erythrocyte buffer capacity and oxygen-linked proton binding to hemoglobin are pH and $[DPG]_T$ dependent.

Disturbances in blood acid–base balance may not be the clinically most important cause of impaired blood gas transport. However, accumulating evidence suggests that in the great majority of clinical situations where hypoxia is present or suspected, there are associated changes in the acid–base status of the blood. It is therefore convenient to start with an analysis of the effect of primary disturbances of the acid–base status of the blood on its respiratory function.

From a purely physicochemical point of view, the effects of abnormal acid–base balance on blood gas transport can be directly related to altered proton and 2,3-DPG activities in red cell water. Plots of required blood flow vs. the respective activities of these species might therefore appear to be the most straightforward demonstration of those effects. On the other hand, from a physiological point of view, changes in proton activity should be regarded as *results* of physiological perturbations that are more fundamental, as it were, and more directly related to diseased states.

Thus, it would seem more realistic to consider the red cell hydrogen activity in light of (1) the partial pressure of carbon dioxide in arterial blood, which is typically a result of lung function, and (2) blood base excess, which is typically a result of metabolic processes. Fortunately, the dependence of proton activity upon pCO_2 and base excess may be derived on the basis of available data (see Chapter 5).

Results of Simulations. A plot of required blood flow at rest vs. base excess for a number of $[DPG]_T$ values and normal hemoglobin concentration and arterial gas tensions is shown in Figure 51. Included are loci of constant average pH^c, which is simply the arithmetic average of the respective values at the capillary's entrance and exit (see Chapter 6). Further details from the simulations of these states are listed in Table XIV.

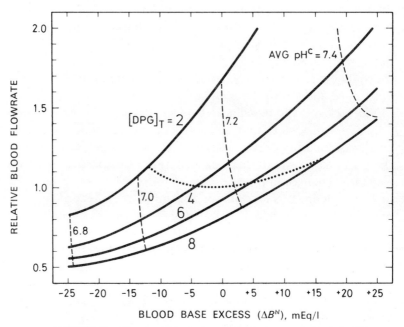

Figure 51. Theoretically required blood flowrate at rest (normalized to the base case value for normal blood) as a function of blood base excess and erythrocyte 2,3-DPG level. Arterial gas tensions and hematocrit normal. Broken curves are loci of constant time-averaged red cell pH. Dotted curve is locus of conditions in which averaged pH^c and $[DPG]_T$ are in agreement.

Table XIV

Details from Simulations of Gas Exchange at Rest with Abnormal Blood Acid–Base Status [a]

ΔB^{bl} (meq/ liter)	$[DPG]_T$	$\overline{pH}^{pl}$	$\overline{pH}^c$	$\overline{p(50)}$	pO_2^v	$\bar{O}_2^a$	$\bar{O}_2^v$	Q_{rel}
−25	2	6.889	6.787	29.8	32.2	95.4	53.0	0.83
	4	6.917	6.793	37.9	30.4	92.9	36.9	0.63
	6	6.946	6.794	43.4	28.7	90.9	26.9	0.55
	8	6.975	6.787	47.7	27.1	89.3	19.8	0.51
−12.5	2	7.158	7.017	25.4	34.9	97.9	66.4	1.11
	4	7.176	7.013	31.7	34.1	96.5	52.6	0.80
	6	7.200	7.008	35.7	33.1	95.5	43.2	0.68
	8	7.223	7.000	38.8	32.2	94.5	36.2	0.61
0	2	7.376	7.203	21.5	36.3	98.9	78.8	1.70
	4	7.388	7.187	26.5	35.6	98.1	67.0	1.10
	6	7.405	7.179	29.7	35.6	97.5	60.0	0.92
	8	7.425	7.165	31.9	34.9	96.9	53.9	0.80
12.5	2	7.552	7.348	18.8	36.4	99.3	84.8	2.40
	4	7.558	7.333	22.8	36.0	98.8	76.5	1.57
	6	7.572	7.313	25.4	35.8	98.3	70.5	1.26
	8	7.589	7.294	27.2	35.5	97.9	66.2	1.10
25	2	7.695	7.462	17.1	36.6	99.5	87.9	3.02
	4	7.698	7.444	20.5	36.3	99.1	81.6	2.00
	6	7.707	7.420	22.7	36.0	98.7	76.9	1.60
	8	7.723	7.396	24.2	35.9	98.4	73.7	1.42

[a] Q_{rel} is calculated blood flowrate relative to that for normal $[DPG]_T$ (5 mM) and base excess ($\Delta B^{bl} = 0$). Overbars denote average of arterial and venous values.

The results show that changes in blood base excess, at constant red cell 2,3-DPG concentration, profoundly affect the oxygen transport properties of the blood. Thus, in order to maintain the oxygen consumption of the model tissue when the base excess increases from, say, −15 to +15 meq/liter, the blood flow must double in the absence of additional compensations. Furthermore, the data show the effect of changes in $[DPG]_T$; the relative effect is, at least in nonalkalotic conditions, rather insensitive to the value of ΔB^{bl} and corresponds to a reduction in blood flow by a factor of about 2 for an increase of $[DPG]_T$ from 2 to 8 mmol/liter. Because of the extremes of alkalosis simulated in these runs, it was found that carbamate compounds are responsible for up to 15% of CO_2 transport by the blood.

The data contained in Figure 51 and Table XIV cover theoretically possible combinations of perturbed variables in primary metabolic acid–base disturbances with normal hemoglobin concentration and arterial gas tensions. More relevant physiological and pathophysiological information can be extracted from such data when one views them in light of the rather strong coupling under steady-state conditions *in vivo* between red cell 2,3-DPG concentration and both the time-averaged red cell pH and hemoglobin oxygen saturation. Moreover, changes in plasma pH are likely to influence pulmonary ventilation and thereby the arterial gas tensions. Regardless of their exact cause-and-effect nature, the very existence of such interactions imposes important restrictions on the variability of the parameters in real-life situations.

The effects of changes in pulmonary ventilation on blood gas transport function are discussed in more detail in a later section. Here we illustrate particular cases in which moderate abnormalities in metabolic acid–base balance are partially pH compensated by such changes. Figure 52 shows the calculated results when a simulated metabolic acidosis is offset to a degree by ventilation increases that lower arterial pCO_2 to values of 30 and 20 mm Hg, respectively, and when a metabolic alkalosis is partly compensated by decreases in ventilation that raise pCO_2^a to 50 and 60 mm Hg, respectively. The simultaneous changes in arterial pO_2 induced by these ventilatory adjustments are also indicated.

The tendency toward normalization of plasma pH through ventilation is seen generally to increase the blood flow demand. In the cases of (metabolic) acidosis, this is due to the adverse effect of (respiratory) alkalosis, while in the (metabolically) alkalotic cases, the explanation is the decrease in arterial pO_2. It is particularly clear from the figure that subjects with metabolic alkalosis, low red cell 2,3-DPG content, and depressed ventilation (e.g., patients with severe trauma who have received large transfusions of stored blood, are on morphine, and have an alkalosis due to vomiting) must—in the absence of additional compensations such as capillary

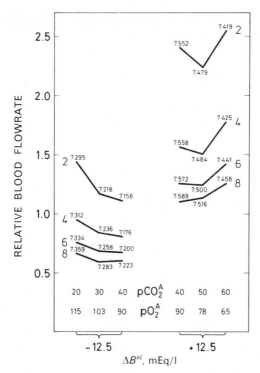

Figure 52. Required blood flow rate at rest (normalized to the base case value for normal blood), with positive and negative base excess, as a function of red cell 2,3-DPG level (2, 4, 6 and 8 mM) and coupled arterial gas tensions. Time-averaged plasma pH indicated at the three discrete points for each ΔB^{bl}–$[DPG]_T$ pair.

recruitment—increase their blood flow quite considerably in order to ensure sufficient tissue oxygenation.

The in Vivo Dependence of Red Cell 2,3-DPG Level, $[DPG]_T$, upon pH and Hemoglobin Oxygen Saturation

In the previous chapter, we outlined mechanisms by which the hydrogen ion activity and state of hemoglobin oxygenation are thought to influence $[DPG]_T$. The pioneering observations with respect to the pH dependence were made by Rapoport and Guest (1939; see also Guest and Rapoport, 1941), who measured the erythrocyte concentrations of acid-soluble phosphorus compounds in experimental rickets, renal insufficiency, pyloric obstruction, gastroenteritis, ammonium chloride acidosis, and diabetic acidosis.

Empirically obtained expressions for the dependence of erythrocyte 2,3-DPG level upon steady-state values of pH and hemoglobin oxygenation are summarized in Table XV. We have presented the data as the average effective slopes of plots of $[DPG]_T$ vs. pH^c or $\bar{O}_2$, i.e., $\Delta[DPG]_T/\Delta pH^c$ or $\Delta[DPG]_T/\Delta\bar{O}_2$. For cases in which the data were obtained from *in vivo* measurements, and where it was possible to do so, we have used the time-averaged pH^c and $\bar{O}_2$ values in the circulating blood (i.e., the weighted averages of arterial and venous values). In addition, wherever it was possible to isolate organic phosphate changes due solely to changes in pH or $\bar{O}_2$, we have reported the data as such. Furthermore, the original data in several cases were reported in terms of plasma rather than erythrocyte pH values, and we have therefore taken the liberty of transforming such data. To do so, we have simply divided the $\Delta[DPG]_T/\Delta pH^{pl}$ values by a constant η value of 0.8. Rigorously speaking, the correction factor is a variable containing terms other than η alone. However, it can be surmised from the data in Table XII that, for the range of $[DPG]_T$ values encountered under most

Table XV

Slopes of Linear Fits to Empirical Correlations of Red Cell 2,3-DPG Concentration with Average Steady State Red Cell pH and Hemoglobin O_2 Saturation, Both in vitro and in vivo

$\dfrac{\Delta[DPG]_T}{\Delta pH^c}$	$\left(\dfrac{\Delta[DPG]_T}{\Delta pH^c}\right)_{\bar{O}_2}$	$-\left(\dfrac{\Delta[DPG]_T}{\Delta\bar{O}_2}\right)_{pH^c}$	Ref.[a]
	10	0.3	1
20			2
20			3
28			4
33–38			5
13	10	2	6
23			7
15			8
20			9
29		2	10

[a]See text.

pathophysiological conditions investigated here, i.e., between 2 and 8 mM, the approximation is small, if not negligible, by comparison with the scatter of the data presented in Table XV.

1. Rörth (1970) measured red cell 2,3-DPG levels once a steady state had been established during *in vitro* incubation of whole blood at various pH values, at both $pO_2 = 0$ and 100 mm Hg. The values in Table XV were calculated from his data points for plasma pH values between 7.0 and 7.5, using a value of 0.032 for $\Delta pH^c(d-0)$ (see Table XI). Above $pH^{pl} = 7.5$, the coefficient $\Delta[DPG]_T/\Delta pH^c$ at constant $\bar{O}_2$ showed a marked decrease, possibly because of substrate limitation.

2. Astrup *et al.* (1970) measured red cell 2,3-DPG concentrations and pH in a number of nonanemic subjects with acid–base disturbances. The value in column 1 of the table is taken from their data points by inspection.

3. Bellingham *et al.* (1970) observed red cell 2,3-DPG levels and plasma pH in subjects administered either acid or base. The value in column 1 in the table is derived from that portion of their figure where a steady state had been reached.

4. Rörth and Bille-Brahe (1971) measured red cell 2,3-DPG and plasma pH in normal pregnant woman.

5. Versmold *et al.* (1973) obtained values of red cell pH and 2,3-DPG concentration in normal infants and children. The values in column 1 are slopes of the respective regression lines for (1) infants and children more than 8 months of age, and (2) infants of 2 days and less.

6. Lichtman *et al.* (1974*a*) observed several blood parameters in a study of myocardial infarction. The value in column 1 of the table is that obtained from the slope of their regression equation of 2,3-DPG level on arterial pH (arterial and venous pH^{pl} were nearly identical in their subjects). The values in columns 2 and 3 are taken from the multiple regression equation given by the authors.

7. Lichtman *et al.* (1974*c*) observed red cell 2,3-DPG levels and plasma pH in normal and anemic subjects. The value in the table is derived from the slope of their regression line of 2,3-DPG vs. plasma pH. Conversion of 2,3-DPG concentrations per weight of hemoglobin to the same values per volume of cells were made on the basis of the following relation between hemoglobin concentration and hematocrit: c_{Hb} (g/liter) $= 4.02PCV - 30.2$ ($PCV = 100h$).

8. Hamasaki (1974) observed red cell 2,3-DPG levels and plasma pH in subjects with respiratory insufficiency. In a subsample of subjects with arterial pH values between 7.35 and 7.45, and hematocrit above 35%, there was a clear-cut negative correlation between red cell 2,3-DPG level and arterial pO_2 to the extent that the former decreased from 6 mM at $pO_2^a = 40$ mm Hg to 4.5 mM at 100 mm Hg. This finding is difficult to evaluate in terms of time-averaged oxygen saturation, but appears to be consistent with the notion of a nonzero value of $\Delta[DPG]_T/\Delta\bar{O}_2$ at constant erythrocyte pH.

9. Vanuxem *et al.* (1975) measured pH^c and $[DPG]_T$ in a large number of subjects suffering from chronic respiratory insufficiency and hypoxia. The value in the table was obtained by inspection of their data points.

10. Versmold *et al.* (1976) determined pH^c and $[DPG]_T$ in infants with acyanotic heart disease and arterial oxygen saturations greater than 90%. The value in column 1 of the table is the slope of their regression line. They also measured the same parameters in children with cyanotic heart disease and an arterial oxygen saturation between 25 and 75%. The value in column 3 was obtained by inspection of the data points for these children.

Tweeddale *et al.* (1977) measured plasma pH and red cell 2,3-DPG levels as well as $\bar{O}_2^a$ in twenty subjects with chronic respiratory failure. Their regression of $[DPG]_T$ on pH^{pl} and $\bar{O}_2^a$ was (personal communication)

$$[DPG]_T = 13.5pH^{pl} - 5.1\bar{O}_2^a - 90$$

Keitt *et al.* (1974) found no significant correlation between $[DPG]_T$ and arterial pH^{pl} in 12 patients with chronic obstructive pulmonary disease, but a significant correlation between $[DPG]_T$ and pO_2^a. They did, however, make the further observation that when these patients were made acutely hypoxemic by withdrawal of supplemental oxygen, the increase in arterial pH was closely associated with an increase in $[DPG]_T$.

The values in columns 1 and 3 in Table XV differ rather considerably, but the discrepancies may be but apparent. First, non-steady-state conditions may have prevailed in many of the subjects within the various studies. Second, several of the values were obtained from regression lines calculated on the assumption of error in the dependent variable only. Third, the coefficients of correlation are rather low, between 0.5 and 0.8, and one is therefore led to suspect the influence of additional factors. An important observation in this respect is one of Versmold *et al.* (1973) that has not been included in the table. They found that the red cell 2,3-DPG level, at a given erythrocyte pH, is about 2 mM larger in infants between 3 and 9 days of age than in younger or older infants. This observation, as well as the difference between values of $\Delta[\text{DPG}]_T/\Delta\bar{\text{O}}_2$ at constant pH^c obtained from *in vitro* and *in vivo* studies, is seemingly impossible to account for without resort to other important factors (see p. 195).

Of the several factors besides pH^c and $\bar{\text{O}}_2$ that are known to influence $[\text{DPG}]_T$, i.e., phosphate and ammonium ions, inosine, and the pyruvate–lactate ratio, the first two have been shown to be clinically important and are pursued in more detail in the following section (p. 239). The relatively large variations about the regressions of erythrocyte 2,3-DPG level both upon pH^c at constant time-averaged $\bar{\text{O}}_2$ and upon the latter at constant pH^c are thus largely explicable by random experimental error and variations in red cell inorganic phosphate and ammonium ion concentrations. Whether or not still other factors play significant roles remains to be ascertained.

Constrained relationships. If we assume a value for $\Delta[\text{DPG}]_T/\Delta\text{pH}^c$ of 20 mM/pH unit, and combine this with normal $[\text{DPG}]_T$ and pH^c values of 5 mM and 7.185, then the dotted curve in Figure 51 may be taken to describe a "constrained relationship" between relative blood flowrate and whole blood base excess. Inasmuch as the curve straddles the unity ordinate value, *we conclude that perturbations in blood O_2 transport associated with the sort of base excess changes depicted are effectively nullified by the response of $[DPG]_T$ to pH alteration.* These same calculated results are replotted in Figure 53 to show more explicitly the changes in $[\text{DPG}]_T$ required to offset metabolic acid–base disturbances.

The half-time for response of red cell 2,3-DPG to perturbations of acid–base status is on the order of $\frac{1}{2}$–1 day (see p. 194). Thus,

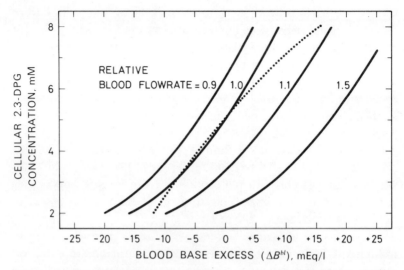

Figure 53. Theoretical results of Figure 51 replotted as curves of $[DPG]_T$ vs. ΔB^{bl} at constant relative blood flowrate. Dotted curve again indicative of cases in which $[DPG]_T$ and pH^c are in agreement.

deviations from the dotted lines in Figures 51 and 53 may be expected to occur frequently in clinical practice.

Abnormal Erythron Function

The term erythron function is used here to cover two aspects of respiratory function that are characteristic of the circulating blood: the whole blood hemoglobin concentration (c_{Hb}) and the oxygen affinity of the hemoglobin, which one measures at fixed levels of pH and pCO_2. Abnormalities of the first aspect of erythron function include anemia and polycythemia, while those with respect to the second include the so-called abnormal hemoglobins, abnormal red cell 2,3-DPG and other organic phosphate concentrations not attributable to acid–base disturbance, and finally abnormal concentrations of carbon monoxide hemoglobin and methemoglobin. In a related vein, red cells stored for transfusion may undergo changes that are not related to the above-mentioned functions but nevertheless impair blood gas transport function.

Anemia

A decrease in hemoglobin concentration, other factors remaining unchanged, requires an increase in blood flowrate to the extent governed by a simple hyperbolic relationship between the two variables. With normal arterial gas tensions, the theoretical influence of red cell 2,3-DPG concentration on such flow requirements is as shown in Figure 54 (see also Table XVI). The relative effects are seen to be largely independent of hematocrit in the range 15–45%; the limited spread at the extremes of $[DPG]_T$ is due to a hematocrit-related dependence of pH^c upon the 2,3-DPG concentration [see equation (5-45)].

As was the case with changing blood base excess, important constraints govern the variations of red cell pH and $[DPG]_T$ with changes in steady-state *in vivo* whole blood hemoglobin concentration. Besides the dependence of $[DPG]_T$ on time-averaged pH^c and $\bar{O}_2$ (as reviewed in the section on acid–base disturbances and quantitated in Table XV), both the red cell pH and 2,3-DPG levels are correlated with c_{Hb}.

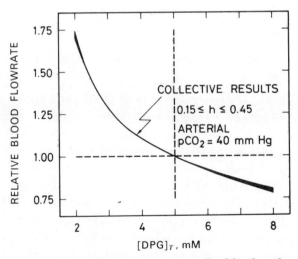

Figure 54. Required blood flowrate at rest (normalized by the value *at the same hematocrit*, but with $[DPG]_T = 5$ mM) as a function of red cell 2,3-DPG concentration. Arterial gas tensions and blood base excess are normal. Results at different hematocrit levels are superimposed.

Table XVI

Effect of Changes in Red Cell 2,3-DPG Level on Hemoglobin Flow Requirements in Anemia[a]

Hematocrit fraction	$[DPG]_T$ (mM)	$\overline{p(50)}$ (mm Hg)	pO_2^v (mm Hg)	$\overline{pH}^c$	Q_{rel}^b
0.15	2	21.1	36.2	7.219	1.75
0.15	4	26.2	35.4	7.203	1.11
0.15	6	29.5	35.4	7.182	0.92
0.15	8	32.1	34.7	7.160	0.78
0.25	2	21.2	36.2	7.213	1.74
0.25	4	26.3	35.7	7.198	1.10
0.25	6	29.7	35.5	7.179	0.92
0.25	8	32.2	34.8	7.159	0.79
0.35	2	21.4	36.3	7.208	1.72
0.35	4	26.4	35.5	7.189	1.10
0.35	6	29.7	35.5	7.179	0.92
0.35	8	32.1	34.9	7.161	0.79
0.45	2	21.5	36.3	7.203	1.70
0.45	4	26.5	35.6	7.187	1.10
0.45	6	29.7	35.6	7.179	0.92
0.45	8	31.9	34.9	7.165	0.80

[a] $pO_2^a = 90$ mm Hg, $HpCO_2^a = 40$ mm Hg. Overbar denotes average of venous and arterial quantities.
[b] Blood flowrate normalized by value *at same hematocrit* with $[DPG]_T = 5$ mM.

The Empirical Correlation between Red Cell pH and Whole Blood Hemoglobin Concentration. The pH of capillary blood is 0.01–0.02 units higher in female than in male subjects under normal resting conditions (Shock and Hastings, 1934; Ipbüker *et al.*, 1973; Siggaard-Andersen, 1974). Furthermore, arterial and capillary CO_2 tensions are about 3 mm Hg greater in men (see Siggaard-Andersen, 1974), and the difference in pH therefore appears to be due to a difference in pulmonary ventilation. The connection between intersexual differences in arterial pCO_2 or pH and in c_{Hb} is not known, but, in light of similarities to the correlations found in anemia (see below), it may well be causal.

Subjects with anemia generally have a lower arterial pCO_2 than normal individuals. The relation between pCO_2^a and c_{Hb} is without doubt greatly dependent upon the subjects' physical activity. At rest, though, it approximates a straight line of slope 15 mm Hg per 100 g/liter (Möller, 1959; Housley, 1967; Lichtman, personal communication) which is consistent with the ~3 mm Hg difference between normal male and female subjects, whose c_{Hb} values differ by ~20 g/liter. Moreover, the variations are recorded together with 0.06–0.10 unit arterial pH^{pl} increases per 100 g/liter decrease of c_{Hb} (Möller, 1959; Housley, 1967) and a similar behavior of venous pH^{pl} (Lichtman, personal communication).

The clear-cut association between plasma pH and whole blood hemoglobin concentration is highly consequential in regard to the clarification of several aspects of whole blood oxygen affinity in anemia. First, it offers a causal explanation for the well-established correlation of $[DPG]_T$ and c_{Hb}; this is discussed in the section immediately following. Second, it suggests a framework for a definitive hypothesis concerning the role of 2,3-DPG in the regulation of blood oxygen affinity over and above that already discussed in relation to blood base excess. This aspect is discussed in detail later in this chapter.

The in Vivo Relation between Red Cell 2,3-DPG Concentration and Whole Blood Hemoglobin Concentration. A highly significant, negative correlation between red cell 2,3-DPG and whole blood hemoglobin levels has been established by several studies of groups of normal and anemic subjects, the first by Eaton and Brewer (1968). The pioneering observation was made by Maizels and Paterson (1937): "In the erythrocyte, part of the cation is combined with Cl^- and HCO_3^- and the rest, about one-third of the total, is combined with Hb^- and X^-. The latter consists of unknown and probably complex ions, which in normal cells bind nearly as much base as does Hb^- and which in anemic cells bind nearly twice as much."

Table XVII summarizes representative data, more detailed and quantitative evaluation of which is precluded by the lack of information concerning individual subjects. Lichtman *et al.* (1974c) and Ninness *et al.* (1974) have, for example, pointed out that the $[DPG]_T$–c_{Hb} relationship in anemic subjects with *uremia* is very different.

Since experimental errors in 2,3-DPG and whole blood hemoglobin determinations are rather small, the relatively low correlation

Table XVII

Relation between Red Cell 2,3-DPG and Whole Blood Hemoglobin Concentration under Normal and Different Anemic Conditions

Regression equation $[DPG]_T$ (mM) $= a - bc_{Hb}$ (g/liter)	Sex	c_{Hb} range	r^a
$13.5-0.064c_{Hb}$	M	120–150	0.65^b
$11.1-0.052c_{Hb}$	F	110–145	0.61^b
$8.9-0.028c_{Hb}$	M,F	40–170	0.76^c
$7.9-0.027c_{Hb}$	M,F	40–160	0.90^d
$8.7-0.024c_{Hb}$	M	50–170	0.65^e
$9.2-0.029c_{Hb}$	F	40–140	0.65^e
$9.2-0.032c_{Hb}$	F	70–160	0.71^f

[a] Coefficient of correlation.
[b] Hjelm (1969): apparently healthy subjects.
[c] Lichtman *et al.* (1974c): apparently healthy subjects and hypoproliferative anemia.
[d] Ninnes *et al.* (1974): nonuremic anemia.
[e] Torrance *et al.* (1970): anemic subjects, including uremia.
[f] Hjelm and Wadman (1974): apparently healthy subjects and iron deficiency anemia (see also Slawsky and Desforges, 1972).

coefficients found in most investigations must be due to extraneous factors, presumably pH and those factors discussed in regard to $[DPG]_T$–pH^c correlations, i.e., hemoglobin O_2 saturation and the concentrations of phosphate and ammonium ions.

In view of the dependence of red cell 2,3-DPG concentration upon red cell pH and of plasma pH upon whole blood hemoglobin concentration, the demonstrated relationship between $[DPG]_T$ and c_{Hb} is most likely ascribable to the common variable pH. In fact, the 15–30 mM change of $[DPG]_T$ per unit change in pH^c plus the 0.06–0.10 unit pH^c change per 100 g/liter c_{Hb} difference requires an increase in red cell 2,3-DPG concentration of 1 to 3 mM for a decrease in the hemoglobin concentration of 100 g/liter. This range just meets the lower limit of the values indicated in Table XVII, which again points to the involvement of other factors in the regulation of $[DPG]_T$ in anemia. Though a precise statement of the relative contributions of all such factors is impossible at this stage, available data do appear to justify the conclusion that red cell pH is the most important.

Compensatory Responses in Anemia. Figure 55 and Table XVIII contain the results of simulated gas exchange in anemia when pulmonary ventilation and hematocrit are assumed to be coupled so as to engender the arterial pCO_2–hematocrit correlation described in the preceding section. The solid curves again depict results for freely varying $[DPG]_T$, while the dotted curve is for the coupling of $[DPG]_T$ to pH^c. The results have been normalized in such a fashion as to essentially eliminate the direct effect upon flow requirements of a change in hematocrit *per se*. As such, the rise in relative flow requirement with progressive anemia (solid curves) is a consequence of the associated alkalosis. The response of red cell 2,3-DPG to the

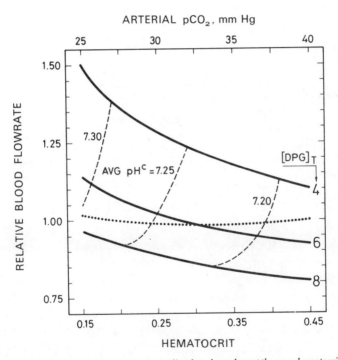

Figure 55. Required blood flowrate (normalized to the value *at the same hematocrit*, but with $[DPG]_T = 5$ mM and normal arterial gas tensions) as a function of red cell 2,3-DPG level and hematocrit. Arterial pCO_2 coupled to hematocrit as indicated (pCO_2^a and pO_2^a also coupled as listed in Table XVIII). Broken curves are loci of constant time-averaged erythrocyte pH. Dotted curve is locus of points at which $[DPG]_T$ and pH^c are in agreement.

Table XVIII

Effects of Changes in Red Cell 2,3-DPG Level on Hemoglobin Flow Requirements in Anemia, Where the Latter Has Induced Responses in pO_2^a and pCO_2^a [a]

$[DPG]_T$ (mM)	$\overline{pH^{pl}}$	$\overline{pH^c}$	$\overline{p(50)}$	pO_2^v	$\bar{O}_2^a$	$\bar{O}_2^v$	Q_{rel}^b
	Hematocrit $= 0.15$, $pCO_2^a = 25$ mm Hg, $pO_2^a = 109$ mm Hg						
2	7.555	7.350	17.4	35.8	99.7	86.1	2.47
4	7.558	7.332	21.9	35.3	99.5	77.2	1.51
6	7.563	7.307	24.9	34.8	99.2	69.9	1.14
8	7.569	7.281	27.3	31.9	99.0	64.1	0.96
	Hematocrit $= 0.25$, $pCO_2^a = 30$ mm Hg, $pO_2^a = 103$ mm Hg						
2	7.481	7.288	19.0	35.9	99.6	83.5	2.11
4	7.485	7.272	23.7	35.3	99.2	73.0	1.30
6	7.495	7.251	26.9	34.9	98.8	65.3	1.02
8	7.505	7.228	29.3	34.9	98.5	60.3	0.90
	Hematocrit $= 0.35$, $pCO_2^a = 35$ mm Hg, $pO_2^a = 96.3$ mm Hg						
2	7.422	7.240	20.3	36.0	99.3	81.1	1.87
4	7.430	7.226	25.2	35.5	98.8	69.7	1.18
6	7.444	7.209	28.4	35.3	98.3	62.4	0.96
8	7.459	7.191	30.8	34.9	97.8	56.6	0.84

[a] pO_2^a calculated from pCO_2^a and respiratory quotient, $q_R (= 0.8)$ according to $pO_2^a = 90 + (40 - pCO_2^a)/q_R$.

[b] Normalized by calculated blood flowrate *at same hematocrit* with normal $[DPG]_T$ (5 mM) and arterial gas tensions.

higher red cell pH—as in acid–base disturbance—is such that the oxygen affinity of the blood is restored to normal, and the same flowrate is therefore required (dotted curve) as calculated for the same hematocrit with normal $[DPG]_T$ and arterial gas tensions.

If we presume that the hypocapnia and/or associated alkalosis serve some purpose in anemic subjects, then the increase in red cell 2,3-DPG level can be regarded as a mechanism to ensure maintenance of the oxygen affinity within normal limits.

In light of the offsetting pH and $[DPG]_T$ effects, the only remaining means of compensation for anemia would seem to be increases in blood flow, tissue capillarization, or the efficiency of tissue metabolism. Though the first mechanism is a dear one in terms of energy usage, it is nonetheless highly appropriate inasmuch as it preserves the natural stimulus to the flow-independent ESF-producing system (see p. 201).

The question naturally arises as to the physiological significance of the respiratory alkalosis in anemia. With the last of the three just-mentioned compensatory mechanisms in mind, one might look for means by which more useful work—in the thermodynamic sense—might be derived per mole of oxygen consumed, i.e., the contents of the transfer function of Box XI in Figure 45. Although there is little experimental data to support these thoughts, a recent paper by Kogure *et al.* (1975) is worth mentioning. These workers showed that with equal steady-state energy reserves in rat brain tissue, the rate of high-energy phosphate use is lower during hypocapnia than in normocapnia. Furthermore, since the hypocapnic and normocapnic brain tissues retained their postdecapitation electroencephalogram patterns for equal periods, such data may well be construed as indicative of more efficient energy transduction of high-energy phosphates in hypocapnia. A similar effect of hypocapnic alkalosis on brain metabolism was also demonstrated by Hrbek *et al.* (1974). With arterial pO_2 values between 10 and 20 mm Hg, the somatosensory-evoked electroencephalogram responses in fetal lambs were markedly depressed at low arterial pH values but much less affected at higher pH.

Oxygen Affinity and Red Cell Age

The chemical composition of red cells varies with cell age (see review articles by Danon, 1968; Fornaini, 1967; and Hjelm, 1974). The oxygen affinity of whole blood containing an excessive fraction of young cells is lower than normal (Edwards and Rigas, 1967; Edwards *et al.*, 1971, 1972) while its 2,3-DPG content is normal. Removal of 250 to 750 ml of blood from normal subjects over a few weeks' time was found to induce a ~ 2 mm Hg increase of whole blood $p(50)$ without a change in $[DPG]_T$, but a significant increase in the red cell activity of glutamic oxalacetic transaminase (Edwards and Canon, 1972), a change known to be closely associated with red cell aging.

Recent work by Lichtman and Murphy (1975) has demonstrated that cells with an average age of 5 days have almost three times the mean concentration of 1 mM ATP, while those averaging 100 days old contain one-third the average. The effect of such variation in red cell ATP upon their oxygen affinity, particularly in light of the experiments of Edwards and Canon (1972), is not clear, nor is it likely to fully explain the observed effect.

Though the above-described findings await chemical and molecular interpretation, they do help to clarify the rather large variations in whole blood oxygen affinity—at standard pH^{pl} and $[DPG]_T$—among patients with clinical conditions that may differ considerably in average red cell age.

Kinetics of Oxygen Transfer in Red Cells with Increased Rigidity

Sirs (1969) found that red cells stored in ACD solution have impaired rates of oxygen egress and that the dissociation rates were well correlated with measures of red cell membrane flexibility. He therefore suggested that increased resistance to O_2 diffusion through the internal medium or red cell membrane might be the cause. Sirs also found that the impairment could be completely relieved by incubation of the stored red cells with adenosine at 37°C.

These studies are particularly interesting in view of the later demonstration by Weed and collaborators (Weed, 1970; Weed *et al.*, 1969; LaCelle and Weed, 1971) that red cell membrane flexibility is closely correlated with erythrocyte ATP content, and that decreased red cell lifetimes in many cases of hemolytic anemia are associated with decreases in red cell flexibility. The precise clinical significance of the phenomenon discovered by Sirs remains unclear, but it most likely provides at least partial explanation for the impaired oxygen transfer in stored red cells (see p. 243).

Polycythemia

Conditions characterized by an abnormally high level of whole blood hemoglobin concentration (c_{Hb}) are often called *polycythemic* and the term *primary polycythemia* is reserved for those with no obvious abnormality in blood oxygen affinity or pO_2^a, nor evidence of increased ESF production. In many cases, the increased hemoglobin level is associated with below normal arterial oxygen tension or above normal hemoglobin oxygen affinity, and the name *secondary polycythemia* is applied to them because the increase in c_{Hb} is a compensation, consistent with the model for its control shown in Figure 48. Secondary polycythemia may also result from an increase in plasma ESF in the absence of any decrease in blood O_2 release capacity.

In secondary polycythemia due to chronic respiratory insufficiency, the whole blood oxygen affinity *in vivo* is normal, as evidenced by the fact that the *in vivo* pO_2^a and oxygen saturation values obtained by Segel and Bishop (1966) fall within the normal limits of the standard oxygen binding curve (Table V).

The greater capacity of polycythemic blood to carry oxygen theoretically allows less blood flow to tissue. However, the greater viscosity of such blood should offset this effect (the latter increase is difficult to estimate because of its dependence upon the actual geometry of the vascular tree; see p. 20). There is good evidence to show that at least in cases of polycythemia *vera* uncomplicated by hypertension, cardiac work is unaffected by viscosity-induced elevations in intravascular pressure, since the latter are largely mitigated by the reduced vascular hindrance associated with an increased blood volume (Segel and Bishop, 1967).

Abnormal Hemoglobins

Abnormal hemoglobins may be defined as tetramers whose chemical structure differs from that of hemoglobin A. Thus the term abnormal may be applied to hemoglobin F and other hemoglobins present during embryonic and fetal life (whose respiratory functions have already been described; see p. 103) as well as HbA_2, HbA_{IA}, HbA_{IB}, and HbA_{IC} (see Table II). The most common abnormal hemoglobins differ with HbA in primary structure of the globin chains as a result of different genetic coding for amino acid assemblage. Others, present in the red blood cells of many individuals, are brought about by chemical modification of the existing structure and are therefore said to have "acquired" hemoglobin abnor-malities. Although a distinction between the two types of modification—genetic and chemical—makes little sense from a physiological point of view, it has certain advantages and so will be maintained here.

Abnormal hemoglobins may affect the respiratory functions of the blood in several ways. Some are unstable within the red cells and exhibit abnormal tetramer–tetramer interaction, globin denatura-tion and precipitation, or other related phenomena that tend to impair erythrocyte viability and often result in hemolytic anemia. Others have abnormal ligand binding properties. In view of the close relationship between hemoglobin structure and function it is not surprising to find molecules that exhibit both types of abnormality.

The discoveries of mutant hemoglobins and those with acquired abnormalities, and identification of their exact chemical makeup, three-dimensional structure, and functional behavior vis-a-vis ligands, are cornerstones in the elucidation of hemoglobin structure–function relationships. Accounts of these fascinating developments can be found in several reviews (Perutz and Lehman, 1968; Antonini and Brunori, 1971; Bunn, 1974; Nagel and Book-chin, 1974, 1975; Pulsinelli, 1974) and so will not be pursued here. The following section deals primarily instead with the consequences of the presence of abnormal hemoglobins for blood respiratory function.

A quantitative analysis of the effects of each abnormal hemoglo-bin upon blood gas transport—apart from the anemia so engendered—would be a rather difficult undertaking, given the lack of accurate O_2 binding data and interaction coefficients for blood with varying proportions of the respective abnormal hemoglobins and HbA. Measurements of $p(50)$, Hill's constant, 2,3-DPG, Bohr effect, etc., have generally been performed on very dilute solutions of the isolated hemoglobins and are therefore of questionable relevance (see p. 98). The same comment applies also to those measurements performed at temperatures and pH values far removed from the physiological. Thus, the available data do not, in general, allow the type of calculations performed in regard to blood containing hemoglobin A only. On the other hand, enough information is available to allow an approximate but meaningful analysis on the basis of principles applied previously in this book.

Mutant Hemoglobins. At the present, it appears that over 190 structurally different human hemoglobin variants have been reported. A recent catalog was prepared by Hunt and Dayhoff (1974), and an up-to-date list is maintained at the U.S. National Biomedical Research Foundation, Georgetown University Medical Center, Washington, D.C.

Mutant hemoglobins arise through errors in coding, which result in (1) single amino acid substitutions, (2) amino acid deletions, (3) improper termination of subunits, and (4) fusion and frame shift mutations. The great majority are of the first type.

All but a handful of the mutants produce minor if any clinical symptoms in the subjects harboring them, and this is because of the mutants' generally low concentrations compared to that of hemoglobin A, and/or a low degree of instability or ligand binding abnormality.

Mutant Hemoglobins Having High Oxygen Affinity. Nagel and Bookchin (1974; see also 1975) have listed 18 essentially stable mutants with high oxygen affinity and discussed the relation of their properties to their structure. Since the publication of their reviews, the following high affinity mutants have been discovered: Hb Deer–Lodge (β2His→Arg) (Bonaventure *et al.*, 1975), Hb Creteil (β89Ser→Asn) (Garel *et al.*, 1974), Hb Abruzzo (β143His→Arg) (Chiarioni *et al.*, 1974), Hb Syracuse (β143His→Pro) (Jensen *et al.*, 1975), Hb Andrew–Minneapolis (β144Lys→Asn), Hb Osler–Nancy (β145Tyr→Asp) (Charache *et al.*, 1975; Gracon *et al.*, 1975), Hb McKees–Rocks (β145Tyr→Term) (Winslow *et al.*, 1976), and Hb York (β 146His→Pro) (Bare *et al.*, 1976). A high oxygen affinity is also exhibited by many of the *unstable* hemoglobins (see below). However, the cause of abnormal function in most of these is rooted in instability rather than abnormal oxygen binding.

A striking feature of most mutants is a low Hill's constant, n, which indicates a low degree of cooperativity in oxygen binding (see p. 60). In fact, the values of 1.0 to 1.1 for Hb Yakima, Hb Syracuse, Hb Bethesda, and Hb McKees Rocks imply a nearly complete absence of cooperativity. The combination of low cooperativity and high oxygen affinity is most readily explained by destabilization of only the T quaternary structure of the mutant (see Chapter 4). In this extreme situation, the process is without cooperativity and characterized by a $p(50)$ equal to $1/K_R$, or ~ 1.5 mm Hg under physiological conditions. Such a high oxygen affinity is indeed found with many of the mutants, in particular those with alterations near the β-carboxyl terminus.

In most instances it has been possible to explain the high oxygen affinity and low cooperativity on molecular grounds (see, for example, the review by Nagel and Bookchin, 1974). The contact regions of the tetramer that are of particular importance for the $T \leftrightarrow R$ transition are the $\alpha_1\beta_2$ and $\beta_1\beta_2$ areas, and most of the mutants have substitutions in one of these. There are, however, questions still unanswered. Particularly interesting are the differences in cooperativity between Hb J Capetown and Hb Chesapeake, and between Hb Little Rock and Hb Syracuse, since both pairs have substitutions at the same residue. Likewise, many of the reported differences in the Bohr effect cannot readily be explained on the basis of present knowledge.

As pointed out by Bellingham (1972, 1974), the "survival" of mutants with the combination of a high oxygen affinity and low cooperativity can be explained on the basis of these oxygen transport properties. This will become evident below as we consider results from simulations of O_2 transport by these species.

Mutant Hemoglobins Having Low Oxygen Affinity. To date, three mutant hemoglobins have been identified whose primary functional abnormality is a reduced affinity for oxygen. They are Hb Kansas (Asn102$\beta \rightarrow$ Thr), which is also reported to have a normal Bohr effect, Hb Agenoni (Glu90$\beta \rightarrow$ Lys), and Hb Yoshizuka (Asn108$\beta \rightarrow Asp$), which has a low Bohr effect. In addition there are more or less unstable hemoglobins that also exhibit a low oxygen affinity, notably Hb Seattle (Ala76$\beta \rightarrow$ Glu) and Hb Peterborough (Val111$\beta \rightarrow$ Phe).

In oxygenated Hb Kansas the substituted threonine residue is incapable of forming the hydrogen bond across the $\alpha_1\beta_2$ interface normally made by asparagine. This protein's abnormally low oxygen affinity is therefore explained by destabilization of the R structure, in conformity with which its Hill's constant is 1.3. The molecular basis of the low oxygen affinity of the two other mutants has not yet been elucidated.

M-Hemoglobins. M-hemoglobins are mutants in which the oxidation–reduction equilibrium of the iron atoms is displaced toward the oxidation state to such an extent that discoloration (cyanosis) of the skin occurs. In the M-hemoglobins, each mutant globin chain (α or β) is characterized by an abnormal microenvironment about the heme moiety that promotes electron donation from the iron.

Table XIX lists characteristic data on the five M-mutants discovered to date. Given the oxidation–reduction state of their iron atoms, it is not surprising that the amino acid substitution in four of the species involves either histidine E7 or F8 (see Figures 5 and 11). The substituted glutamate residue in Hb Milwaukee occupies the sixth coordination position of the iron. All the M-hemoglobins have a low Hill constant, and three have a high oxygen affinity. It is probably significant that both α chain variants have a high oxygen affinity and low Bohr effect, while the two β variants with histidine replacement have a normal oxygen affinity and Bohr effect.

Unstable Hemoglobins. There are at least 39 structurally different mutant hemoglobins that are unstable in the environment of the red cell interior, and therefore decrease red cell viability so as to

Table XIX
Human M-Hemoglobins[a]

Mutant	Substitution	$p(50)$	n	Bohr effect
Hb M Boston	$\alpha 58$(E7)His $\rightarrow$ Tyr	Low	1.2	Low
Hb M Iwate	$\alpha 87$(F8)His $\rightarrow$ Tyr	Low	1.1	Low
Hb M Saskatoon	$\beta 63$(E7)His $\rightarrow$ Tyr	N	1.2	N
Hb M Milwaukee	$\beta 67$(E11)Val $\rightarrow$ Glu	Low	1.2	N
Hb M Hyde Park	$\beta 92$(F8)His $\rightarrow$ Tyr	N	1.3	N

[a] For references, see Nagel and Bookchin (1974).

cause hemolysis and anemia. Most of them are listed in the review by Nagel and Bookchin (1975). Their molecular and clinical pathology has been reviewed by White and Dacie (1971; see also Bunn, 1974).

The effect of unstable hemoglobins on blood gas transport depends mainly on the degree of anemia associated with them. This does not seem to be strongly related to the proportion of mutant in the cells, which may vary from a few percent in the cases of Hb Ann Arbor (Leu80α → Arg) and Hb Bibba (Leu136α → Pro) to about 40% with Hb BrynMawr (Phe85β → Ser) and Hb Toulouse (Lys66β → Glu). The blood oxygen affinity of subjects with unstable hemoglobins is well correlated with the relative number of reticulocytes in the circulation (see p. 227) and also with the proportion of mutant hemoglobin since several of them have been shown to have abnormal oxygen affinity.

Acquired Hemoglobin Abnormalities. Hemoglobin A_{IC}, one of the two "minor" components of normal adult blood (see Table I), is a hemoglobin A molecule to which hexose is bound by Shiff linkage at the N-terminal α-amino groups of the β chains. Its intrinsic oxygen affinity is normal (Steinmeier and Parkhurst, 1975), but, as might be expected (see p. 87), its 2,3-DPG affinity is not (Bunn and Briehl, 1970). This hemoglobin is present at above normal concentrations in subjects with diabetes mellitus (Rahbar, 1968; Trivelli *et al.*, 1971). The *in vivo* blood oxygen affinity in controlled diabetic subjects is, however, normal (Ditzel *et al.*, 1973; Arturson *et al.*, 1974c) because of the high 2,3-DPG level in their red cells (see p. 241), presumably a compensation for the increased amounts of HbA_{IC}.

Subjects on acetylsalicylic acid—aspirin—therapy have elevated levels of a minor hemoglobin component that has a lower isoelectric point than hemoglobin A and that comigrates in electrophoresis with HbA_{IB} (Bridges *et al.*, 1975). This component is a hemoglobin A molecule acetylated at the ε-amino groups of several lysine residues (Shamsuddin *et al.*, 1974), the α and β chains to roughly equal extents. The acetylated hemoglobin has only a slightly greater oxygen affinity (Bridges *et al.*, 1975) and, since it rarely amounts to more than 10% of the total hemoglobin present, this explains the normal oxygen affinity of blood hemolysates from subjects given even fairly large doses of aspirin.

Charache and Weatherall (1966) reported the presence of a minor hemoglobin with abnormal electrophoretic mobility in children with lead poisoning. Its nature and functional characteristics have not yet been determined.

Fetal blood contains, in addition to HbF ($\alpha_2\gamma_2$), a minor component, HbF^{acetyl}. This is an $\alpha_2\gamma_2$ tetramer acetylated at the NH$_2$-termini of the γ chains. It constitutes 15–20% of the total fetal hemoglobin, shows no oxygen-linked binding of 2,3-DPG (Bunn and Briehl, 1970), and forms less oxylabile carbamate than HbF (Bauer *et al.*, 1975).

Results of Simulations of Abnormal Oxygen Binding. As already pointed out, the gas transport function of blood containing abnormal hemoglobins may be abnormal for a number of reasons: anemia, abnormal acid–base balance, abnormal 2,3-DPG levels, etc. Here we focus upon those abnormalities in O_2 transport function that arise because of the shape of the associated binding curve and oxygen affinity—$p(50)$—intrinsic to a particular species of hemoglobin molecule. For the simulations whose results are described below, we have used the simplified numerical method based on the Hill equation, which was described and applied to exercise in Chapter 6.

Figure 56 shows the relationship between the required flow of hemoglobin under resting conditions and $p(50)$, with the Hill constant n as parameter (see also Table XX). For n values in the investigated range of 1.0 to 3.0, an increase in $p(50)$ is beneficial up to 50 mm Hg. In the low-affinity range, i.e., $10 \leqslant p(50) \leqslant 25$ mm Hg, the apparently optimum value of n varies with $p(50)$. With $p(50)$ equal to 27 mm Hg, i.e., the normal standard value, it is interesting to note than an n value between 1.5 and 2.0 is more favorable than the normal value between 2.5 and 3.0.

The situation is changed during heavy exercise (as defined in Chapter 6) by the correspondingly lower venous blood O_2 tensions (see Figure 57 and Table XXI). Greater O_2 extraction makes an increase of n up to 3 beneficial at the normal standard $p(50)$ and higher $p(50)$ caused by the lower pH and higher temperature of exercise.

Also illustrated in Figure 57 is the advantage of a lower n value in the event of a high O_2 affinity [i.e., low $p(50)$]. This result would

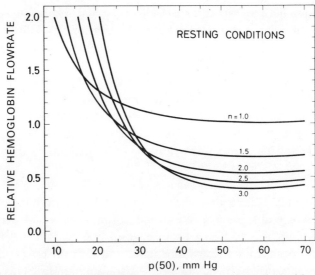

Figure 56. Relative hemoglobin flowrate at rest (i.e., the product of hemoglobin concentration and blood volumetric flowrate normalized to the value at $p(50) =$ 27.4 mm Hg, $n = 2.95$) as a function of $p(50)$ and Hill's constant n.

seem to explain the survival of mutants with high oxygen affinity and decreased cooperativity, in accordance with the ideas put forward by Bellingham (1972, 1974). They furthermore suggest that the hemoglobin-A molecule was becoming fixed at a time in evolution when what we now consider to be heavy exercise was a natural situation.

Abnormal Red Cell Organic Phosphate Concentration

Primary disorders of their metabolic system or alterations in their chemical environment may cause red cells to contain abnormal amounts of organic phosphates. Increases in the latter as a rule induce decreases in whole blood oxygen affinity (as discussed in Chapters 4 and 5), both through a direct (allosteric) effect upon the hemoglobin molecule, and through changes in the pH^c–pH^{pl} difference: Accumulation of red cell organic phosphate lowers the red cell pH at a given plasma pH, and this enhances the decrease in oxygen affinity.

Table XX
Effect of Changes in Hill's Constant n and p(50) on Blood Flow Requirements at Rest[a]

n	$p(50)$:	10	15	20	25	30	35	40
1.0	$\bar{O}_2^a$	90.0	85.7	81.8	78.3	75.0	72.0	69.2
	$\bar{O}_2^v$	75.7	67.1	60.1	54.3	49.4	45.3	41.8
	pO_2^v	31.1	30.7	30.2	29.8	29.3	28.9	28.6
	Q_{rel}	2.02	1.55	1.32	1.21	1.13	1.08	1.05
1.5	$\bar{O}_2^a$	96.4	93.6	90.5	87.2	82.9	80.5	77.1
	$\bar{O}_2^v$	85.8	76.3	66.9	58.4	50.8	44.2	38.5
	pO_2^v	33.2	32.7	32.0	31.4	30.6	30.0	29.3
	Q_{rel}	2.94	1.66	1.23	1.00	0.87	0.71	0.75
2.0	$\bar{O}_2^a$	98.8	97.3	95.3	92.8	90.0	86.8	83.5
	$\bar{O}_2^v$	92.4	84.2	74.1	63.6	53.6	44.3	36.3
	pO_2^v	34.9	34.6	33.9	33.1	32.2	31.2	30.2
	Q_{rel}	4.54	2.20	1.37	0.99	0.79	0.68	0.61
2.5	$\bar{O}_2^a$	99.6	98.9	97.9	96.1	94.0	91.4	89.4
	$\bar{O}_2^v$	96.2	89.9	80.7	69.5	57.3	45.5	34.9
	pO_2^v	36.3	36.1	35.5	34.8	33.8	32.5	31.2
	Q_{rel}	8.47	3.24	1.70	1.09	0.79	0.63	0.54
3.0	$\bar{O}_2^a$	99.9	99.5	98.9	97.9	96.4	94.5	91.9
	$\bar{O}_2^v$	98.0	93.8	86.2	75.1	61.8	47.7	34.5
	pO_2^v	37.3	37.1	36.8	36.2	35.2	33.9	32.3
	Q_{rel}	16.6	5.06	2.26	1.27	0.83	0.62	0.50

[a] Q_{rel} is required hemoglobin flowrate relative to that calculated for $n = 2.95$ and $p(50) = 27.4$ mm Hg.

Very high concentrations of fructose-1,6-diphosphate in specially stored blood are responsible for the latter's low O_2 affinity, mostly because of an influence upon the pH^c–pH^{pl} difference (Duhm, 1971). In all other cases studied to date, 2,3-DPG and ATP have been the only organic phosphates found to influence significantly the oxygen affinity under physiological and pathophysiological circumstances.

ATP is a hemoglobin effector molecule like 2,3-DPG (Rörth, 1968; Garby et al., 1969; Lo and Schimmel, 1969; Udkow et al., 1973; Hamasaki and Rose, 1974), though its intrinsic effect appears to be

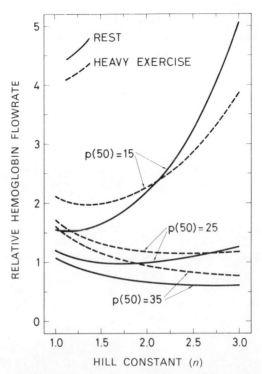

Figure 57. Relative hemoglobin flow rate (i.e., the product of hemoglobin concentration and blood volumetric flow rate normalized to the value at $p(50) = 27.4$ mm Hg, $n = 2.95$) as a function of Hill's constant n and $p(50)$. Solid curves are adapted from the data in Figure 56 for rest. Broken curves are for heavy exercise in the presence of myoglobin ($[Mb]_T = 5$ mM, $D_{Mb} = 2.5 \times 10^{-7}$ cm^2 sec^{-1}).

somewhat smaller. Its preferential binding to *deoxygenated* hemoglobin is markedly decreased by 2,3-DPG (Garby *et al.*, 1969; Udkow *et al.*, 1973) and thus one would not expect moderate changes in red cell ATP concentration, $[ATP]_T$, at normal 2,3-DPG levels, to influence significantly the oxygen affinity. The effects of ATP upon hemoglobin proton and carbon dioxide binding and the pH^c–pH^{pl} difference have not yet been worked out, but one could estimate the last effect by considering the charges per ATP and DPG molecule and the known effect of the latter upon the pH^c–pH^{pl} difference.

The relationship between whole blood oxygen affinity and $[ATP]_T$ in chronic renal disease with anemia was examined by

Table XXI
Effects of Changes in Hill's Constant n and p(50) on Blood Flow Requirements during Heavy Exercise[a]

n	$p(50)$:	10	15	20	25	30	35	40
1.0	$\bar{O}_2^a$	90.0	85.7	81.8	78.3	75.0	72.0	69.2
	$\bar{O}_2^v$	64.3	53.3	44.9	38.5	33.4	29.3	25.9
	pO_2^v	18.0	17.1	16.3	15.7	15.0	14.5	14.0
	Q_{rel}	2.67	2.12	1.85	1.72	1.65	1.60	1.58
1.5	$\bar{O}_2^a$	96.4	93.6	90.5	87.2	83.9	80.5	77.1
	$\bar{O}_2^v$	74.5	59.4	46.5	35.8	27.7	21.2	16.1
	pO_2^v	20.4	19.3	18.2	16.9	15.6	14.5	13.3
	Q_{rel}	3.13	2.00	1.55	1.33	1.22	1.15	1.12
2.0	$\bar{O}_2^a$	98.8	97.3	95.3	92.8	90.0	86.9	83.5
	$\bar{O}_2^v$	83.4	67.3	50.6	35.6	23.5	14.7	8.4
	pO_2^v	22.5	21.5	20.2	18.6	16.7	14.5	12.1
	Q_{rel}	4.51	2.28	1.53	1.20	1.03	0.95	0.91
2.5	$\bar{O}_2^a$	99.6	98.9	97.7	96.1	94.0	91.4	88.4
	$\bar{O}_2^v$	90.0	75.0	56.0	37.1	21.3	10.0	2.9
	pO_2^v	24.0	23.2	22.1	20.2	17.8	14.5	9.8
	Q_{rel}	7.08	2.87	1.65	1.12	0.94	0.84	0.80
3.0	$\bar{O}_2^a$	99.9	99.5	98.9	97.9	96.4	94.5	91.9
	$\bar{O}_2^v$	94.1	81.9	62.3	40.1	20.3	6.5	0.1
	pO_2^v	25.2	24.8	23.7	21.9	19.0	14.4	1.2
	Q_{rel}	12.0	3.88	1.87	1.19	0.90	0.78	0.75

[a] Q_{rel} as defined in Table XX. $[Mb] = 0.5$ mM, $D_{Mb} = 2.5 \times 10^{-7}$ cm^2/sec, average $r_{tis} = 45\mu$m.

Lichtman *et al.* (1974*b*). Values of $[DPG]_T$ and $[ATP]_T$ in their subjects exceeded those of normal controls by 0.5 and 0.9 mM, respectively, whereas their $p(50)$ values were 0.5 mm Hg *lower* at the same plasma pH. This unexpected finding indicates the influence of unrecognized factors upon $p(50)$.

Low 2,3-DPG concentrations are found in subjects with:

1. Rare cases of red cell hexokinase deficiency and 2,3-DPG mutase deficiency. Accounts of their biochemical pathology and clinical manifestations can be found in review articles by Waller and Benöhr (1974) and Mentzer (1974). In one case of hexokinase deficiency, described in detail by Delivoria-Papadopoulos *et al.*

(1969) and Oski *et al.* (1971), $[DPG]_T$ was 2.7 mM and the whole blood $p(50)$ was, as might be expected, only 19 mm Hg. The subject responded to excercise with a much greater increase in cardiac output than should have been warranted by his relatively mild anemia.

2. Hypophosphatemia, e.g., after hyperalimentation with low phosphate nutrients or anion resin therapy for hyperphosphatemia. Travis *et al.* (1971) studied five such subjects with plasma inorganic phosphate concentrations of 0.40 to 0.70 mg/100 ml, i.e., 5 to 10 times below normal. They found $[DPG]_T$ values of 2.2 to 3.2 mM and $p(50)$ values of 17 to 23 mm Hg.

3. Panhypopituitarism, polycythemia vera, and hyperbaric hyperoxia.

Abnormally high levels of red cell 2,3-DPG are found in subjects with:

1. Pyruvate kinase deficiency. The oxygen affinity of the blood of such subjects has been demonstrated to be low as expected (Delivoria-Papadopoulos *et al.*, 1969; Oski *et al.*, 1971).

2. Cirrhosis of the liver (Hurt and Chanutin, 1965; Astrup and Rörth, 1973). The explanation is not clear since the same patients often have anemia and metabolic alkalosis as well. Of specific interest is the association of high $[DPG]_T$ with high plasma ammonium ion levels, as already discussed in Chapter 7. Astrup and Rörth (1973) have provided experimental data showing an increase in $[DPG]_T$ of ~1.5 mmol/liter of cells for each millimole of NH_4^+ per liter of plasma. The high red cell 2,3-DPG content of these subjects is associated with an expectedly low blood oxygen affinity (Keys and Snell, 1938; Mulhausen *et al.*, 1967; Thomas *et al.*, 1974).

High $[DPG]_T$ values have been reported in subjects with hyperthyroidism, while tri-iodothyronine has been reported to increase red cell 2,3-DPG both *in vitro* and *in vivo*. Other investigators found no effect in animal experiments. The conflicting data have been discussed by Duhm and Gerlach (1974).

Low, normal, and high $[DPG]_T$ values have all been reported for subjects with diabetes mellitus. Such results are highly sensitive to the patients' acid–base status during the period preceding the observation (see p. 215). In subjects free of acid–base disturbance, slightly elevated levels have been reported (Arturson *et al.*, 1974*c*) together with normal blood oxygen affinity (see also p. 234).

Simulations of the isolated effect of abnormal $[DPG]_T$ on blood O_2 transport function have been described in the previous section (see Figure 54).

Carboxyhemoglobin and Methemoglobin

Under normal conditions, carboxyhemoglobin and methemoglobin constitute below 2 and 1%, respectively, of total blood hemoglobin and their significance is accordingly negligible. In heavy smokers and in subjects exposed to ambient carbon monoxide concentrations of more than 10–20 ppm, a much larger fraction of the hemoglobin exists in the form of COHb, and its effect on oxygen transport may not be negligible.

An evaluation of carbon monoxide's effect on blood oxygen transport may be performed on the basis of the conventional analysis of simultaneous hemoglobin O_2 and CO binding presented in Chapter 4, and the assumption that the concentration of COHb is constant throughout the peripheral circulation. The latter assumption derives from the facts that: (1) as O_2 is released to tissue in the steady state, blood carbon monoxide content remains unchanged, but CO redistributes itself between physically dissolved and hemoglobin-bound forms; (2) the decrease in $\overline{O}_2$ causes $\overline{CO}$ to increase, but to a degree made negligible by the exceedingly small amount of physically dissolved CO.

We have applied the above-described data and assumption to the simulation of O_2 transport under resting conditions, using the simplified numerical method based on the Hill equation and applied to exercise in Chapter 6. Figure 58 shows the calculated results when the atmospheric carbon monoxide concentration was allowed to vary between zero and 400 ppm. An additional curve that shows the relative blood flowrate required by an anemia of magnitude defined by the concentration of carboxyhemoglobin is included for comparison. The hazards of CO are seen to overshadow those of a comparable anemia, which, as discussed by Roughton (1964), is due to the

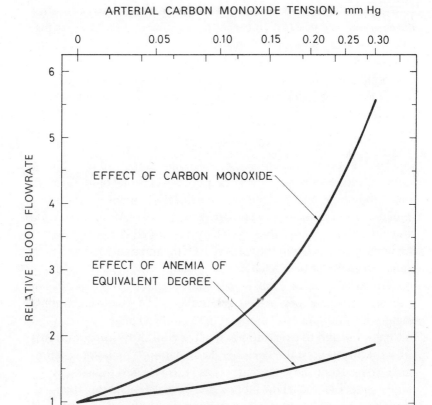

ARTERIAL CARBON MONOXIDE TENSION, mm Hg

Figure 58. Upper curve: relative blood flowrate at rest (normalized to the base case value for normal blood) as a function of $\overline{CO}$ or the corresponding pCO^a value; hematocrit = 45%. Lower curve: the same relative blood flowrate when the $\overline{CO}$ value is translated into an equivalent anemia.

decreasing sigmoidicity of the effective oxyhemoglobin dissociation curve with increasing levels of CO (Figure 29).

As expected on theoretical grounds and shown by Darling and Roughton (1942), the effect of methemoglobin on oxygen binding to hemoglobin is quite similar to that of carboxyhemoglobin. Thus, for evaluation of the former effect, the oxygen binding curve of whole blood containing methemoglobin may be taken to equal that of whole blood containing the same fraction of carboxyhemoglobin. Clinical conditions with methemoglobinemia are, however, often associated with accelerated red cell destruction; the decrease in oxygen affinity associated with the decrease of mean red cell age (see p. 227) may well compensate for the direct effect of methemoglobin on O_2 affinity.

Stored Red Cells

Red cells stored in acid citrate dextrose media at 4°C for later transfusion are known to have abnormal oxygen binding properties. The pioneering observations were made by Valtis and Kennedy (1954), who demonstrated the high oxygen affinity of stored blood and maintenance of this increase several hours after transfusion. Some 15 years passed before it was realized that the effect was due to the marked decrease in red cell 2,3-DPG concentration during storage.

Another factor responsible for the high oxygen affinity of stored red cells is the large concentration of citrate ions typically employed in the storage media. These ions are impermeable to the red cell membrane (Garby, 1965) and therefore markedly affect the distribution of diffusible ions across the red cell membrane, whence a low erythrocyte hydrogen ion activity (Funder and Wieth, 1966b; Minakami *et al.*, 1975). Upon transfusion of stored red cells, their proton activity rapidly approaches that prescribed by the respective concentrations of membrane-impermeable charged species within them and the citrate-free plasma.

Since the oxygen affinity of stored red cells after transfusion is determined by their 2,3-DPG concentration, their gas transport function may, in principle, be evaluated by means of Figure 54. However, recent studies by Yhap *et al.* (1975) and Harken and Woods (1976) strongly indicate the importance of factors other than red cell 2,3-DPG in this context. Yhap and co-workers measured oxygen uptake by isolated dog hindlimbs perfused with constantly flowing fresh blood or blood stored for 21 days in ACD solution.

Before and during perfusion, the plasma pH of each blood was brought to 7.40 by administration of sodium bicarbonate. The concentrations of 2,3-DPG in the stored red cells were about half those in fresh, so that the $p(50)$ values were respectively 20 and 26 mm Hg. Oxygen consumption by the limbs perfused with fresh blood was between 1.5 and 2.3 times higher, but results of individual experiments differed by factors of up to 5. Essentially the same results were reported by Harken and Woods (1976) from a similar experimental study.

Although the above differences in oxygen consumption are undoubtedly related to those in oxygen affinity, additional factors must be identified before the size of the differences can be explained. The previously mentioned results of Sirs (1969; see p. 228), show that the egress of oxygen from stored red cells is relatively slow. The significance of this effect merits consideration.

Abnormal Lung Function and Ambient Air

Introduction

The main function of the lung in respiration is to ensure that the partial pressures of oxygen and carbon dioxide in arterial blood be maintained in the vicinities of 90 and 40 mm Hg, respectively. This function is accomplished by (1) the mechanical work of breathing, which maintains the alveolar gas tensions at values close to these, and (2) the design of the alveolar–capillary interphase, which ensures that the relaxation times for gas equilibration are smaller than the residence time of the blood in the capillaries.

Insufficient ventilation results in alveolar oxygen and carbon dioxide tensions that are, respectively, lower and higher than those required. Furthermore, the relaxation times for gas equilibration may be prolonged to the detriment of gas transfer because of increased alveolar–capillary interphase resistance to diffusion. Venoarterial shunting of pulmonary blood may be regarded as the extreme example of the latter type of disturbance. Finally, a shortened blood residence time in otherwise normal capillaries—as in severe exercise—also may preclude attainment of gas equilibration. Insufficient ventilation, impaired permeability and venoarterial shunting may combine in different proportions and vary from one part of the lung to another. To a minor extent, all these phenomena prevail in the lungs of apparently healthy subjects.

Disturbances in ventilation produce alveolar gas tensions that differ appreciably from normal values. Such deviations of pO_2^A and pCO_2^A are, however, governed by a number of physical constraints, among them that the sum of all partial pressures (pO_2, pCO_2, pN_2, pH_2O, etc.) in the alveoli must equal ambient pressure. For a thorough review of these relationships, see Otis (1964).

Disturbances in gas transfer from alveolus to lung capillary, arising from the above-mentioned causes, widen the alveolar-to-arterial oxygen tension gradient, which in the healthy lung amounts to 5–15 mm Hg. In disease, this pO_2 gradient can reach 50 mm Hg when breathing ambient air at sea level, whereas the alveolar–arterial gradient of pCO_2 rarely exceeds 5 mm Hg (see Rahn and Farhi, 1964).

A detailed discussion of the mechanisms of such derangement of lung function is beyond the scope of this work; suffice it to say that pO_2^a can vary from 40 to 120 mm Hg, and pCO_2^a from 30 to 90 mm Hg when the subject, albeit diseased, is breathing air at sea level, and that such alterations in blood tensions conform to patterns dictated by the underlying functional disturbances.

In primary hypoventilation as may arise from narcotic poisoning, severe neuromuscular disease, or central respiratory depression, a fall in arterial pO_2 is associated with a rise in pCO_2^a to a degree dictated by the alveolar air equation (see Otis, 1964). On the other hand, when gas transfer is primarily impaired by lung disease, a low arterial pO_2 is usually associated with a *low* pCO_2^a. However, in adult clinical practice, hypoxemia frequently results from chronic bronchitis and emphysema, and in the more advanced cases of this disease, a secondary, though poorly understood, disturbance of ventilatory control compounds the problem, so that arterial blood gas analysis reveals low pO_2 with *high* pCO_2 and a variable degree of respiratory acidosis.

Subjects with chronic arterial hypoxia compensate through a number of different mechanisms. Those operating in subjects living at high altitude have recently been reviewed by Frisancho (1975). An increase in hemoglobin concentration is generally the rule, and this is mediated through the ESF system. Hyperventilation decreases the ambient-to-alveolar oxygen tension gradient and thus facilitates oxygen exchange. The consequently low arterial pCO_2 induces but slight alkalosis, and so the whole blood oxygen affinity *in vivo* is normal or nearly so. During the initial days of adaptation to high altitude, there is a pronounced hyperventilation and concomitant alkalosis. At least during the first hours and days, there is a simultaneous increase in whole blood oxygen affinity *in vivo*, the importance of which may rest in its maintenance of high arterial oxygen saturation. The alkalosis causes increased red cell 2,3-DPG synthesis by means of which the whole blood oxygen affinity *in vivo* eventually decreases back to normal. The mechanisms of red cell adaptation to high altitude have been reviewed by Rörth (1972).

Simulation of the Effects of Abnormal Arterial Gas Tensions

Results of simulations of blood gas transport under resting conditions with freely varying arterial pO_2 and pCO_2 and red cell 2,3-DPG concentration are shown in Figure 59, for which details are provided in Tables XXII–XXIV. The ranges of arterial gas tensions employed cover theoretically imaginable situations in both health and disease, with the broken portions of the curves corresponding to cases in which the ambient air definitely contains abnormally high tensions of one or both gases.

Under the given circumstances of fixed capillary density, the blood flow requirement is clearly rather sensitive to arterial oxygen tension. Thus in subjects with pO_2^a values below 60 mm Hg, i.e., in the majority of patients requiring therapy, compensation by blood flow (and/or hemoglobin concentration) is neither a desirable nor realistic mechanism. Decreases in blood oxygen affinity due to either the pCO_2-mediated pH (Bohr) effect or to 2,3-DPG are estimated to provide appreciable compensation in the given pO_2^a range of 60 to 120 mm Hg, but, as noted in the earlier sections on acid–base disturbances and anemia, the *in vivo* coupling of pH^c and $[DPG)_T$ works to nullify such effects.

Subjects with chronic hypoxic lung disease have essentially normal blood oxygen affinity *in vivo* (Segel and Bishop, 1966;

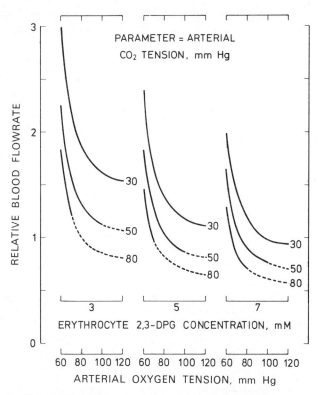

Figure 59. Relative blood flowrate at rest (normalized to the base case value for normal blood) as a function of $[DPG]_T$, pO_2^a, and pCO_2^a, with all three varying freely. Broken portions of curves denote cases in which $pO_2^a + pCO_2^a > 150$ mm Hg.

Flenley *et al.*, 1975; Tweeddale *et al.*, 1977), although the variation about the mean affinity is considerably larger than found with normal subjects. These patients have also essentially normal O_2 consumption at rest, and their cardiac output does not differ much from that of normal subjects (Flenley *et al.*, 1975).

The effect of increased tissue capillary density upon the blood flow requirements of the model tissue at rest is shown in Figure 60, further details for which are provided in Table XXV (note that the average capillary density assumed in the calculations for Figure 59 and all previous simulations of resting conditions in this chapter was 14.1 vessels/mm^2). With an arterial pO_2 of 50 mm Hg, a $\sim 15\%$

Table XXII

Effect of Changes in pO_2^a and pCO_2^a on Blood Flow Requirements at Rest[a]
$([DPG]_T = 3\ mM)^a$

pO_2^a	$\overline{pH}^{pl}$	$\overline{pH}^{c}$	$\overline{p(50)}$	pO_2^v	$\bar{O}_2^a$	$\bar{O}_2^v$	Q_{rel}
			$pCO_2^a = 30$ mm Hg				
60	7.464	7.266	21.7	40.7	94.9	84.1	3.25
70	7.463	7.263	21.8	38.2	97.0	81.2	2.22
90	7.463	7.261	21.8	36.0	98.9	78.4	1.71
120	7.462	7.260	21.9	35.0	99.6	76.9	1.54
			$pCO_2^a = 50$ mm Hg				
60	7.323	7.150	25.6	40.4	92.4	76.9	2.25
75	7.321	7.147	25.7	37.0	96.3	71.5	1.41
100	7.319	7.143	25.8	35.0	98.8	67.8	1.13
120	7.319	7.142	25.8	34.3	99.4	66.6	1.07
			$pCO_2^a = 80$ mm Hg				
60	7.183	7.041	29.2	40.9	88.8	69.6	1.84
70	7.183	7.037	29.4	37.9	93.0	64.2	1.23
90	7.181	7.030	29.7	34.9	97.3	58.1	0.90
120	7.180	7.028	29.3	32.9	99.1	55.7	0.81

[a] Q_{rel} is flow relative to that calculated at normal arterial gas tensions and red cell 2,3-DPG.

Table XXIII

Effect of Changes in pO_2^a and pCO_2^a on Blood Flow Requirements at Rest[a]
$([DPG]_T = 5\ mM)^a$

pO_2	$\overline{pH}^{pl}$	$\overline{pH}^{c}$	$\overline{p(50)}$	pO_2^v	$\bar{O}_2^a$	$\bar{O}_2^v$	Q_{rel}
			$pCO_2^a = 30$ mm Hg				
60	7.480	7.254	25.3	40.4	92.7	78.0	2.37
70	7.477	7.250	25.4	37.8	95.5	74.1	1.64
90	7.475	7.247	25.5	35.6	98.3	70.2	1.25
120	7.475	7.246	25.6	34.4	99.4	68.1	1.12
			$pCO_2^a = 50$ mm Hg				
60	7.341	7.140	29.4	40.6	89.4	70.2	1.84
75	7.336	7.136	29.6	36.9	94.8	63.5	1.13
100	7.335	7.132	29.8	34.0	98.3	57.7	0.86
120	7.333	7.131	29.8	33.4	99.2	56.2	0.82
			$pCO_2^a = 80$ mm Hg				
60	7.200	7.038	33.8	40.6	85.0	60.7	1.45
70	7.198	7.031	34.0	36.9	90.5	53.8	0.96
90	7.196	7.024	34.3	33.5	96.0	47.1	0.72
120	7.196	7.019	33.9	31.5	98.8	44.7	0.65

[a] Q_{rel} is flow relative to that calculated at normal arterial gas tensions and red cell 2,3-DPG.

Table XXIV

Effect of Changes in pO_2^a and pCO_2^a on Blood Flow Requirements at Rest[a]
$([DPG]_T = 7 \ mM)^a$

pO_2^a	$\overline{pH^{pl}}$	$\overline{pH^c}$	$\overline{p(50)}$	pO_2^v	$\bar{O}_2^a$	$\bar{O}_2^v$	Q_{rel}
			$pCO_2^a = 30$ mm Hg				
60	7.498	7.239	27.6	40.2	91.0	73.4	1.99
70	7.495	7.235	27.7	38.1	94.3	69.9	1.44
90	7.494	7.233	27.8	35.0	97.7	64.3	1.05
120	7.492	7.230	27.8	33.8	99.3	62.0	0.94
			$pCO_2^a = 50$ mm Hg				
60	7.321	7.131	31.9	40.6	87.0	65.6	1.65
75	7.356	7.124	32.2	36.3	93.6	57.2	0.97
100	7.353	7.119	32.4	33.7	97.8	51.6	0.76
120	7.351	7.117	32.5	32.6	99.0	49.1	0.70
			$pCO_2^a = 80$ mm Hg				
60	7.220	7.030	36.9	40.1	82.0	54.4	1.29
70	7.217	7.021	37.3	36.3	88.6	46.8	0.84
90	7.213	7.012	37.6	32.6	95.0	39.3	0.63
120	7.215	7.006	37.1	30.6	98.5	37.1	0.57

[a] Q_{rel} is flow relative to that calculated at normal arterial gas tensions and red cell 2,3-DPG.

increase in capillary density *halves* the blood flow requirement. The seemingly excessive magnitude of this effect is a consequence of the particular circumstances chosen for simulation, i.e., a normal capillary density at rest, which implies tissue diffusional distances so high that only a slight arteriovenous pO_2^{bl} difference can be tolerated once pO_2 has fallen below 60 mm Hg. In any event, capillary recruitment certainly appears to be an extremely efficient means of compensation. It is, in fact, so efficient in theory that one is led to doubt whether tissue hypoxia in chronic ventilatory insufficiency is at all related to mitochondrial oxygen consumption—unless, of course, there are specific limitations within the processes leading to and maintaining capillarization.

On the other hand, it can be reasoned that vessel recruitment cannot be nearly as efficient a means of compensation for diminished pO_2^a with respect to O_2-consuming reactions characterized by a very *high* apparent K_m value for oxygen. Such reactions

Table XXV
Effect of Changes in Capillary Density on Blood Flow Requirements in Arterial Hypoxia at Rest[a]

$[DPG]_T$	$\overline{pH^{pl}}$	$\overline{pH^c}$	$\overline{p(50)}$	pO_2^v	$\bar{O}_2^a$	$\bar{O}_2^v$	$Q_{rel}{}^b$
		$\bar{r}_{tis} = 140\mu\text{m}, pO_2^a = 60$ mm Hg					
2	7.378	7.203	21.3	32.8	95.2	74.7	1.72
4	7.391	7.193	26.1	32.2	92.2	62.6	1.19
6	7.411	7.181	29.0	31.5	90.0	54.6	1.00
8	7.432	7.168	31.0	31.3	88.0	49.7	0.92
		$\bar{r}_{tis} = 140\mu\text{m}, pO_2^a = 50$ mm Hg					
2	7.377	7.210	21.3	35.6	91.6	78.6	2.71
4	7.398	7.204	26.2	35.2	86.6	67.6	1.83
6	7.408	7.195	29.3	35.0	83.0	60.7	1.58
8	7.430	7.186	31.3	35.0	80.0	56.3	1.49
		$\bar{r}_{tis} = 130\mu\text{m}, pO_2^a = 50$ mm Hg					
2	7.379	7.202	21.3	27.4	91.7	64.3	1.28
4	7.393	7.193	26.1	26.7	86.9	50.2	0.96
6	7.415	7.183	29.0	26.3	83.0	42.6	0.87
8	7.438	7.172	30.9	25.8	80.7	37.4	0.81
		$\bar{r}_{tis} = 130\mu\text{m}, pO_2^a = 40$ mm Hg					
2	7.378	7.215	21.3	30.8	84.9	71.1	2.53
4	7.391	7.212	26.1	30.7	77.0	59.4	2.00
6	7.410	7.206	29.2	30.7	71.6	52.5	1.84
8	7.433	7.198	31.3	30.7	67.9	47.9	1.76

[a] Arterial $pCO_2 = 40$ mm Hg.
[b] Calculated blood flowrate in tissue, relative to case of normal arterial gas tensions, $[DPG]_T = 5$ mM, and capillary density (i.e., $\bar{r}_{tis} = 150\ \mu$m, 14.1 vessels/mm^2); i.e., Q_{rel} is an index of blood flow per unit *volume* of tissue.

include hydroxylation and oxygenation of substrate with molecular oxygen, and are essential in the metabolism of, for example, amino acids and steroids. They are responsible for only a tiny fraction of total oxygen consumption; therefore, a substantial decrease in their oxygen consumption rate would not readily be detected by conventional methods. The possibility must therefore be considered that part of the symptoms in chronic hypoxic lung disease are related to derangement in those metabolic pathways which depend upon this particular class of reactions.

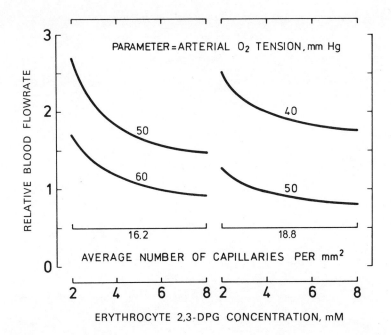

Figure 60. Relative blood flowrate at rest (normalized to the base case value for normal blood *and capillary density*) as a function of $[DPG]_T$, pO_2^a, and capillary density, $pCO_2^a = 40$ mm Hg.

Chapter 9

Concluding Remarks

Present-day scientific writing has been accused of being neutral and noncommital to an extent that has lowered the quality of its information content. It has been argued that writers of reviews, texts, and monographs should be less hesitant to express their personal opinions on issues of scientific endeavor. We find such criticism not to be without justification and so attempt in these final pages a summary of our views on the present status of the field and an outlook toward future work.

With regard to the phenomenological aspects of *equilibrium* binding of oxygen, protons, carbon dioxide, and 2,3-DPG in blood containing primarily hemoglobin A, present knowledge appears rather adequate for the purpose of determining and understanding the macroscopic events likely to occur under most physiological and pathophysiological conditions. The work commenced by the early masters of the field now seems to be concluded. The next few decades will doubtless witness further clarification of these events on the molecular scale, but such advances, though of unpredictable consequence for other fields of biology and medicine, are not likely to change our current understanding of blood gas transport at this level.

The mechanisms underlying cooperativity in oxygen binding to hemoglobin have been clarified to a very considerable degree. Although details remain to be worked out, the general principles are clear. From a physiological point of view, it is interesting to note that the significance of this phenomenon, for which evolution may be held responsible, is not obvious when one considers human beings at rest and in light exercise. In heavy exercise, though, its importance is clear. We find that in order to sustain mitochondrial oxygen consumption when the oxygen binding curve is made less sigmoidal by a reduction of Hill's constant from 3 to 1, the blood flow or hemoglobin concentration must increase by 50%, all other parameters remaining unchanged.

The physiological role of the interaction between protons and oxygen molecules in relation to their binding to hemoglobin appears to be clear. It is, however, remarkable how relatively unimportant it appears to be at rest in regard to the progressive rightward shift in the O_2 dissociation curve as the blood flowing through a systemic capillary becomes more acid. On the other hand, changes in the pH of the circulating blood due to changes in arterial pCO_2 or base excess can be far more important. For example, abolishing the Bohr effect engendered by the lactic acidosis of heavy exercise can be compensated at constant capillary density only by an increase in blood flow or hemoglobin concentration, amounting in the model system to a factor of about 1.5.

The effect of carbamino formation on oxygen affinity and its reciprocal phenomenon is intriguing: Even under extreme conditions of alkalosis, high pCO_2, and low red cell 2,3-DPG, it is quantitatively so small that one wonders about the significance of its evolution.

At least one important physiological role of red cell 2,3-DPG appears to be firmly established. Long-term changes in the blood's oxygen affinity due to changes in blood pH, whether respiratory or metabolic, are largely reversed by simultaneous changes in erythrocyte 2,3-DPG. The biochemical and physiological mechanisms behind this control have also been clarified appreciably. Such compensation, e.g., in alkalosis, is calculated to be responsible for reductions in blood flow or hemoglobin concentration requirements by as much as a factor of 2. Whether or not this is the sole or main role of red cell 2,3-DPG is uncertain. There are instances in which its steady state *in vivo* concentration cannot be fully explained by previously established factors. The role of circulating nucleosides in this regard may well be worth exploring.

Hemoglobin–hemoglobin interaction is not well understood and must be clarified in order to arrive at a more detailed understanding of hemoglobin–ligand interaction as well as the phenomenon of sickling of HbS-containing erythrocytes.

Many of the available data suggest that the rates of chemical reaction and species translocation within the blood do not significantly limit the supply of oxygen to tissues under normal conditions. However, there are insufficient data to make this a generalization and the possibility cannot be excluded that there exist appreciable disequilibria between red cells and plasma, or within the erythrocytes as a result of, say, relatively short capillary transit times. Of even greater importance in this vein may be the effects of increased rigidity and internal diffusion resistance of abnormal red cells. This area of investigation merits further work in light of recent results with stored red cells.

Following conventional wisdom, we too have assumed that the integrated gas transport system consisting of the lungs, the circulation, and the blood responds so as to fulfill those tissue oxygen requirements that derive from reactions of the mitochondrial respiratory chain, i.e., reactions that account for nearly all the body's oxygen uptake and that exhibit extremely low K_m values. It should be kept in mind, however, that this generalization lacks solid experimental support.

The possibility must seriously be entertained that other aerobic reactions, in which oxygen is incorporated into other molecules and for which the apparent K_m values for oxygen far exceed those of the respiratory chain, may be involved in the regulation of not only the blood flow but also blood gas transport properties. If this indeed is so, then hypoxia may well be present in tissues whose energy-producing reactions proceed at essentially normal rates. The tiny fraction of the total oxygen consumption attributable to these other reactions prevents the detection of such hypoxia with conventional methods and thus makes the total consumption appear normal. Although there is evidence in support of the importance of these metabolic pathways in circulatory control, there is also much work to be done.

A detailed analysis of blood gas transport in relation to tissue oxygen demands requires data not only on the intrinsic kinetics of tissue oxygen consumption, but also on capillary–tissue geometry and organization. Although clearly recognized by Krogh more than 50 years ago, this field of research has been revived only recently, and a long series of questions remain unanswered. When this area of research has been much more fully developed, more specific questions concerning the blood's gas transport properties can be asked.

Clinical studies together with simulation of gas transport dynamics strongly suggest that in subjects with low arterial oxygen tension there must exist adaptive mechanisms over and above those involving blood flow and gas transport properties. One that quickly comes to mind is increased capillary density. However, the apparent ease with which such adaptations may restore normal oxygen consumption to the respiratory chain of reactions—a moderate recruitment of capillaries would suffice to offset even the lowest of observed arterial oxygen tensions—makes it somewhat difficult to maintain that "mitochondrial hypoxia" is the main cause of dysfunction in acute or chronic respiratory insufficiency. The etiology of dysfunction in such cases, however, may readily be understood if one instead assumes that the hypoxia is related to the "high K_m reactions"; the effect of a low arterial pO_2 on these reactions can be eliminated only to a limited extent by an increase in capillary density.

References

Ackers, G. K., Johnson, M. L., Mills, F. C., Halvorsen, H. R., and Shapiro, S. (1975), The linkage between oxygenation and subunit dissociation in human hemoglobin. Consequences for the analysis of oxygenation curves, *Biochemistry* **14**, 5128–5134.

Ackers, G. K., Johnson, M. L., Mills, F. C., and Ip, S. H. C. (1976), Energetics of oxygenation-linked subunit interactions in human hemoglobin, *Biochem. Biophys. Res. Commun.* **69**, 135–142.

Adair, G. S. (1923), Thermodynamic proof of the reciprocal relation of oxygen and carbon dioxide in blood, *J. Physiol. (London)* **58**, iv–v.

Adair, G. S. (1925), The hemoglobin system. VI. The O_2 dissociation curve of hemoglobin, *J. Biol. Chem.* **63**, 529–545.

Adair, G. S. (1928), A theory of partial osmotic pressures and membrane equilibria, with special reference to the application of Dalton's law to hemoglobin solutions in the presence of salts, *Proc. Roy. Soc. (London) A* **120**, 573–603.

Allen, D. W., Wyman, J., and Smith, C. A. (1953), The oxygen equilibrium of fetal and adult human hemoglobin, *J. Biol. Chem.* **203**, 81–87.

Andreasson, K., de Verdier, C.-H., and Åkerblom, O. (1973), Biochemical variables influencing the storage ability of erythrocytes at 4°C. II. Inter- and intraindividual variations, *Abhandl. Akad. Wissenschaft. DDR, Jahrgang* 1973, 461.

Antonini, E., and Brunori, M. (1970), On the rate of reaction of an organic phosphate (ATP) with deoxyhemoglobin, *FEBS Lett.* **7**, 351–352.

Antonini, E., and Brunori, M. (1971), *Hemoglobin and Myoglobin in Their Interactions with Ligands.* North Holland Publ. Co., Amsterdam.

Antonini, E., Wyman, J., Brunori, M., Fronticelli, C., Bucci, E., and Rossi-Fanelli, A. (1965), Studies on the relations between molecular and functional properties of hemoglobin. V. The influence of temperature on the Bohr effect in human and in horse hemoglobin, *J. Biol. Chem.* **240**, 1096–1103.

Arnone, A. (1972), X-ray diffraction study of binding of 2,3-diphosphoglycerate to human deoxyhemoglobin, *Nature* **237**, 146–148.

Arnone, A. (1974), X-ray studies of the interaction of CO_2 with human deoxyhemoglobin, *Nature* **247**, 143–145.

Arturson, G., Garby, L., Robert, M., and Zaar, B. (1974a), The oxygen dissociation curve of normal human blood with special reference to the influence of physiological effector ligands, *Scand. J. Clin. Lab. Invest.* **34**, 9–13.

Arturson, G., Garby, L., Robert, M., and Zaar, B. (1974b), Determination of the oxygen affinity of human blood *in vivo* and under standard conditions, *Scand. J. Clin. Lab. Invest.* **34**, 15–18.

Arturson, G., Garby, L., Robert, M., and Zaar, B. (1974c), Oxygen affinity of whole blood *in vivo* and under standard conditions with diabetes mellitus, *Scand. J. Clin. Lab. Invest.* **34**, 19–22.

Arturson, G., Garby, L., Wranne, B., and Zaar, B. (1974d), Effect of 2,3-diphosphoglycerate on the oxygen affinity and on the proton- and carbamino-linked oxygen affinity of hemoglobin in human whole blood, *Acta Physiol. Scand.* **92**, 332–340.

Asmussen, E. (1965), Muscular exercise, in: *Handbook of Physiology, Respiration, Sect.* 3 (Fenn, W. O., and Rahn, H., eds.), Ch. 36, pp. 939–978. Amer. Physiol. Soc., Washington, D.C.

Astrup, P. (1969), Oxygen dissociation curves in some diseases. *Försvarsmed.* **5**, 199–204.

Astrup, P., and Rörth, M. (1973), Oxygen affinity of hemoglobin and red cell 2,3-diphosphoglycerate in hepatic cirrhosis, *Scand. J. Clin. Lab. Invest.* **31**, 311–317.

Astrup, P., Engel, K., Severinghaus, J., and Munson, E. (1965), The influence of temperature and pH on the dissociation curve of oxyhemoglobin of human blood, *Scand. J. Clin. Lab. Invest.* **17**, 515–523.

Astrup, P., Rörth, M., and Thorshauge, C. (1970), Dependency on acid–base status of oxyhemoglobin dissociation and 2,3-diphosphoglycerate level in human erythrocytes. II. *In vivo* studies, *Scand. J. Clin. Lab. Invest.* **26**, 47–52.

Bansil, R., Herzfeld, J., and Stanley, E. (1976), Kinetics of cooperative ligand binding in proteins: the effects of organic phosphates on hemoglobin oxygenation, *J. Mol. Biol.* **103**, 89–126.

Barcroft, J. (1914), *The Respiratory Functions of the Blood*, 1st ed. Cambridge Univ. Press, Cambridge. The second edition appeared in two volumes from the same publisher: Volume I: *Lessons from High Altitudes* (1925); Volume II: *Hemoglobin* (1928).

Bare, G. H., Bromberg, P. A., Alben, J. O., Brimhall, B., Jones, R. T., Mintz, S., and Rother, J. (1976), Altered C-terminal salt bridges in hemoglobin York cause high oxygen affinity, *Nature* **259**, 155–156.

Bauer, C. (1969), Antagonistic influence of CO_2 and 2,3-diphosphoglycerate on the Bohr effect of human haemoglobin, *Life Sci.* **8**, 1041–1046.

Bauer, C. (1970), Reduction of the carbon dioxide affinity of human hemoglobin solutions by 2,3-diphosphoglycerate, *Resp. Physiol.* **10**, 10–19.

Bauer, C. (1974), On the respiratory function of hemoglobin, *Rev. Physiol. Biochem. Pharmacol.* **70**, 1–31.

Bauer, C., Ludwig, J., and Ludwig, M. (1968), Different effects of 2,3-diphosphoglycerate and adenosine triphosphate on the oxygen affinity of adult and foetal human haemoglobin, *Life Sci.* **7**, 1339–1343.

Bauer, C., Klocke, R. A., Kamp, D., and Forster, R. E. (1973), Effect of 2,3-diphosphoglycerate and H^+ on the reaction of O_2 and hemoglobin, *Am. J. Physiol.* **224**, 838–847.

Bauer, C., Baumann, R., Engels, U., and Pacyna, B. (1975), The carbon dioxide affinity of various human hemoglobins, *J. Biol. Chem.* **250**, 2173–2176.

Bauer, C., and Schröder, E. (1972), Carbamino compounds of haemoglobin in human adult and fetal blood, *J. Physiol.* **227**, 457–471.

Baumann, R., Bauer, C., and Haller, E. A. (1975), Oxygen-linked CO_2 transport in sheep blood. *Am. J. Physiol.* **229**, 334–339.

Bellingham, A. J. (1972), The physiological significance of the Hill parameter "*n*," *Acta Haematol. Scand.* **9**, 552–556.

Bellingham, A. J. (1974), The red cell in adaptation to anaemic hypoxia, *Clinics in Haematol.* **3**, 577–594.

Bellingham, A., Detter, M., and Lenfant, C. (1970), The role of hemoglobin affinity for oxygen and red-cell 2,3-diphosphoglycerate in the management of diabetic ketoacidosis, *Trans. Am. Soc. Physicians* **33**, 113–120.

Benesch, R., and Benesch, R. E. (1967), The effect of organic phosphates from the human erythrocyte on the allosteric properties of hemoglobin, *Biochem. Biophys. Res. Commun.* **26**, 162–167.

Benesch, R. E., and Benesch, R. (1974), The mechanism of interaction of red cell organic phosphates with hemoglobin, *Adv. Prot. Chem.* **28**, 211–237.

Benesch, R. E., Benesch, R., and Yu, C. I. (1969), The oxygenation of hemoglobin in the presence of 2,3-diphosphoglycerate. Effect of temperature, pH, ionic strength and hemoglobin concentration, *Biochemistry* **8**, 2567–2571.

Berger, H., Jänig, G.-R., Gerber, G., Ruckpaul, K., and Rapoport, S. (1973), Interaction of hemoglobin with ions, *Eur. J. Biochem.* **38**, 553–562.

Beutler, E., and Wood, L. A. (1969), The *in vivo* regeneration of red cell 2,3-diphosphoglyceric acid (DPG) after transfusion of stored blood, *J. Lab. Clin. Med.* **94**, 300–304.

Biörck, G. (1949), On myoglobin and its occurrence in man, *Acta Med. Scand., Supp.* 226, 1–216.

Böning, D., Meier, U., Schweigart, U., and Kunze, M. (1975*a*), Diurnal changes of the 2,3-diphosphoglycerate concentration in human red cells under influence of posture, *Eur. J. Appl. Physiol.* **34**, 11–17.

Böning, D., Schweigart, U., Tibes, U., and Hemmer, B. (1975*b*), Influences of exercise and endurance training on the oxygen dissociation curve of the blood under *in vivo* and *in vitro* conditions, *Eur. J. Appl. Physiol.* **34**, 1–10.

Bohr, C., Hasselbalch, K. A., and Krogh, A. (1904), Über einen in biologischer Beziehung wichtigen Einfluss, den die Kohlensäure-Spannung des Blutes auf dessen Sauerstoffbindung übt. *Skand. Arch. Physiol.* **16**, 402–412.

Bonaventura, J., Bonaventura, C., Sullivan, B., and Godette, G. (1975), Hemoglobin Deer Lodge ($\beta 2$ His → Arg). Consequences of altering the 2,3-DPG binding site, *J. Biol. Chem.* **250**, 9250–9255.

Booth, U. H. (1938), Carbonic anhydrase activity inside corpuscles. Enzyme substrate accessibility factors, *J. Physiol.* **93**, 117–128.

Boulton, F. E., and Holly, J. M. P. (1975), The oxygen affinity of horse and human myoglobins, *J. Physiol. (London)* **248**, 32P–33P.

Bourdeau-Martini, J., Odoroff, C. L., and Honig, C. R. (1974), Dual effect of oxygen on magnitude and uniformity of coronary intercapillary distance, *Am. J. Physiol.* **226**, 800–810.

Bridges, K. R., Schmidt, G. J., Jensen, M., Cerami, A., and Bunn, H. F. (1975), The acetylation of hemoglobin by aspirin, *J. Clin. Invest.* **56**, 201–207.

Bromberg, P. A., Theodore, J., Robin, E. D., and Jensen, W. N. (1965), Anion and hydrogen ion distribution in human blood. *J. Lab. Clin. Med.* **66**, 464–475.

Bunn, H. F. (1974), The structure and function of normal and abnormal hemoglobins, *in : Hematology of Infancy and Childhood* (Nathan, D. G. and Oski, F. A., eds.), pp. 390–418. W. B. Saunders, Philadelphia.

Bunn, H. F., and Briehl, R. W. (1970), The interaction of 2,3-diphosphoglycerate with various human hemoglobins. *J. Clin. Invest.* **49**, 1088–1095.

Bunn, H. F., and Guidotti, G. (1972), Stabilizing interactions in hemoglobin, *J. Biol. Chem.* **247**, 2345–2350.

Bunn, H. F., and Jandl, J. H. (1966), Exchange of heme among hemoglobin molecules, *Proc. Nat. Acad. Sci. U.S.A.* **56**, 974–978.

Bunn, H. F., and Jandl, J. H. (1968), Exchange of heme among hemoglobins and between hemoglobin and albumin, *J. Biol. Chem.* **243**, 465–475.

Card, R. T., and Brain, M. C. (1973), The "anemia" of childhood: Evidence for physiologic response to hyperphosphatemia, *New Engl. J. Med.* **288**, 388–392.

Chance, B., Williamson, J. R., Jamieson, D., and Schoener, B. (1965), Properties and kinetics of reduced pyridine nucleotide fluorescence of the isolated and *in vivo* rat heart, *Biochem. J.* **341**, 357–377.

Chanutin, A., and Curnish, P. (1967), Effect of organic and inorganic phosphate on the oxygen equilibrium of human erythrocytes, *Arch. Biochem. Biophys.* **121**, 96–102.

Charache, S., and Weatherall, D. J. (1966), Fast hemoglobin in lead poisoning, *Blood* **28**, 377–386.

Charache, S., Brimhall, B., and Jones, R. T. (1975), Polycythemia produced by hemoglobin Osler (β 145 Tyr $\rightarrow$ Asp), *Johns Hopkins Med. J.* **136**, 132–136.

Chiancone, E., Norne, J. E., Forsén, S., Bonaventura, J., Brunori, M., Antonini, E., and Wyman, J. (1975), Identification of chloride-binding sites in hemoglobin by nuclear-magnetic-resonance quadruple-relaxation studies of hemoglobin digests, *Eur. J. Biochem.* **55**, 385–390.

Chiarioni, T., Nardi, E., Papa, G., Sasso, G. F., and Tentori, L. (1974), A new hemoglobin (Hb Abruzzo, β 193 His $\rightarrow$ Arg) with increased oxygen affinity in two brothers with hemolytic syndrome of the "Mediterranean" type and marked erythrocytosis, *Nouv. Rev. Franc. Hematol.* **14**, 543–549.

Chotia, C., and Janin, J. (1975), Principles of protein–protein recognition, *Nature* **256**, 705–708.

Christiansen, J., Douglas, C. G., and Haldane, J. S. (1914), The absorption and dissociation of carbon dioxide by human blood, *J. Physiol.* **48**, 244–271.

Clark, J. B., Nicklas, W. J., and Degn, H. (1976), The apparent K_m for oxygen of rat brain mitochondrial respiration, *J. Neurochem.* **26**, 409–411.

Coburn, R. F., and Mayers, L. B. (1971), Myoglobin O_2 tension determined from measurements of carboxymyoglobin in skeletal muscle, *Am. J. Physiol.* **220**, 66–74.

Coburn, R. F. (1973), Mean myoglobin oxygen tension in skeletal and cardiac muscle, *Adv. Exp. Med. Biol.* **37a**, 571–577.

Constantine, H. P., Craw, M. R., and Forster, R. E. (1965), Rate of the reaction of carbon dioxide with human red blood cells, *Am. J Physiol.* **208**, 801–811.

Coryell, C. D., Pauling, L., and Stitt, F. (1937), The magnetic properties and structure of ferrihemoglobin (methemoglobin) and some of its compounds, *J. Am. Chem. Soc.* **59**, 633–642.

Crandall, E. D., Klocke, R. A., and Forster, R. E. (1971), Hydroxyl ion movements across the human erythrocyte membrane, *J. Gen. Physiol.* **57**, 665–683.

Dalmark, M. (1975), Chloride and water distribution in human red cells, *J. Physiol.* **250**, 65–84.

Damaschun, G., Damaschun, H., Gedicke, C., Müller, J. J., Pürschel, H.-V., Ruckpaul, K., and Zinke, M. (1975), Über die supramolekulare Organisation des Oxyhämoglobins in Erythrozyten. Eine Röntgen–Kleinwinkelstreuungs-Studie, *Acta Biol. Med. Germ.* **34**, 391–398.

Danon, D. (1968), Biophysical aspects of red-cell ageing, *Bibl. Haematol.* **29**, 178–188.

Darling, R. C., and Roughton, F. J. W. (1942), The effect of methemoglobin on the equilibrium between oxygen and hemoglobin, *Am. J. Physiol.* **137**, 56–68.

Davenport, H. W. (1974), *The ABC of Acid–Base Chemistry*, 6th ed., Univ. of Chicago Press, Chicago.

Davis, J. N., Carlsson, A., MacMillan, V., and Siesjö, B. K. (1972), Brain tryptophan hydroxylation: Dependence on arterial oxygen tension, *Science* **182**, 72–74.

de Bruin, S. H., and Janssen, L. H. M. (1973), The interaction of 2,3-diphosphoglycerate with human hemoglobin. Effects on the alkaline and acid Bohr effect, *J. Biol. Chem.* **248**, 2774–2777.

de Bruin, S. H., Janssen, L. H. M., and van Os, G. A. J. (1973), The interaction of 2,3-diphosphoglycerate on human deoxy and oxyhemoglobin, *Biochem. Biophys. Res. Commun.* **55**, 193–199.

de Bruin, S. H., Rollema, H. S., Janssen, L. H. M., and van Os, G. A. J. (1974a), The interaction of 2,3-diphosphoglycerate with human deoxy- and oxyhemoglobin, *Biochem. Biophys. Res. Commun.* **58**, 204–209.

de Bruin, S. H., Rollema, H. S., Janssen, L. H. M., and van Os, G. A. J. (1974b), The interaction of chloride ions with human hemoglobin, *Biochem. Biophys. Res. Commun.* **58**, 210–215.

Delivoria-Papadopoulos, M., Oski, F. A., and Gottlieb, A. J. (1969), Oxygen–hemoglobin dissociation curve: effect of inherited enzyme defects of the red cell, *Science* **165**, 601–602.

Delivoria-Papadopoulos, M., Poncevic, N. P., and Oski, F. A. (1971), Postnatal changes in oxygen transport of term, premature and sick infants: The role of red cell 2,3-diphosphoglycerate and adult hemoglobin, *Pediatr. Res.* **5**, 235–245.

Dell, R. B., and Winters, R. W. (1970), A model for the *in vivo* CO_2 equilibration curve, *Am. J. Physiol.* **219**, 39–44.

Deuticke, B., Duhm, J., and Dierkesmann, R. (1971), Maximal evelation of 2,3-diphosphoglycerate concentrations in human erythrocytes: Influence on glycolytic metabolism and intracellular pH, *Pflugers Arch.* **326**, 15–34.

de Verdier, C.-H., and Garby, L. (1969), Low binding of 2,3-diphosphoglycerate to haemoglobin F. A contribution to the knowledge of the binding site and an explanation for the high oxygen affinity of foetal blood, *Scand. J. Clin. Lab. Invest.* **23**, 149–151.

Dickerson, R. E., and Geis, I. (1969), *The Structure and Action of Proteins*, Harper & Row, New York.

Dill, D. B., Edwards, H. J., and Consolazio, W. V. (1937), Blood as a physiochemical system, *J. Biol. Chem.* **118**, 635–648.

Ditzel, J., Andersen, H., and Peters, N. D. (1973), Increased haemoglobin A_{1C} and 2,3-diphosphoglycerate in diabetes and their effects on red-cell oxygen releasing capacity, *Lancet* **II**, 1034.

Donnan, F. G., and Guggenheim, E. A. (1932), Exact thermodynamics of membrane equilibrium, *Z. Phys. Chem. A* **162**, 346–360.

Douglas, C. G., Haldane, J. S., and Haldane, J. B. S. (1912), The laws of combination of haemoglobin with carbon monoxide and oxygen, *J. Physiol.* **44**, 275–304.

Duhm, J. (1971), Effect of 2,3-diphosphoglycerate and other organic phosphate compounds on oxygen affinity and intracellular pH of human erythrocytes, *Pflugers Arch.* **326**, 341–356.

Duhm, J. (1973), 2.3-Diphosphoglycerate metabolism of erythrocytes and oxygen transport function of blood, *in Erythrocytes, Thrombocytes and Leukocytes* (Gerlach, E., Moser, K., Deutsch, E., and Wilmanns, W., eds.), pp. 149–157, Georg Thieme, Stuttgart.

Duhm, J., and Gerlach, E. (1971), On the mechanism of hypoxia-induced increase of 2,3-diphosphoglycerate in erythrocytes, *Pflugers Arch.* **326**, 254–269.

Duhm, J., and Gerlach, E. (1974), Metabolism and function of 2,3-diphosphoglycerate in red blood cells, *in The Human Red Cell in Vitro* (Greenwalt, T. J., and Jamieson, G. A., eds.), pp. 111–148, Grune and Stratton, New York.

Duling, B. R., and Byrne, R. M. (1971), Oxygen and the local regulation of blood flow: possible significance of longitudinal gradients in arterial blood oxygen tension, *Circ. Res. Supp. I*, 65–68.

Durán, W. N., and Renkin, E. M. (1974), Oxygen consumption and blood flow in resting mammalian skeletal muscle, *Am. J. Physiol.* **226**, 173–177.

Eaton, J., and Brewer, G. (1968), The relationship between red cell 2,3-diphosphoglycerate and levels of hemoglobin in the human, *Proc. Nat. Acad. Sci. USA* **61**, 756–760.

Edelstein, S. J. (1971), Extensions of the allosteric model for hemoglobin, *Nature* **230**, 224–227.

Edelstein, S. J. (1975), Cooperative interactions of hemoglobin, *Ann. Rev. Biochem.* **44**, 209–232.

Edelstein, S. J., and Gibson, Q. H. (1975), The effect of functional differences in the α and β chains on the cooperativity of the oxidation–reduction reaction of hemoglobin, *J. Biol. Chem.* **250**, 961–965.

Edsall, J. (1972), Blood and hemoglobin: The evolution of knowledge of functional adaptation in a biochemical system. Part I. The adaptation of chemical structure to function in hemoglobin, *J. Hist. Biol.* **5**, 205–257.

Edwards, M. J., and Canon, B. (1972), Oxygen transport during erythropoietic response to moderate blood loss, *New Engl. J. Med.* **287**, 115–119.

Edwards, M. J., and Rigas, D. A. (1967), Electrolyte-labile increase of oxygen affinity during *in vivo* aging of hemoglobin, *J. Clin. Invest.* **46**, 1579–1588.

Edwards, M. J., Canon, B., Albertson, J., and Bigley, R. H. (1971), Mean red cell age as a determinant of blood oxygen affinity, *Nature* **230**, 583–584.

Edwards, M. J., Canon, B., Albertson, J., and Bigley, R. H. (1972), Mean red cell age and 2,3-diphosphoglycerate, separate determinants of blood oxygen affinity, *in*: *Oxygen Affinity of Hemoglobin and Red Cell Acid–Base Status* (Rörth, M., and Astrup, P., eds.), pp. 680–690, Munksgaard, Copenhagen.

Eigen, M., and DeMaeyer, L. (1963), Investigations of rates and mechanisms of reactions, *in*: *Techniques of Organic Chemistry* (Weissberger, A., ed.), pp. 901–1034. Interscience, New York.

Eriksson, E., and Myrhage, R. (1972), Microvascular dimensions and blood flow in skeletal muscle, *Acta Physiol. Scand.* **86**, 211–222.

Fåhraeus, R., and Lindquist, T. (1931), The viscosity of the blood in narrow capillary tubes, *Am. J. Physiol.* **96**, 562–568.

Fermi, G. (1975), Three-dimensional Fourier synthesis of human deoxyhaemoglobin at 2.5 Å resolution: Refinement of the atomic model, *J. Mol. Biol.* **97**, 237–256.

Fitzsimons, E. J., and Sendroy, J. (1961), Distribution of electrolytes in human blood, *J. Biol. Chem.* **236**, 1595–1601.

Flenley, D. C., Fairweather, L. J., Cooke, N. J., and Kirby, B. J. (1975), Changes in haemoglobin binding curve and oxygen transport in chronic hypoxic lung disease, *Brit. Med. J.* **1**, 602–604.

Fornaini, G. (1967), Biochemical modifications during the life span of the erythrocyte, *G. Biochim.* **16**, 267–328.

Forster, R. E. (1967), Oxygenation of the muscle cell, *Circ. Res.* **20**, *Supp.* 1, 115–121.

Forster, R. E. (1971), The transport of water in erythrocytes, *in* : *Curr. Top. Membr. Transp.* **2**, 41–98.

Forster, R. E., and Crandall, E. D. (1975), Time course of exchanges between red cells and extracellular fluid during CO_2 uptake, *J. Appl. Physiol.* **38**, 710–718.

Forster, R. E., Roughton, F. J. W., Kreuzer, F., and Briscoe, W. A. (1957), Photocolorometric determination of rate of uptake of CO and O_2 by reduced human red cell suspensions at 37°C, *J. Appl. Physiol.* **11**, 260–268.

Forster, R. E., Constantine, H. P., Craw, M. R., Rotman, H. H., and Klocke, R. A. (1968), Reactions of CO_2 with human hemoglobin solutions, *J. Biol. Chem.* **243**, 3317–3326.

Frisancho, A. R. (1975), Functional adaptation to high altitude hypoxia, *Science* **187**, 313–319.

Funder, J., and Wieth, J. O. (1966a), Potassium, sodium and water in normal human red blood cells, *Scand. J. Clin. Lab. Invest.* **18**, 167–180.

Funder, J., and Wieth, J. O. (1966b), Chloride and hydrogen ion distribution between human red cells and plasma, *Acta Physiol. Scand.* **68**, 234–245.

Funder, J., and Wieth, J. O. (1974a), Human red cell sodium and potassium in metabolic alkalosis, *Scand. J. Clin. Lab. Invest.* **34**, 49–59.

Funder, J., and Wieth, J. O. (1974b), Combined effects of digitalis therapy and of plasma bicarbonate on human red cell sodium and potassium, *Scand. J. Clin. Lab. Invest.* **34**, 153–160.

Garby, L. (1965), Citrationenpermeabilität der roten Blutkörperchen. *Folia Haematol.* **78**, 295–298.

Garby, L. (1970), The normal hemoglobin level, *Brit. J. Haematol.* **19**, 429–434.

Garby, L., and de Verdier, C.-H. (1971), Affinity of human hemoglobin A to 2,3 diphosphoglycerate: Effect of hemoglobin concentration and of pH, *Scand. J. Clin. Lab. Invest.* **27**, 345–350.

Garby, L., Irnell, L., and Werner, J. (1967), Iron deficiency in women of fertile age in a Swedish community. I. Distribution of packed cell volume and the effect of iron supplementation, *Acta Soc. Med. Upsal.* **72**, 91–101.

Garby, L., Gerber, G., and de Verdier, C.-H. (1969), Binding of 2,3-diphosphoglycerate and adenosine triphosphate to human hemoglobin A, *Eur. J. Biochem.* **10**, 110–115.

Garby, L., Robert, M., and Zaar, B. (1972), Proton- and carbamino-linked oxygen affinity of normal human blood, *Acta Physiol. Scand.* **84**, 482–492.

Garel, M. C., Cohen Solal, M., Bluoquit, Y., and Rosa, J. (1974), A method for isolation of abnormal haemoglobins with high oxygen affinity due to a frozen quaternary R-structure. Application to Hb Creteil $\alpha_2^A \beta_2$ (F5) 89 Asn, *FEBS Lett.* **43**, 93–96.

Garg, L. C., and Maren, T. H. (1972), The rates of hydration of carbon dioxide and dehydration of carbonic acid at 37°C, *Biochim. Biophys. Acta* **261**, 70–76.

Garner, M. H., Bogardt, R. A., Jr., and Gurd, F. R. N. (1975), Determination of the pK values for the α-amino groups of human hemoglobin, *J. Biol. Chem.* **250**, 4398–4404.

Gary-Bobo, C. M. (1967), Non-solvent water in human erythrocytes and hemoglobin solutions, *J. Gen. Physiol.* **50**, 2547–2564.

Gary-Bobo, C. M., and Solomon, A. K. (1968), Properties of hemoglobin solutions in red cells, *J. Gen. Physiol.* **52**, 825–853.

Gary-Bobo, C. M., and Solomon, A. K. (1971), Hemoglobin charge dependence on hemoglobin concentration *in vitro, J. Gen. Physiol.* **57**, 283–289.

Gerber, G., Berger, H., Jänig, G.-R., and Rapoport, S. M. (1973), Interactions of hemoglobin with ions, *Eur. J. Biochem.* **38**, 563–571.

Gibson, Q. H. (1959), The kinetics of reactions between haemoglobin and gases, *Progr. Biophys. Biophys. Chem.* **9**, 1–53.

Gibson, Q. H. (1970), The reaction of oxygen with hemoglobin and the kinetic basis of the effect of salt on binding of oxygen, *J. Biol. Chem.* **245**, 3285–3288.

Gibson, Q. H. (1973), The contribution of the α and β chains to the kinetics of oxygen binding to and dissociation from hemoglobin, *Proc. Nat. Acad. Sci. U.S.A.* **70**, 1–4.

Gibson, Q. H., Kreuzer, F., Meda, E., and Roughton, F. J. W. (1955), The kinetics of human haemoglobin in solution and in the red cell at 37°C, *J. Physiol.* **129**, 65–89.

Goethe, J. W. von (1963), *Faust, Verse* 1740. Christian Wegner Verlag, Hamburg.

Goldfischer, S. (1966), The cytochemical localization of myoglobin in striated muscle of man and walrus, *J. Cell. Biol.* **34**, 398–403.

Goldman, D. E. (1943), Potential, impedance, and rectification in membranes, *J. Gen. Physiol.* **27**, 37–60.

Goodman, M., Moore, G. W., and Matsuda, G. (1975), Darwinian evolution in the genealogy of haemoglobin, *Nature* **253**, 603–608.

Gracon, G., Wajcman, H., Labie, D., and Vigneron, C. (1975), Structural and functional study of Hb Nancy β145 (HC2)Tyr→Asp. A high oxygen affinity hemoglobin, *FEBS Lett.* **56**, 39–42.

Gros, G., Forster, R. E., and Lin, L. (1976), The carbamate reaction of glycylglycine, plasma, and tissue extracts evaluated by a pH stopped flow apparatus, *J. Biol. Chem.* **251**, 4398–4407.

Guest, G. M., and Rapoport, S. M. (1941), Organic acid-soluble phosphorus compounds of the blood, *Physiol. Rev.* **21**, 410–437.

Guillez, A. (1976), Sur la diffusion de l'oxygéne á partir des vaisseaux capillaires, *Math. Biosci.* **29**, 59–83.

Haldane, J. B. S. (1912), The dissociation of oxyhaemoglobin in human blood during partial CO poisoning, *J. Physiol.* **45**, xxii.

Haldane, J. B. S., and Priestley, J. G. (1935), *Respiration.* Clarendon Press, Oxford.

Hamasaki, N., and Rose, Z. B. (1974), The binding of phosphorylated red cell metabolites to human hemoglobin A, *J. Biol. Chem.* **249**, 7896–7901.

Hamasaki, N., Matsuda, Y., Hamano, S., Hara, T., and Minakami, S. (1974), Respiratory insufficiency and red cell 2,3 diphosphoglycerate. The correlation of 2,3-diphosphoglycerate with arterial pH, oxygen tension and hematocrit value, *Clin. Chim. Acta* **50**, 385–391.

Hammersen, F. (1968), The pattern of the terminal vascular bed and the ultrastructure of capillaries in skeletal muscle, *in*: *Oxygen Transport to Blood and Tissue* (Lübbers, D.-W., Luft, U. C., Thews, G., and Witzleb, E., eds.), pp. 184–197. Georg Thieme, Stuttgart.

Harken, A. H., and Woods, M. (1976), The influence of oxyhemoglobin affinity on tissue oxygen consumption, *Ann. Surgery* **183**, 130–135.

Hartridge, H., and Roughton, F. J. W. (1923), The kinetics of haemoglobin. II. The velocity with which oxygen dissociates from its combination with haemoglobin, *Proc. Roy. Soc. (London)* **104**, 395–430.

Hasselbalch, K. A. (1917), Wasserstoffzahl und Sauerstoffbindung des Blutes, *Biochem. Z.* **82**, 282–288.

Haurowitz, F. (1938), Das Gleischgewicht zwischen Hämoglobin und Sauerstoff, *Z. Physiol. Chem.* **254**, 266–274.

Hedlund, B. E., and Lovrien, R. (1974), Thermodynamics of 2,3-diphosphoglycerate association with human oxy- and deoxy-hemoglobin, *Biochem. Biophys. Res. Commun.* **61**, 859–867.

Henderson, L. J. (1928), *Blood: A Study in General Physiology.* Yale Univ. Press, New Haven.

Hensley, C. P., Edelstein, S. J., Wharton, D. C., and Gibson, Q. H. (1975), Conformation and spin states in methemoglobin, *J. Biol. Chem.* **250**, 952–960.

Herzfeld, J., and Stanley, H. E. (1974), A general approach to cooperativity and its application to the oxygen equilibrium of hemoglobin and its effectors, *J. Mol. Biol.* **82**, 231–265.

Hill, A. V. (1910), The possible effects of aggregation of the molecules of haemoglobin on its dissociation curve, *J. Physiol.* **40**, 4P.

Hill, A. V. (1928), The diffusion of oxygen and lactic acid through tissues, *Proc. Roy. Soc. (London) B* **104**, 39–96.

Hill, A. V. (1965), *Trails and Trials in Physiology.* Edward Arnold, London.

Hill, E. P., Power, G. G., and Longo, L. D. (1973*a*), A mathematical model of carbon dioxide transfer in the placenta and its interaction with oxygen, *Am. J. Physiol.* **224**, 283–299.

Hill, E. P., Power, G. G., and Longo, L. D. (1973b), Mathematical simulation of pulmonary O_2 and CO_2 exchange, *Am. J. Physiol.* **224**, 904–917.

Hjelm, M. (1969), The content of 2,3-diphosphoglycerate and some other phosphocompounds in human erythrocytes from healthy adults and subjects with different types of anaemia, *Forsvarsmed.* **5**, 219–226.

Hjelm, M. (1974), Methodological aspects of current procedures to separate erythrocytes into age groups, *in: Cellular and Molecular Biology of Erythrocytes* (Yoshikawa, H., and Rapoport, S. M., eds.), pp. 427–444. Univ. of Tokyo Press, Tokyo.

Hjelm, M., and Wadman, B. (1974), Clinical symptoms, haemoglobin concentration and erythrocyte biochemistry, *Clinics in Haematol.* **3**, 689–703.

Hlastala, M. P. (1973), Significance of the Bohr and Haldane effects in the pulmonary capillary, *Respir. Physiol.* **17**, 81–92.

Hlastala, M. P., and Woodson, R. D. (1975), Saturation dependency of the Bohr effect: interactions among H^+, CO_2 and DPG, *J. Appl. Physiol.* **38**, 1126–1131.

Ho, C. (1974), Modulation of hemoglobin function by small molecules, *Ann. N.Y. Acad. Sci.* **241**, 545–548.

Hoard, J. L. (1966), Stereochemistry of porphyrins, *in: Hemes and Hemoproteins* (Chance, B., Estabrook, R. W., and Yonetani, T., eds.), pp. 9–24. Academic Press, New York.

Holland, R. A. B., and Forster, R. E. (1975), Effect of temperature on rate of CO_2 uptake by human red cell suspensions, *Am. J. Physiol.* **228**, 1589–1596.

Honig, C. R., Frierson, J. L., and Nelson, C. (1971), O_2 transport and $\dot{V}_{O_2}$ in resting muscle: significance for tissue–capillary exchange, *Am. J. Physiol.* **220**, 357–363.

Housley, E. (1967), Respiratory gas exchange in chronic anemia, *Clin. Sci.* **32**, 19–26.

Hrbek, A., Karlsson, K., Kjellmer, J., Olsson, T., and Riha, M. (1974), Cerebral reactions during intrauterine asphyxia in the sheep. II. Evoked electroencephalogram responses, *Pediat. Res.* **8**, 58–63.

Hsieh, H.-S., and Jaffé, E. R. (1975), The metabolism of methemoglobin in human erythrocytes, *in: The Red Blood Cell* (Surgenor, D. MacN., ed.), 2nd ed., pp. 800–824. Academic Press, New York.

Huehns, E. R., and Farooqui, A. M. (1975), Oxygen dissociation properties of human embryonic red cells, *Nature* **254**, 335–337.

Hunt, L. T., and Dayhoff, M. O. (1974), Table of abnormal human globins, *Ann. N.Y. Acad. Sci.* **241**, 722–735.

Hurt, G. A., and Chanutin, A. (1965), Organic phosphate compounds of erythrocytes from individuals with cirrhosis of the liver, *Proc. Soc. Exp. Biol. (N.Y.)* **118**, 167–169.

Ilgenfritz, G., and Schuster, T. M. (1974), Kinetics of oxygen binding to human hemoglobin, *J. Biol. Chem.* **249**, 2959–2973.

Ipbüker, A., Deckert, T., and Aaby, P. (1973), *Changes in aB-pH and AB-pCO₂ in Diabetics and Normals in Relation to Change in Posture.* Niels Steensen Hospital, Copenhagen.

Imai, K., and Yonetani, T. (1975), Thermodynamic studies of oxygen equilibrium of hemoglobin, *J. Biol. Chem.* **250**, 7093–7098.

Jacobasch, G., Minakami, S., and Rapoport, S. M. (1974), Glycolysis of the erythrocyte, *in: Cellular and Molecular Biology of Erythrocytes* (Yoshikawa, H., and Rapoport, S. M., eds.), pp. 55–92. Univ. of Tokyo Press, Tokyo.

Jänig, G.-R., Gerber, G., and Jung, W. (1973), Interaction of haemoglobin with ions. Binding of inorganic phosphate to human oxyhaemoglobin, *Acta Biol. Med. Germ.* **30**, 171–175.

Jaffé, E. R. (1974), The formation and reduction of methemoglobin in human erythrocytes, *in*: *Cellular and Molecular Biology of Erythrocytes* (Yoshikawa, H., and Rapoport, S. M., eds.), pp. 345–376. Univ. of Tokyo Press, Tokyo.

Janssen, L. H. M., de Bruin, S. H., and van Os, G. A. J. (1972), Titration behavior of histidines in human, horse and bovine hemoglobins, *J. Biol. Chem.* **247**, 1743–1749.

Janssen, L. H. M., Willekens, F. L. A., de Bruin, S. H., and van Os, G. A. J. (1974), Quaternary-structure-dependent proton dissociation of tyrosines, lysines and cysteins in human hemoglobin, *Eur. J. Biochem.* **45**, 53–56.

Jensen, M., Oski, F. A., Nathan, D. G., and Bunn, H. F. (1975), Hemoglobin Syracuse ($\alpha_2\beta_2$, 143His $\rightarrow$ Pro), a new high-affinity variant detected by special electrophoretic methods, *J. Clin. Invest.* **55**, 469–477.

Joels, N., and Pugh, L. G. C. E. (1958), The carbon monoxide dissociation curve of human blood, *J. Physiol.* **142**, 63–77.

Kawashiro, T., and Scheid, P. (1976), Measurement of Krogh's diffusion constant of CO_2 in respiring muscle at various CO_2 levels: evidence for facilitated diffusion, *Pflugers Arch.* **362**, 129–133.

Kawashiro, T., Nüsse, W., and Scheid, P. (1975), Determination of diffusivity of oxygen and carbon dioxide in respiring tissue: results in rat skeletal muscle, *Pflugers Arch.* **359**, 231–251.

Keitt, A. S. (1972), Hereditary methemoglobinemia with deficiency of NADH methemoglobin reductase, *in*: *The Metabolic Basis of Inherited Disease*, 3rd ed. Stanbury, J. B., Wyngaarden, J. B., and Fredrickson D. S., eds.), p. 1389. McGraw-Hill, New York.

Keitt, A. S., Hinkes, C., and Block, A. J. (1974), Comparison of factors regulating red cell 2,3-diphosphoglycerate (2,3-DPG) in acute and chronic hypoxemia, *J. Lab. Clin. Med.* **84**, 275–280.

Kernohan, J. C., and Roughton, F. J. W. (1968), Thermal studies of the reactions of carbon dioxide in concentrated hemoglobin solutions and in red blood cells. A. The reactions catalyzed by carbonic anhydrase. B. The carbamino reactions of oxygenated haemoglobin, *J. Physiol.* **197**, 345–361.

Kessler, M. (1974), Oxygen supply to tissue in normoxia and in oxygen deficiency, *Microvasc. Res.* **8**, 283–290.

Kety, S. S. (1957), Determinants of tissue oxygen tension, *Fed. Proc.* **16**, 666–670.

Keys, A., and Snell, A. M. (1938), Respiratory properties of the arterial blood in normal man and in patients with disease of the liver: position of the oxygen dissociation curve, *J. Clin. Invest.* **17**, 59–67.

Kilmartin, J. V. (1973), The interaction of inositol hexaphosphate with methaemoglobin, *Biochem. J.* **133**, 725–733.

Kilmartin, J. V. (1974), The alkaline Bohr effect of human hemoglobin, *Ann. N.Y. Acad. Sci.* **241**, 465–471.

Kilmartin, J. V., and Rossi-Bernardi, L. (1969), Inhibition of CO_2 combination and reduction of the Bohr effect in haemoglobin chemically modified at its α-amino groups, *Nature* **222**, 1243–1246.

Kilmartin, J. V., and Rossi-Bernardi, L. (1971), The binding of carbon dioxide by horse haemoglobin, *Biochem. J.* **124**, 31–45.

Kilmartin, J. V., and Rossi-Bernardi, L. (1973), Interaction of hemoglobin with hydrogen ions, carbon dioxide and organic phosphates, *Physiol. Rev.* **53**, 836–915.

Kilmartin, J. V., Breen, J. J., Roberts, G. C. K., and Ho, C. (1973*a*), Direct measurement of the p*K* valves of an alkaline Bohr group in human hemoglobin, *Proc. Nat. Acad. Sci. USA* **70**, 1246–1249.

Kilmartin, J. V., Fogg, J., Luzzana, M., and Rossi-Bernardi, L. (1973*b*), Role of the α-amino groups of the α and β chains of human hemoglobin in oxygen-linked binding of carbon dioxide, *J. Biol. Chem.* **248**, 7039–7043.

Klinger, R., Zahn, D., Brox, D., and Frunder, H. (1971), Interaction of hemoglobin with ions. Binding of ATP to human hemoglobin under simulated *in vivo* conditions, *Eur. J. Biochem.* **18**, 171–177.

Klocke, R. A. (1973), Mechanism and kinetics of the Haldane effect in human erythrocytes, *J. Appl. Physiol.* **35**, 673–681.

Klocke, R. A. (1976), Rate of bicarbonate–chloride exchange in human red cells at 37°C, *J. Appl. Physiol.* **40**, 707–714.

Kogure, K., Busto, R., Matsumoto, A., Scheinberg, P., and Reinmuth, O. M. (1975), Effect of hyperventilation on dynamics of cerebral energy metabolism, *Am. J. Physiol.* **228**, 1862–1867.

Koshland, D. E., Nemethy, G., and Filmer, D. (1966), Comparison of experimental binding data and theoretical models in proteins containing subunits, *Biochemistry* **5**, 365–385.

Kreuzer, F. (1970), Facilitated diffusion of oxygen and its possible significance: A review, *Respir. Physiol.* **9**, 1–30.

Kreuzer, F., de Koning, J., van Haren, R., and Hoofd, L. J. C. (1976), Oxygen diffusion facilitated by myoglobin in the chicken gizzard smooth muscle. Paper presented at *IXth World Conf. Eur. Microcirc. Soc., Antwerpen*, proceedings in press.

Krogh, A. (1918–1919*a*), The rate of diffusion of gases through animal tissues, with some remarks on the coefficient of invasion, *J. Physiol. (London)* **52**, 391–408.

Krogh, A. (1918–1919*b*), The number and distribution of capillaries in muscles with calculations of the oxygen pressure head necessary for supplying the tissue, *J. Physiol. (London)* **52**, 409–415.

La Celle, P. L., and Weed, R. J. (1971), The contributions of normal and pathological erythrocytes to blood rheology. *Progr. Hematol.* **7**, 1–31.

Landis, E. M., and Pappenheimer, J. R. (1963), Exchange of substances through the capillary walls, *in*: *Handbook of Physiology, Sect. 2, Circulation*, Ch. 29, pp. 961–1034. Amer. Physiol. Soc., Washington, D.C.

Lassen, U. V., and Steen-Knudsen, O. (1968), Direct measurements of membrane potential and membrane resistance of human red cells, *J. Physiol.* **195**, 681–696.

Lassen, U. V., Nielsen, A.-M. T., Pape, L., and Simonsen, L. O. (1971), The membrane potential of Ehrlich ascites tumor cells. Microelectrode measurements and their critical evaluation, *J. Membrane Biol.* **6**, 269–288.

Lawson, W. H., and Forster, R. E. (1967), Oxygen tension gradients in peripheral capillary blood, *J. Appl. Physiol.* **22**, 970–973.

Leonard, E. F., and Bay Jørgensen, S. (1974), The analysis of convection and diffusion in capillary beds, *Ann. Rev. Biophys. Bioeng.* **3**, 293–339.

Lichtman, M. A., and Murphy, M. S. (1975), Red cell adenosine triphosphate in hypoproliferative anemia with and without chronic renal disease: Relationship to hemoglobin deficit and plasma inorganic phosphate, *Blood Cells* **1**, 467–484.

Lichtman, M. A., and Weed, R. J. (1972), Divalent cation content of normal and ATP-depleted erythrocytes and erythrocyte membranes, *in: Red Cell Shape* (Weed, R. J., and Leblond, P. F., eds.), pp. 79–93. Springer-Verlag, New York.

Lichtman, M. A., Cohen, J., Young, J., Whitbeck, A. A., and Murphy, M. S. (1974a), The relationships between arterial oxygen flow rate, oxygen binding by hemoglobin, and oxygen utilization after myocardial infarction, *J. Clin. Invest.* **54**, 501–513.

Lichtman, M. A., Murphy, M. S., Byer, B. J., and Freeman, R. B. (1974b), Hemoglobin affinity for oxygen in chronic renal disease: The effect of hemodialysis, *Blood* **43**, 417–424.

Lichtman, M. A., Murphy, M. S., Whitbeck, A. A., and Kearney, E. A. (1974c), Oxygen binding to hemoglobin in subjects with hypoproliferative anaemia with and without chronic renal disease: Role of pH, *Brit. J. Haematol.* **27**, 439–452.

Lichtman, M. A., Murphy, M. S., Whitbeck, A. A., Pogal, M., and Lipchik, E. O. (1975), Acidification of plasma by the red cell due to radiographic contrast materials, *Circulation* **52**, 943–950.

Lightfoot, E. N. (1974), *Transport Phenomena and Living Systems*. Wiley (Interscience), New York.

Lionetti, F. J. (1974), Pentose phosphate pathway in human erythrocytes, *in: Cellular and Molecular Biology of Erythrocytes* (Yoshikawa, H., and Rapoport, S. M., eds.), pp. 143–166. Univ. of Tokyo Press, Tokyo.

Lloyd, B. B., and Michel, C. C. (1966), A theoretical treatment of the carbon dioxide dissociation curve of the plasma *in vitro*, *Resp. Physiol.* **1**, 107–120.

Lo, H. H., and Schimmel, P. R. (1969), Interaction of human hemoglobin with adenine nucleotides, *J. Biol. Chem.* **244**, 5084–5086.

Lowy, P. H. (1970), Preparation and chemistry of erythropoietin. *Regul. Hematopoiesis* **1**, 395–412.

Luckner, H. (1939), Über die Geschwindigkeit des Austasches der Atemgase im Blut, *Pflugers Arch. Ges. Physiol.* **241**, 753–778.

McConaghey, P. D., and Maizels, M. (1961), The osmotic coefficients of haemoglobin in red cells under varying conditions, *J. Physiol.* **155**, 28–45.

Maizels, M., and Paterson, J. L. H. (1937), Base binding in erythrocytes, *Biochem. J.* **31**, 1642–1656.

Mansouri, A., and Winterhalter, K. H. (1973), Nonequivalence of chains in hemoglobin oxidation, *Biochemistry* **12**, 4946–4949.

Maxwell, J. C., and Caughey, W. S. (1976), An infrared study of NO bonding to heme B and hemoglobin A. Evidence for inositol hexaphosphate induced cleavage of proximal histidine to iron bonds, *Biochemistry* **15**, 388–396.

Meier, U., Böning, D., and Rubenstein, H. J. (1974), Oxygenation dependent variations of the Bohr coefficient related to whole blood and erythrocyte pH, *Pflüg. Arch.* **349**, 203–213.

Meldon, J. H. (1976), The theoretical role of myoglobin in steady-state oxygen transport to tissue and its impact upon cardiac output requirements, *Acta Physiol. Scand., Supp.* 440, 93 (abstract).

Meldon, J. H., An evaluation of blood gas transport properties through simulated *in vivo* function (in preparation).

Meldon, J. H., and Garby, L. (1975), The blood oxygen transport system. A numerical simulation of capillary–tissue respiratory gas exchange, *Acta Med. Scand., Supp.* 578, 19–29.

Meldon, J. H., and Garby, L. (1976), A theoretical model of the respiratory function of the blood, *Adv. Exp. Med. Biol.* 75, 241–250.

Mentzer, W. C. (1974), Pyruvate kinase deficiency and disorders of glycolysis, *in*: *Hematology of Infancy and Childhood* (Nathan, D. G., and Oski, F. A., eds.), pp. 315–345. W. B. Saunders, Philadelphia.

Middleman, S. (1972), *Transport Phenomena in the Cardiovascular System*. Wiley (Interscience), New York.

Miller, M. E., Rörth, M., Parving, H. H., Howard, D., Reddington, J., Valeri, L. R., and Stohlman, F. (1973), pH effect on erythropoietin response to hypoxia, *New Engl. J. Med.* 288, 706–710.

Millikan, G. (1937), Experiments on muscle haemoglobin *in vivo*. The instantaneous measurement of muscle metabolism, *Proc. Roy. Soc. (London) B* 123, 218–241.

Minakami, S., Tomeda, A., and Tsuda, S. (1975), Effect of intracellular pH (pH_i) change on red cell glycolysis, *in*: *Erythrocyte Structure and Function* (Brewer, G., ed.), pp. 149–162. Alan R. Liss, New York.

Mochizuki, M. (1970), Oxygenation velocity of the red cell and pulmonary diffusing capacity, *in*: *Blood Oxygenation* (Hershey, D., ed.), pp. 24–61. Plenum, New York.

Möller, B. (1959), The hydrogen ion concentration in arterial blood. A clinical study of patients with diabetes mellitus and diseases of the kidneys, lungs, and heart, *Acta Med. Scand. Supp.* 348, 1–238.

Moll, W. (1968), The diffusion coefficient of myoglobin in muscle homogenate, *Pflugers Arch.* 299, 247–251.

Monod, J., and Jacob, F. (1961), General conclusions: Teleonomic mechanisms in cellular metabolism, growth and differentiation, *Cold Spring Harbor Symp. Quant. Biol.* 26, 389–401.

Monod, J., Wyman, J., and Changeaux, J.-P. (1965), On the nature of allosteric transitions: A plausible model, *J. Mol. Biol.* 12, 88–118.

Morrow, J. S., Matthew, J. B., Wittebort, R. J., and Gurd, F. R. N. (1976), Carbon 13 resonances of $^{13}CO_2$ carbamino adducts of α and β chains in human adult hemoglobin, *J. Biol. Chem.* 251, 477–484.

Mulhausen, R., Astrup, P., and Kjeldsen, K. (1967), Oxygen affinity of hemoglobin in patients with cardiovascular diseases, anemia and cirrhosis of the liver, *Scand. J. Clin. Lab. Invest.* 19, 291–297.

Murayama, M. (1971), Molecular mechanism of human red cell (with HbS) sickling, *in*: *Molecular Aspects of Sickle Cell Hemoglobin* (Nalbandian, R. M., ed.). Charles E. Thomas, Springfield, Illinois.

Murray, J. D. (1974), On the role of myoglobin in muscle respiration, *J. Theor. Biol.* 47, 115–126.

Myrhage, R., and Hudlická, O. (1976), The microvascular dimensions and capillary surface area in rat extensor hallucis proprius muscle (EPH), *Microvasc. Res.* 11, 315–323.

Naccache, D., and Sha'afi, R. F. (1973), Patterns of nonelectrolyte permeability in human red blood cell membrane, *J. Gen. Physiol.* 62, 714–736.

Næraa, N., Strange Petersen, E., and Boye, E. (1963), The influence of simultaneous independent changes in pH and carbon dioxide tension on the *in vitro* oxygen tension—saturation relationship of human blood, *Scand. J. Clin. Lab. Invest.* 15, 141–151.

Næraa, N., Strange Petersen, E., Boye, E., and Severinghaus, J. W. (1966), pH and molecular CO_2 components of the Bohr effect in human blood, *Scand. J. Clin. Lab. Invest.* 18, 96–102.

Nagel, R. L., and Bookchin, R. M. (1974), Human hemoglobin mutants with abnormal oxygen binding, *Sem. Hematol.* 11, 385–403.

Nagel, R. L., and Bookchin, R. M. (1975), Molecular aspects of structural mutants of human hemoglobins, *in: Molecular Pathology* (Good, R. A., Day, S. B., and Yunis, J. J., eds.), pp. 547–582. Charles C. Thomas, Springfield, Illinois.

Naylor, B. A., Welch, M. H., Shafer, A. W., and Guenter, C. A. (1972), Blood affinity for oxygen in hemorrhagic and endotoxic shock, *J. Appl. Physiol.* 32, 829–833.

Ninnes, J. R., Kimber, R. W., and McDonald, J. W. D. (1974), Erythrocyte 2,3-DPG, ATP and oxygen affinity in hemodialysis patients, *Can. Med. Ass. J.* 111, 661–665.

Okada, Y., Tyuma, J., Ueda, Y., and Sugimoto, T. (1976), Effect of carbon monoxide on equilibrium between oxygen and hemoglobin, *Am. J. Physiol.* 230, 471–475.

Oski, F. A., Marshall, B. E., Cohen, P. J., Sugerman, H. J., and Miller, L. D. (1971), Exercise with anemia: The role of the left-shifted or right-shifted oxygen–hemoglobin equilibrium curve, *Ann. Intern. Med.* 74, 44–46.

Otis, A. B. (1964), Quantitative relationships in steady-state gas exchange, *in: Handbook of Physiology, Section 3, Respiration, Vol. I* (Fenn, W. O., and Rahn, H., eds.), Ch. 27, pp. 681–698. Amer. Physiol. Soc., Washington, D.C.

Paganelli, C. V., and Solomon, A. K. (1957), The rate of exchange of tritiated water across the red cell membrane, *J. Gen. Physiol.* 41, 259–277.

Pauling, L. (1935), The oxygen equilibrium of hemoglobin and its structural interpretation, *Proc. Nat. Acad. Sci. USA* 21, 186–191.

Perella, M., Bresciano, D., and Rossi-Bernardi, L. (1975*a*), The binding of CO_2 to human hemoglobin, *J. Biol. Chem.* 250, 5413–5418.

Perella, M., Kilmartin, J. V., Fogg, J., and Rossi-Bernardi, L. (1975*b*), Identification of the high and low affinity CO_2-binding sites of haemoglobin, *Nature* 256, 759–761.

Perutz, M. F. (1964), The hemoglobin molecule. *Sci. Am.* 211, 64–76.

Perutz, M. F. (1969), Structure and function of hemoglobin, *Harvey Lectures*, 1967–1968, *Ser.* 63, 213–261.

Perutz, M. F. (1970), Stereochemistry of cooperative aspects in haemoglobin, *Nature* 228, 726–739.

Perutz, M. F. (1972), Nature of haem–haem interaction, *Nature* 237, 495–499.

Perutz, M. F. (1976), Structure and mechanism of haemoglobin, *Brit. Med. Bull.* 32, 195–208.

Perutz, M. F., and Lehmann, H. (1968), Molecular pathology of human haemoglobin, *Nature* **219**, 902–909.

Perutz, M. F., and TenEyck, L. F. (1971), Stereochemistry of cooperative effects in hemoglobin, *Cold Spring Harbor Symp. Quant. Biol.* **36**, 295–310.

Perutz, M. F., Muirhead, H., Mazzarella, L., Crowther, R. A., Greer, J., and Kilmartin, J. V. (1969), Identification of residues responsible for the alkaline Bohr effect in haemoglobin, *Nature* **222**, 1240–1243.

Perutz, M. F., Ladner, J. E., Simon, S. R., and Ho, C. (1974a), Influence of globin structure on the state of the heme. I. Human deoxyhemoglobin, *Biochemistry* **13**, 2163–2173.

Perutz, M. F., Fersht, A. R., Simon, S. R., and Roberts, G. C. K. (1974b), Influence of globin structure on the state of the heme. II. Allosteric transitions in methemoglobin, *Biochemistry* **13**, 2174–2186.

Perutz, M. F., Heidner, E. J., Ladner, J. E., Beetlestone, J. G., Ho, C., and Slade, E. F. (1974c), Influence of globin structure on the state of the heme. III. Changes in heme spectra accompanying allosteric transitions in methemoglobin and their implications for heme–heme interaction, *Biochemistry* **13**, 2187–2200.

Perutz, M. F., Kilmartin, J. V., Nagai, K., Szabo, A., and Simon, S. R. (1976), Influence of globin structures on the state of the heme. Ferrous low spin derivatives, *Biochemistry* **15**, 378–387.

Pulsinelli, P. D. (1974), The manifestations of abnormal hemoglobin of man: Hemoglobins M, *Ann. N.Y. Acad. Sci.* **241**, 456–464.

Plyley, M. J., and Groom, A. C. (1975), Geometrical distribution of capillaries in mammalian striated muscle, *Am. J. Physiol.* **228**, 1376–1383.

Prewitt, R. L., and Johnson, P. C. (1976), The effect of oxygen on arterial red cell velocity and capillary density in the rat cremaster muscle, *Microvasc. Res.* **12**, 59–70.

Rahbar, S. (1968), An abnormal hemoglobin in red cells of diabetics, *Clin. Chim. Acta* **22**, 296–298.

Rahn, H., and Farhi, L. E. (1964), Ventilation, perfusion and gas exchange—the V_A/Q concept, *in*: *Handbook of Physiology, Section 3: Respiration*, Vol. I (Fenn, W. O., and Rahn, H., eds.), Ch. 30, pp. 735–766. Amer. Physiol. Soc., Washington, D.C.

Rahn, H., Reeves, R. B., and Howell, B. J. (1975), Hydrogen ion regulation, temperature and evolution, *Am. Rev. Resp. Dis.* **112**, 165–172.

Rand, R. P., and Burton, A. C. (1964), Mechanical properties of the red cell membrane. I. Membrane stiffness and intracellular pressure, *Biophys. J.* **4**, 115–135.

Rapoport, J., Berger, H., Rapoport, S. M., Elsner, R., and Gerber, G. (1976), Response of the glycolysis of human erythrocytes to the transition from the oxygenated to the deoxygenated state at constant intracellular pH, *Biochim. Biophys. Acta* **428**, 193–204.

Rapoport, S. M. (1968), The regulation of glycolysis in mammalian erythrocytes, *Essays Biochem.* **4**, 69–103.

Rapoport, S. M., and Guest, G. (1939), The role of diphosphoglyceric acid in the electrolyte equilibrium of blood cells: studies of pyloric obstruction in dogs, *J. Biol. Chem.* **131**, 675–689.

Reeves, R. B. (1976a), Temperature-induced changes in blood acid–base status: pH and pCO_2 in a binary buffer, *J. Appl. Physiol.* **40**, 752–761.

Reeves, R. B. (1976b), Temperature-induced changes in blood acid–base status: Donnan r_{Cl} and red cell volume, *J. Appl. Physiol.* **40**, 762–767.

Reich, J. G., and Zinke, J. (1974), Analysis of kinetic and binding measurements. IV. Redundancy of model parameters, *Stud. Biophys.* **43**, 91–107.

Reneau, D. D., Bruley, D. F., and Knisely, M. H. (1967), A mathematical simulation of oxygen release, diffusion and consumption in the capillaries and tissue of the human brain, *in*: *Chemical Engineering in Medicine* (Hershey, D., ed.), pp. 135–241. Plenum, New York.

Rifkind, R. A., Bank, A., and Marks, P. A. (1974), Erythropoiesis, *in*: *The Red Blood Cell* (Surgenor, D. MacN., ed.), 2nd ed., pp. 800–824. Academic Press, New York.

Riggs, T. E., Shafer, A. W., and Guenter, C. A. (1973), Acute changes in oxyhemoglobin affinity. Effects on oxygen transport and utilization, *J. Clin. Invest.* **52**, 2660–2663.

Roepke, R. R., and Baldes, E. J. (1942), Osmotic properties of erythrocytes, *J. Cell. Comp. Physiol.* **20**, 71–93.

Rörth, M. (1968), Effects of some organic phosphate compounds on the oxyhemoglobin dissociation curve in human erythrolysate, *Scand. J. Clin. Lab. Invest.* **22**, 208–210.

Rörth, M. (1970), Dependency on acid–base status of blood of oxyhemoglobin dissociation and 2,3-diphosphoglycerate level in human erythrocytes. I. *In vitro* studies on reduced and oxygenated blood, *Scand. J. Clin. Lab. Invest.* **26**, 43–46.

Rörth, M. (1972), Hemoglobin interactions and red cell metabolism, *Ser. Haematol,* **5**, 1–104.

Rörth, M., and Bille-Brahe, N. E. (1971), 2,3-Diphosphoglycerate and creatine in the red cell during human pregnancy, *Scand. J. Clin. Lab. Invest.* **28**, 271–276.

Rollema, H. S., de Bruin, S. H., Janssen, L. H. M., and van Os, G. A. J. (1975), The effect of potassium chloride on the Bohr effect of human hemoglobin, *J. Biol. Chem.* **250**, 1333–1339.

Rollema, H. S., de Bruin, S. H., and van Os, G. A. J. (1976), The influence of organic phosphates on the Bohr effect of human hemoglobin valency hybrids, *Biophys. Chem.* **4**, 223–228.

Rossi-Bernardi, L., and Roughton, F. J. W. (1967), The specific influence of carbon dioxide and carbamate compounds on the buffer power and Bohr effects in human haemoglobin solutions, *J. Physiol.* **189**, 1–29.

Rossi-Fanelli, A., and Antonini, E. (1958), Oxygen and carbon monoxide equilibriums of human myoglobin, *Arch. Biochem. Biophys.* **77**, 478–492.

Roughton, F. J. W. (1935), Recent work on carbon dioxide transport by the blood, *Physiol. Rev.* **15**, 241–296.

Roughton, F. J. W. (1943), Some recent work on the chemistry of carbon dioxide transport by the blood, *Harvey Lectures* **29**, 96–142.

Roughton, F. J. W. (1959), Diffusion and chemical reaction velocity in hemoglobin solutions and red cell suspensions, *Progr. Biophys. Biophys. Chem.* **9**, 55–104.

Roughton, F. J. W. (1964), Transport of oxygen and carbon dioxide, *in*: *Handbook of Physiology, Section 3, Respiration, Vol. I* (Fen , W. O., and Rahn, H., eds.), Ch. 31, pp. 767–825. Amer. Physiol. Soc., Washington, D.C.

Roughton, F. J. W. (1965), The oxygen equilibrium of mammalian hemoglobin, *J. Gen. Physiol.* **49**, 105–124.

Roughton, F. J. W. (1970), The equilibrium of carbon monoxide with human hemoglobin in whole blood, *Ann. N.Y. Acad. Sci.* **174**, 177–188.

Roughton, F. J. W. (1972), Comparison of the O_2Hb and COHb dissociation curves of human blood, *in*: *Oxygen Affinity of Hemoglobin and Red Cell Acid–Base Status*, (Rörth, M., and Astrup, P., eds.), pp. 84–92. Munksgaard, Copenhagen.

Roughton, F. J. W., and Darling, R. C. (1944), The effect of carbon monoxide on the oxyhemoglobin dissociation curve, *Am. J. Physiol.* **141**, 17–31.

Roughton, F. J. W., and Severinghaus, J. W. (1973), Accurate determination of O_2 dissociation curve of human blood above 98.7% saturation with data on O_2 solubility in unmodified human blood from 0° to 37°C, *J. Appl. Physiol.* **35**, 861–869.

Salhany, J. M. (1972), Effect of carbon dioxide on human hemoglobin. Kinetic basis for the reduced oxygen affinity, *J. Biol. Chem.* **247**, 3799–3801.

Salhany, J. M., Eliot, R. S., and Mizukami, H. (1970), The effect of 2,3-diphosphoglycerate on the kinetics of deoxygenation of human hemoglobin, *Biochem. Biophys. Res. Commun.* **39**, 1052–1057.

Salling, N., and Siggaard-Andersen, O. (1971), Liquid-junction potentials between plasma erythrolysate and KCl-solutions, *Scand. J. Clin. Lab. Invest.* **28**, 33–40.

Savitz, D., Sidel, V. W., and Solomon, A. K. (1964), Osmotic properties of human red cells, *J. Gen. Physiol.* **48**, 79–94.

Schindler, F. J. (1964), *Oxygen kinetics in the cytochrome system*, Ph.D. thesis, Univ. of Pennsylvania.

Segel, N., and Bishop, J. M. (1966), The circulation in patients with chronic bronchitis and emphysema at rest and during exercise, with special reference to the influence of changes in blood viscosity and blood volume on the pulmonary circulation, *J. Clin. Invest.* **45**, 1555–1568.

Segel, N., and Bishop, J. M. (1967), Circulatory studies in polycythaemia vera at rest and during exercise, *Clin. Sci.* **32**, 527–549.

Severinghaus, J. W. (1966), Blood gas calculator, *J. Appl. Physiol.* **21**, 1108–1116.

Severinghaus, J. W., Roughton, F. J. W., and Bradley, A. F. (1972), Oxygen dissociation curve analysis at 98.7–99.0% saturation, *in*: *Oxygen Affinity of Hemoglobin and Red Cell Acid–Base Status* (Rörth, M., and Astrup, P., eds.), pp. 65–72. Munksgaard, Copenhagen.

Shamsuddin, M., Mason, R. G., Ritchey, J. M., Honig, G. R., and Klotz, J. M. (1974), Sites of acetylation of sickle cell hemoglobin by aspirin, *Proc. Nat. Acad. Sci. USA* **71**, 4693–4697.

Shaw, L. A., and Messer, A. C. (1932), The transfer of bicarbonate between the blood and tissues caused by alterations of the carbon dioxide concentration in the lungs, *Am. J. Physiol.* **100**, 122–136.

Shock, N. W., and Hastings, A. B. (1934), Studies of the acid–base balance of the blood. III. Variation in the acid–base balance of the blood in normal individuals, *J. Biol. Chem.* **104**, 585–600.

Shulman, R. G., Hopfield, J. J., and Ogawa, S. (1975), Allosteric interpretation of hemoglobin properties, *Quart. Rev. Biophys.* **8**, 325–420.

Siggaard-Andersen, O. (1971), Oxygen-linked hydrogen-ion binding of human hemoglobin. Effects of carbon dioxide and 2,3-diphosphoglycerate, *Scand. J. Clin. Lab. Invest.* **27**, 351–360.

Siggaard-Andersen, O. (1974), *The Acid–Base Status of the Blood*, 4th ed. Munksgaard, Copenhagen.

Siggaard-Andersen, O., and Salling, N. (1971), Oxygen-linked hydrogen-ion binding of human hemoglobin. Effects of carbon dioxide and 2,3 diphosphoglycerate. II. Studies on whole blood, *Scand. J. Clin. Lab. Invest.* **27**, 361–366.

Siggaard-Andersen, O., Salling, N., Nörgaard-Pedersen, B., and Rörth, M. (1972*a*), Oxygen-linked hydrogen-ion binding of human hemoglobin. Effects of carbon dioxide and 2,3 diphosphoglycerate. III. Comparison of the Bohr effect and the Haldane effect, *Scand. J. Clin. Lab. Invest.* **29**, 185–193.

Silverman, D. N., Tu, C., and Wynns, G. C. (1976), Depletion of ^{18}O from $C^{18}O_2$ in erythrocyte suspensions, *J. Biol. Chem.* **251**, 4428–4435.

Sinet, M., Joubin, C., Lachia, L., and Pocidalo, J. J. (1976), Effect of osmotic changes on intra-cellular pH and haemoglobin oxygen affinity of human erythrocytes, *Biomedicine* **25**, 66–69.

Sirs, J. A. (1967), The egress of oxygen from human HbO_2 in solution and in the erythrocyte, *J. Physiol.* **189**, 461–473.

Sirs, J. A. (1969), The respiratory efficiency and flexibility of erythrocytes stored in acid–citrate–dextrose solutions. *J. Physiol.* **203**, 93–109.

Sirs, J. A. (1974), The kinetics of the reaction of carbon monoxide with fully oxygenated hemoglobin in solution and erythrocytes, *J. Physiol.* **236**, 387–401.

Slawsky, P., and Desforges, J. F. (1972), Erythrocyte 2,3-diphosphoglycerate in iron deficiency, *Arch. Int. Med.* **129**, 914–917.

Snyder, G. K. (1973), Erythrocyte evolution: the significance of the Fåhraeus–Lindquist phenomenon, *Respir. Physiol.* **19**, 271–278.

Stahrlinger, H., and Lübbers, D. W. (1973), Polarographic measurements of the oxygen pressure performed simultaneously with optical measurements of the redox state of the respiratory chain in suspensions of mitochondria under steady-state conditions at low oxygen tensions, *Pflugers Arch.* **341**, 15–22.

Stainsby, W. N., and Otis, A. B. (1964), Blood flow, blood oxygen tension, oxygen uptake and oxygen transport in skeletal muscle, *Am. J. Physiol.* **206**, 858–866.

Staub, N. C., Bishop, J. M., and Forster, R. E. (1961), Velocity of O_2 uptake by human red blood cells, *J. Appl. Physiol.* **16**, 511–516.

Steinmeier, R. C., and Parkhurst, L. J. (1975), Kinetic studies on the five principal components of normal adult human hemoglobin, *Biochemistry* **14**, 1564–1572.

Tenney, S. M. (1974), A theoretical analysis of the relationship between venous blood and mean tissue oxygen pressures, *Resp. Physiol.* **20**, 283–296.

Thomas, H. M., Lefrak, S. S., Irwin, R. S., Fritts, H. W., and Caldwell, P. R. B. (1974), The oxyhemoglobin dissociation curve in health and disease, *Am. J. Med.* **57**, 331–348.

Thomson, J. M., Dempsey, J. A., Chosy, L. W., Shahid, N. T., and Reddan, W. G. (1974), Oxygen transport and oxyhemoglobin dissociation during prolonged muscle work, *J. Appl. Physiol.* **37**, 658–664.

Torrance, J., Jacobs, P., Restrepo, A., Eschbach, J., Lenfant, C., and Finch, C. A. (1970), Intraerythrocytic adaptation to anemia, *New Engl. J. Med.* **283**, 165–169.
Travis, S. F., Sugermann, H. J., Ruberg, R. L., Dudrick, S. J., Delivoria-Papadopoulos, M., Miller, L. D., and Oski, F. A. (1971), Alterations of red cell glycolytic intermediates and oxygen transport as a consequence of hypophosphatemia in patients receiving intravenous hyperalimentation, *New Engl. J. Med.* **285**, 763–768.
Trivelli, L. A., Ranney, H. M., and Lai, H. T. (1971), Hemoglobin components in patients with diabetes mellitus, *New Engl. J. Med.* **284**, 353–357.
Tweeddale, P. M., Leggett, R. J. E., and Flenley, D. C. (1976), Effect of age on oxygen-binding in normal human subjects, *Clin. Sci. Mol. Med.* **51**, 185–188.
Tweeddale, P. M., Leggett, R. J. E., and Flenley, D. C. (1977), Oxygen affinity *in vivo* and *in vitro* in chronic ventilatory failure, *Clin. Sci.*, in press.
Tyuma, I., and Ueda, Y. (1975), Non-linear relationship between oxygen saturation and proton release, and equivalence of the Bohr and Haldane coefficients in human hemoglobin, *Biochem. Biophys. Res. Commun.* **65**, 1278–1283.
Tyuma, I., Shimizu, K., and Imai, K. (1971), Effect of 2,3-diphosphoglycerate on the cooperativity in oxygen binding to human adult hemoglobin, *Biochem. Biophys. Res. Commun.* **43**, 423–428.
Udkow, M. P., Lacelle, P. L., and Weed, R. J. (1973), The effects of pH, oxygen tension and 2,3-diphosphoglycerate concentration upon the binding of adenosine triphosphate to concentrated hemoglobin A solutions, *Nouv. Rev. Franc. Hematol.* **13**, 817–834.
Valeri, C. R., and Hirsch, N. M. (1969), Restoration *in vivo* of erythrocyte adenosine triphosphate, 2,3-diphosphoglycerate, potassium ion and sodium ion concentration following transfusion of acid citrate–dextrose-stored human red blood cells, *J. Lab. Clin. Med.* **73**, 722–733.
Valtis, D. J., and Kennedy, A. C. (1954), Defective gas-transport function of stored red blood cells, *Lancet* **1**, 119–125.
van Os, G. A. J. (1976), personal communication.
van Slyke, D. D. (1922), The carbon dioxide carriers of the blood, *Physiol. Rev.* **1**, 141–176.
Vanuxem, D., Fornaris, E., Delpierre, S., and Grimaud, Ch. (1975), Role de l'équilibre acido-basique dans les modifications de l'affinité de l'hémoglobine pour l'oxygène dans l'hypoxémie artérielles, *Bull. Physiopath. Resp.* **11**, 305–314.
Versmold, H., Seifert, G., and Riegel, K. P. (1973), Blood oxygen affinity in infancy: the interaction of fetal and adult hemoglobin, oxygen capacity, and red cell hydrogen ion and 2,3-DPG concentration, *Respir. Physiol.* **18**, 14–25.
Versmold, H., Linderkamp, O., Doehlemann, C., and Riegel, K. P. (1976), Oxygen transport in congenital heart disease: influence of fetal hemoglobin, red cell pH and 2,3-DPG, *Pediat. Res.* **10**, 566–570.
von Restorff, W., Höfling, B., Holtz, J., and Bassenge, E. (1975), Effect of increased blood fluidity through hemodilution on general circulation at rest and during exercise in dogs, *Pflugers Arch.* **357**, 25–34.
Wade, O. L., and Bishop, J. M. (1962), *Cardiac Output and Regional Blood Flow.* Blackwell, Oxford.
Wagner, P. D., and West, J. B. (1972), Effects of diffusion impairment on O_2 and CO_2 time courses in pulmonary capillaries, *J. Appl. Physiol.* **33**, 62–71.

Waller, H. D., and Benöhr, H. C. (1974), Metabolic disorders in red blood cells, *in*: *Cellular and Molecular Biology of Erythrocytes* (Yoshikawa, H., and Rapoport, S. M., eds.), pp. 377–408. Univ. of Tokyo Press, Tokyo.

Wang, J. H. (1958), Hemoglobin studies. II. A synthetic material with hemoglobin-like property, *J. Am. Chem. Soc.* **80**, 3168–3169.

Wang, J. H., Nakahara, A., and Fleischer, E. B. (1958), Hemoglobin studies. I. The combination of carbon monoxide with hemoglobin and related model components, *J. Am. Chem. Soc.* **80**, 1109–1113.

Wasserman, K., and Whipp, (1975), Exercise physiology in health and disease, *Am. Rev. Respir. Disease* **112**, 219–249.

Watkins, G. M., Rabelo, A., Bevilacqua, R. G., Brennan, M. F., Dmochowski, J. R., Ball, M. R., and Moore, F. D. (1974), Bodily changes in repeated hemorrhage, *Surg. Gynecol. Obst.* **139**, 161–175.

Weed, R. J. (1970), The importance of erythrocyte deformability, *Am. J. Med.* **49**, 147–150.

Weed, R. J., LaCelle, P. L., and Merrill, E. W. (1969), Metabolic dependence of red cell deformability, *J. Clin. Invest.* **48**, 795–809.

Whalen, W. J., Buerk, D., and Thuning, C. (1973), Blood flow-limited oxygen consumption in resting cat muscle, *Am. J. Physiol.* **224**, 763–768.

White, J. M., and Dacie, J. V. (1971), The unstable hemoglobins—molecular and clinical features, *Progr. Hematol.* **7**, 69–109.

Whittaker, S. R. F., and Winton, F. R. (1933), The apparent viscosity of blood flowing in the isolated hindlimb of the dog, and its variation with corpuscular concentration, *J. Physiol.* (*London*), **78**, 339–369.

Williams, T. F., Fordham, C. C., Hollander, W., and Welt, L. G. (1959), A study of the osmotic behaviour of the human erythrocyte, *J. Clin. Invest.* **38**, 1587–1598.

Winslow, R. M., Swenberg, M. L., Gross, E., Chervenick, P. A., Buchman, R, M., and Anderson, W. F. (1976), Hemoglobin McKees Rocks ($\alpha_2\beta_2$ 145Tyr-Term). A human "nonsense" mutation leading to a shortened β-chain, *J. Clin. Invest.* **57**, 772–781.

Winterhalter, K. H., and Colosimo, A. (1971), Chromatographic isolation and characterization of isolated chains from hemoglobin after regeneration of sulfhydryl groups, *Biochemistry* **10**, 621–624.

Winterhalter, K. H., and Deranleau, D. (1967), The structure of a hemoglobin carrying only two hemes, *Biochemistry* **6**, 3136–3143.

Wittenberg, B. A., Wittenberg, J. B., and Caldwell, P. R. B. (1975), Role of myoglobin in the oxygen supply to red skeletal muscle, *J. Biol. Chem.* **250**, 9038–9043.

Wittenberg, J. B. (1959), Oxygen transport—a new function proposed for myoglobin, *Biol. Bull.* **117**, 402–403.

Wittenberg, J. B. (1970), Myoglobin-facilitated oxygen diffusion: role of myoglobin in oxygen entry into muscle, *Physiol. Rev.* **50**, 559–636.

Woodbury, J. W. (1974), Body acid–base state and its regulation, *in*: *Physiology and Biophysics, II, Circulation, Respiration and Fluid Balance* (Ruch, T. C., and Patton, H. D., eds.), pp. 480–524. Saunders, Philadelphia.

Woodson, R. D., Wranne, B., and Detter, J. C. (1974), Effect of osmotic shrinking and swelling of red cells on whole blood oxygen affinity, *Scand. J. Clin. Lab. Invest.* **33**, 261–267.

Wyman, J. (1948), Heme proteins, *Adv. Prot. Chem.* **4**, 407–531.

Wyman, J. (1964), Linked functions and reciprocal effects in hemoglobin: a second look, *Adv. Prot. Chem.* **19**, 223–286.

Wyman, J. (1966), Facilitated diffusion and the possible role of myoglobin as a transport mechanism, *J. Biol. Chem.* **241**, 115–121.

Wyman, J. (1967), Allosteric linkage, *J. Am. Chem. Soc.* **89**, 2202–2218.

Wyman, J. (1968), Regulation in macromolecules as illustrated by haemoglobin, *Quart. Rev. Biophys.* **1**, 35–80.

Yhap, E., Wright, C. B., Popovic, N. A., and Alix, E. C. (1975), Decreased oxygen uptake with stored blood in the isolated hindlimb, *J. Appl. Physiol.* **38**, 882–885.

Index